SURVIVAL
IN TOXIC
ENVIRONMENTS

Academic Press Rapid Manuscript Reproduction

MECHANISMS OF SURVIVAL IN TOXIC ENVIRONMENTS
A Symposium Organized by the
American Society of Zoologists
(Division of Comparative Physiology and Biochemistry)
December 28, 29 and 30, 1973

SURVIVAL
IN TOXIC
ENVIRONMENTS

Edited by

M. A. Q. KHAN

Department of Biological Sciences
University of Illinois

JOHN P. BEDERKA, Jr.

Department of Pharmacognosy and Pharmacology
University of Illinois

ACADEMIC PRESS, INC.

NEW YORK   SAN FRANCISCO   LONDON   1974
A Subsidiary of Harcourt Brace Jovanovich, Publishers

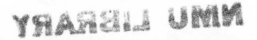

ACADEMIC PRESS, INC.
111 Fifth Avenue, New York, New York 10003

United Kingdom Edition published by
ACADEMIC PRESS, INC. (LONDON) LTD.
24/28 Oval Road, London NW1

Library of Congress Cataloging in Publication Data
Main entry under title:

Survival in toxic environments.

        Papers presented at a symposium held in Houston,
Dec. 1973, and organized by the American Society of
Zoologists, Division of Comparative Physiology and Biochemistry.
        Bibliography: p.
        Includes index.
        1.   Pollution–Physiological effect–Congresses.
2.   Toxicology–Congresses.   3.   Adaptation (Physiology)
–Congresses.   I.   Khan, Mohammed Abdul Quddus,
Date   ed.   II.   Bederka, John P., ed.   III.   Ameri-
can Society of Zoologists. Division of Comparative
Physiology and Biochemistry.   [DNLM: 1.   Environ-
mental pollution–Congresses.   2.   Toxicology–Congresses.   WA670 S963 1973]
QP82.2.P6S87   574.5'222   74-23467
ISBN 0–12–406050–1

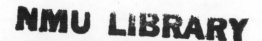

CONTENTS

SECTION III
Role of Mixed-Function Oxidase and Its
Components in Survival in Toxic Environments
Ernest Hodgson, presiding

SECTION IV
Recent Trends in Pesticide Research
F. W. Plapp, Jr., presiding

CONTENTS

FOREWORD

Elmer B. Hadley
Department of Biological Sciences
University of Illinois at Chicago Circle

Ecologists and some governmental and private planners have long been aware of the global nature of our environment and the limits of some of our precious environmental resources. The recent shortage of one of these resources, petroleum, has demonstrated that even the most viable national economies and comfortable lifestyles are still subject to the availability of those resources.

It is appropriate that man, through his technology, be recognized as a major force for change on this planet. Because of his great capacity to control and modify habitat, man can, for better or worse, truly change environment. Certainly we must recognize that this capacity has established man as one of the most successful species on this planet; however, such success has almost of necessity involved an exploitative and wasteful attitude towards our limited resources. Uncontrolled population growth, non-recycling of non-renewable resources, contamination of air, water and food resources through inadequate waste disposal techniques are but symptoms of that attitude.

Professor Eugene Odum has drawn the analogy between living systems and cybernetic systems. The latter systems are composed of interdependent parts that function together and exist in two states, a transient state and a steady state. The transient state is equated with the youthful state, a state of rapid growth in which growth itself is necessary for the survival of the system. ·This transient state with its positive feedback contributes to further rapid growth associated necessarily with environmental exploitation.

Growth in natural systems, whatever the level of those systems, cannot continue at an uncontrolled rate indefinitely. Either internal mechanisms or the external environment must of necessity ultimately trigger diminishing growth and hopefully lead to a steady state system characterized by slower growth rates with emphasis on quality maintenance of the system. Thus, the strategy of unrestricted growth and wasteful exploitation of the environment must ultimately be replaced by the strategy of survival.

The impact of our youthful exploitive attitude to the environment is experienced to an ever-increasing degree in our daily lives. Daily we are confronted with the reality that our natural ecosystems and environment are limited in their abilities to absorb and detoxify our waste products. Daily we are confronted by a spectrum of biologically degradable and non-degradable waste contaminants, many of which have proved harmful to man and some of which have triggered chain reactions within the natural ecosystems which compose our biosphere and have previously rendered that biosphere a suitable habitat for man.

The intelligent utilization of our limited resources would require a fundamental knowledge of the impact of man on his environment. Included would be a knowledge of the synergistic effects of waste contaminants upon the natural ecosystems. Yet we as scientists can provide at this time only fragmentary evidence of the environmental impact and consequences of any one of these contaminants, and knowledge of the synergistic interactions of contaminants is almost totally lacking.

As Professor Khan has pointed out, the chlorinated hydrocarbon pesticides can be long lived in our natural ecosystems. Certainly an extensive literature now exists on the production, application and ecological consequences of these chlorinated hydrocarbon pesticides. For example, the fate of DDT in our ecosystems and its biological consequences have been examined in several recent studies. Yet in spite of this literature we continue to use this substance in enormously large quantities on this planet. This course of action is risky at best since the effects of long-term exposure to these chemicals have not yet been established in man or natural ecosystems. It is not the purpose of this introduction to present arguments for the elimination of such pesticide usage, and indeed such a discussion is beyond the scope of the present paper. Needless to say, both pest control and pesticide control are ecological problems of prime importance that require our immediate attention. It is our purpose to spotlight the fragmentary nature of our knowledge of the effects of environmental contaminants. We as scientists have been occupied elsewhere and have only recently turned our attention to these major ecological questions.

As indicated above, I believe that the transition from the transient to the steady state, from the youthful-exploitive to the mature-quality maintenance state will require considerably greater understanding of the environmental impact of waste contaminants on our natural ecosystem. It is extremely opportune, then, that Professor Khan has organized this major symposium on "Mechanisms of Survival in Toxic Environments." The contributions in this symposium should allow us to assess more fully the state of our knowledge with regard to the effects of selected environmental contaminants, and hopefully allow us to make better judgments as to the directions of our future ecological efforts.

CONTRIBUTORS

Richard H. Adamson, Laboratory of Chemical Pharmacology, National Cancer Institute, N.I.H., Bethesda, Maryland

J. W. Anderson, Department of Biology, Texas A & M University, College Station, Texas

N. Ash, Department of Biological Sciences, University of Illinois at Chicago Circle, Chicago, Illinois

J. P. Bederka, Jr., Department of Pharmacognosy and Pharmacology, University of Illinois at the Medical Center, Chicago, Illinois

W. F. Coello, Department of Biological Sciences, University of Illinois at Chicago Circle, Chicago, Illinois

Robert B. Craig, Department of Zoology, University of California, Davis, California

George C. Decker, Principal Scientist and Head, Emeritus Section of Economic Entomology, Illinois Natural History Survey and Illinois Agricultural Experiment Station, Urbana, Illinois

Harry V. Gelboin, Laboratory of Chemical Pathology, Cancer Research Institute, N. I. H., Bethesda, Maryland

Nancy Goodman, Department of Entomology and Section of Ecology and Systematics, Cornell University, Ithaca, New York

I. C. Gunsalus, School of Chemical Sciences, University of Illinois, Urbana, Illinois

E. B. Hadley, Dean, College of Liberal Arts and Sciences, University of Illinois at Chicago Circle, Chicago, Illinois

R. Haque, Department of Agricultural Chemistry, Environmental Health Sciences Center, Oregon State University, Corvallis, Oregon

Ernest Hodgson, Department of Entomology, North Carolina State University, Raleigh, North Carolina

T. Earl Kaiser, U. S. Bureau of Sport Fisheries and Wildlife, Patuxent Wildlife Research Center, Laurell, Maryland

H. M. Khan, Department of Biological Sciences, University of Illinois at Chicago Circle, Chicago, Illinois

M. A. Q. Khan, Department of Biological Sciences, University of Illinois at Chicago Circle, Chicago, Illinois

Erwin E. Klaas, U. S. Bureau of Sport Fisheries and Wildlife, Patuxent Wildlife Research Center, Laurell, Maryland

Charles O. Knowles, Department of Entomology, University of Missouri, Columbia, Missouri

V. P. Marshall, Fermentation Products, Upjohn Company, Kalamazoo, Michigan

Fumio Matsumura, Department of Entomology, University of Wisconsin, Madison, Wisconsin

J. S. McLellan, Department of Pharmacognosy and Pharmacology, University of Illinois at the Medical Center, Chicago, Illinois

J. M. Neff, Department of Biology, Texas A & M University, College Station, Texas

Harry M. Ohlendorf, U. S. Bureau of Sport Fisheries and Wildlife, Patuxent Wildlife Research Center, Laurell, Maryland

D. G. Penney, Department of Biological Sciences, University of Illinois at Chicago Circle, Chicago, Illinois

Albert S. Perry, Vector Biology and Control Branch, Tropical Disease Program, Center for Disease Control, U.S.P.H.S., Atlanta, Georgia

S. R. Petrocelli, Department of Biology, Texas A & M University, College Station, Texas

David Pimentel, Department of Entomology and Section of Ecology and Systematics, Cornell University, Ithaca, New York

F. W. Plapp, Jr., Department of Entomology, Texas A & M University, College Station, Texas

G. Reddy, Department of Biological Sciences, University of Illinois at Chicago Circle, Chicago, Illinois

Robert L. Rudd, Department of Zoology, University of California, Davis, California

Z. A. Saleem, Departments of Geological Sciences, University of Illinois at Chicago Circle, Chicago, Illinois

Susan M. Sieber, Laboratory of Chemical Pharmacology, National Cancer Institute, Bethesda, Maryland

R. H. Stanton, Department of Biological Sciences, University of Illinois at Chicago Circle, Chicago, Illinois

D. J. Sutherland, Department of Entomology and Economic Zoology, Rutgers – The State University of New Jersey, New Brunswick, New Jersey

Craig B. Warren, Agricultural Division, Monsanto Chemical Company, St. Louis, Missouri

James P. Whitlock, Jr., Laboratory of Chemical Pathology, Cancer Research Institute, N.I.H., Bethesda, Maryland

Friedrich J. Wiebel, Laboratory of Chemical Pathology, Cancer Research Institute, N.I.H., Bethesda, Maryland

James D. Yarbrough, Department of Zoology, Mississippi State University, State College, Mississippi

PREFACE

The material presented in this volume addresses itself to chemical environmental pollutants in general, their fate and disposition in our environment, and their bio-environmental effects. Toward these goals the textual topics have been divided into five categories as shown below. The specific pollutants and/or toxicants include the following: pesticides (insecticides, herbicides, nematocides, fungicides, acaricides), crude and refined oils, polychlorinated biphenyls, polycyclic aromatic hydrocarbons (carcinogens), nitrilotriacetic acid, lead, carbon monoxide and other supposedly less ominous xenobiotics. The dispositions of these substances and the effects of certain of them were studied in either ecosystems and/or organisms, or components thereof.

I. Impact of chemical pollutants on the biology of organisms –
   DDT–The clear lake ecosystem model
   Pesticides–Population biology and evolution of species
   Halogenated Hydrocarbons–Concentrations in estuarine birds and reproduction
   Oils, Mercury, PCB's–Adaptation and survival of clams crabs, oysters and shrimps
II. Detoxication mechanisms of survival in toxic environments—
   Halogenated Hydrocarbons–Fate in microbes, houseflies, and fish.
III. Role of the mixed-function oxidase and its components in survival in toxic environments –
   Cytochrome P-450–Pesticide interactions and genetics in insects and microbes
   Aryl Hydrocarbon Hydroxylase – Effects upon mammalian cells in culture

IV. Recent trends in pesticide research —
   Current Research — Physicochemical considerations, photolysis,
                resistance (research, ecologic and economic
                aspects), costs and benefits.
V. Non-Pesticidal Pollutants —
   Secondary Effects — NTA (a detergent builder), lead and carbon
                monoxide (from molecules to microbes,
                man, and the environment)

In Section I various pollutants are considered in relation to the following ecosystems: Clear Lake, CA; East Coast South of New York; Tidewater Marsh; Global. The considerations span the chasm from the computer-assisted modeling by Drs. Craig and Rudd and considerations of population dynamics by Drs. Pimentel and Goodman to the tissue concentrations of toxicants that are discussed by Drs. Ohlendorf and Anderson and colleagues. This section convincingly documents the global nature of environmental pollution by synthetic chemicals and describes the evolutionary and more short-term effects of these toxicants. Section II on the other hand covers the molecular modifications of the pesticides and other xenobiotics that are produced by the environmental constituents. These two initial sections thus describe our ability to create toxic environments and the abilities of the environments and residents therein to adapt to the toxic insults. Section III extends this latter aspect via coverage of one system (P-450, mixed-function oxygenase), detailing its role in altering the toxicities of chemical environmental pollutants and the genetic control and expression of this metabolic function. The topics in Section IV afford a view of several current areas of research on environmental pollutants from the molecular to the organismic with an emphasis on resistance to the effects of insecticides. The humanistic and monetary costs and human economic and ecologic benefits of pesticides are herein covered by Dr. Decker. His perspective in the form of an overview certainly presents a sound case for our continued dependence upon synthetic chemicals, and, thus, our need for the most advanced information and planning in this area of human endeavor. In the terminal section (V), the life-cycles of environmental chemicals are detailed as per their origins and fates in some environmental life-cycles and ecosystems. The terminal paper in the volume deals with lead in plant and animal environments including the human, and changes in a cardiovascular system as a result of exposure to a toxic environment composed of graded amounts of carbon monoxide.

The scope of the information thus presented is very broad as is our concept of environmental toxicology. However, we feel that the individual topics that are presented toward this broad coverage are very detailed and, in fact, represent the current research and conceptual conditions in the areas. Thus, the volume is appropriate to the needs of the novice in this area of toxicology where a general appreciation is desired and will satisfy the needs of teachers and research workers and administrators involved in considerations of toxicants in OUR environment.

The purposes for preparing this volume were few and seemingly not complicated:

To present in a comprehensive and useful manner reports on chemically contaminated ecosystems and organisms thus affording documentation of the existence of toxic environments

To describe in the available and necessary detail the origins, extent, and some consequences of chemical environmental pollution

To detail the evolutionary aspects of existence in toxic environments with emphasis on and specific reference to pesticide effects both toxic or lethal and resistance to pesticides in insects and many organisms other than the human.

To indicate some previous and current directions in pesticide and non-pesticidal research and their economic, ecologic, and humanistic costs and benefits.

To these ends, the editors and authors trust that they have been at least partially successful. If the material presented herein contributes to our arriving at an environment that affords minimal toxicity to humankind, then our efforts will have been even more rewarding.

Waxing strictly editorially, we have taken considerable lattitude and allowed same in terms of the overall composition of the book. For example, the letter u and the character μ are used in different places to indicate the same concept relating to amounts of materials (micro), the legends and titles to the figures and tables are not strictly placed in the same relative position even within a single report due to considerations of emphasis and space, literature citations are of a generally accepted format except that those references that we considered more obscure were presented in greater detail. Other and similar examples of commission and any omissions are strictly attributable to the editors. Special acclaim must be given to Pat Feeley McDonald and Mary Anderson for their compositional skills in the actual preparation of the textual materials for the camera-ready format.

M. A. Q. Khan
J. P. Bederka

INTRODUCTION

M. A. Q. KHAN

The greatest contribution of scientific knowledge to human health and comfort has come from the use of chemicals. The production and usage of synthetic organic chemicals has enormously increased during the last thirty-four years (10 billion pounds produced in 1943 and 138 billion pounds in 1970) (Pitts and Metcalf, 1969; Stoker and Seager, 1972). The use of synthetic organic chemicals in agriculture, medicine, nutrition, hygiene, etc., has resulted in an increased mean human longevity and thus caused population explosions in most countries. This has put demands on increased food and fiber production and has made man become more dependent on the use of synthetic chemicals.

Unfortunately, the knowledge that enabled man to use the resources of the biosphere to his advantage, somehow, allowed us to overlook the effects that these synthetic chemicals could cause on the biota. These chemicals, after their application, are not confined to the target organism because they are not taken up and degraded completely by the target organism. The non-target organisms can become directly contaminated if the chemical is applied to an open field, forest, a body of water or indirectly by eating contaminated food (pesticides, industrial effluents, fertilizers, etc.). If the particular chemical is refractive to physicochemical and biochemical degradation it can persist in various living and nonliving components of the environment for several years, e.g., DDT, dieldrin, polychlorinated biphenyls, lead and mercury. Biological effects of these chemical contaminants become intensified if they are toxic against living organisms at low concentrations. This is true of certain broad–spectrum residual pesticides.

The U. S. A. alone produces about one billion pounds of approximately 1,000 pesticidal chemicals which are used in 60,000 different formulations (Kearney, 1973). All of the environmental pollution with these toxicants has occurred after 1941 when their industrial synthesis began. The contamination of soils, water, and living organisms, with pesticides such as DDT and dieldrin has greatly concerned scientists, regulatory agencies and the general public.

Besides pesticides, the U. S. A. alone produced 137 billion pounds of synthetic organic chemicals in 1970, and their number is increasing by at least 10 per cent each year. Of these, fertilizers account for 29 billion pounds and detergents 5 billion pounds (Stoker and Seager, 1972). At least 75 billion gallons of gasoline are used every year in this country, thus, releasing, through the automobile exhaust 300 million pounds of lead, 100 million tons of carbon monoxide, 4 million tons of oxides of nitrogen, and several million tons of other pollutants into the environment (Anonymous, 1968). HOW THESE CHEMICALS AFFECT LIVING ORGANISMS AND HOW THEY ARE DEGRADED ARE THE SUBJECTS OF THIS VOLUME. The fate of the environmental contaminants in living organisms is examined at the population, organismal and molecular level. Emphasis has been placed on the pathways and mechanisms of detoxication of the toxic chemical pollutants which enable organisms to dispose of these toxic xenobiotics. The scientists who are participating in this symposium have reviewed the current status of knowledge in various biochemical and ecological aspects of environmental contamination. Since no single book or conference can encompass the problems of environmental pollution, more conferences and more knowledge is needed before conclusions can be made about the ability of living organisms to succumb to or to accomodate the chemical contaminants in their environments.

I am grateful to the Division of Comparative Physiology and Biochemistry of the American Society of Zoologists for assistance in organizing this symposium. Special thanks are due to Drs. Ann E. Kammer, Michael J. Greenberg and L. B. Kirshner for their encouragement and constant support.

The success of this symposium is due to the participating scientists whose courage and wisdom inspired me throughout the symposium. I am confident that the knowledge which took us to outer space will not fail us in our understanding and solving the problems created by the usage of synthetic chemicals. I am especially grateful to Drs. R. L. Rudd, R. W. Estabrook, E. Hodgson, R. H. Adamson and D. Pimentel who in spite of difficulties in traveling here are at this symposium. Their constant advice and guidance has been greatly appreciated. I am highly honored by the help that Dr. Elmer B. Hadley offered me and by his presence here to inaugurate the symposium.

Anonymous 1968, U. S. Dept. of Health, Education and Welfare, *Nationwide Inventory of Air Pollution Emissions,* (1968).

J. N. Pitts and R. L. Metcalf, 1969, *Advances in Environmental Sciences,* Vol. 1, Willey-Interscience, New York.

H. S. Stoker and S. L. Seager, 1972, *Environmental Chemistry:* Air and Water Pollution, Scott, Foresman and Co., Glenview, Illinois, 186 pp.

C. W. Kearney, 1973, In: Significance of Pesticide Metabolites, A Symposium Organized by The American Chemical Society, Chicago, Illinois, August, 1973.

THE ECOSYSTEM APPROACH TO TOXIC CHEMICALS IN THE BIOSPHERE

Robert B. Craig and Robert L. Rudd

Department of Zoology, University of California

Abstract

The intrusion of synthetic chemicals into ecological systems has been the subject of public contention and has caused difficulty in making decisions by regulatory and political agencies. This paper is an attempt to present a modular means of presentation to those agencies. The paper rests upon physical, chemical, biological, and ecological data. Aquatic systems are treated at length using the Clear Lake, California, example. Presented are computer analyses of the DDT-R "load" throughout the lacustrine ecosystem together with descriptive and predictive models of the pesticide residue values to be found in fishes and one fish-eating bird. The bird is the western grebe (Aechmophorus occidentalis) in which adult death followed by reproductive failure in the remaining population has been ascribed to chlorinated hydrocarbon accumulation in tissues. This effect continues in part. Projections indicate no "relief" from partial reproductive inhibition for several years. We extend the ecokinetic analysis of chemical residues to a terrestrial ecosystem whose complexities are reduced by intensive agriculture. More specifically, we are analyzing material flow and pesticide residue distribution in the simplified agricultural ecosystem obtaining in the San Joaquin Valley, California. Predictability of the "fate" and biological consequences of persistent pesticide residues is one purpose; we recognize, however, the transferability of models of the sort we describe to all persistent chemicals from whatever source in living systems.

Introduction

Some synthetic chemicals and elemental by-products of

1

industrialization have produced unexpected consequences following their discharge into the biosphere. Although the toxic nature of the chemicals was known, their total environmental effects were not. Many of the important consequences that have thus far resulted from toxic chemicals could not have been predicted from usual toxicological techniques. Not only was the toxic effect to unintended organisms expressed at the level of the individual, but disruptive consequences at the levels of species populations, restricted communities, and entire ecosystems were also manifest (Moore, 1967). Organochlorine pesticides, heavy metals, and polychlorinated biphenyls are classes of chemicals which show this sequence of effects in the biosphere.

Pimentel (1961) has pointed out that since each species in a community is affected differently (please also see the article on p.25) by an introduced toxic chemical, the entire community organization changes, often resulting in outbreak and general instability. Other authors have also argued that the problem of predictability of chemical "side-effects" is one of ecological-ecosystem nature, not singly toxicological (Rudd, 1964, 1972; Herman, Rudd and Garrett, 1969; Hurtig, 1972). Translated to the effects of toxic chemicals on community structure, two basic aspects concern us. The first is the immediate, differential mortality of species within the community. Feeding and competitive relationships, and ultimately ecosystemic stability, are thus altered. These results can be effected by both short- and long-lived insecticides, and by both biodegradable and non-biodegradable kinds of chemicals. Individual reactions to these insecticides vary with species character and consequent ecological effects are difficult to predict fully. The best pragmatic means of analysis and prediction is to combine knowledge of chemical toxicity with some simple ecological concepts.

The second general ecological effect is the long-term accumulation of residues in body tissue, often causing reduced reproduction, mortality of offspring, and reduction in numbers -- and possible extinction -- of vulnerable species at the top of the food-web. The major mode of residue up-take (trophic accumulation) in this case is by feeding on contaminated prey (Risebrough, Menzel, Martin, and Olcott, 1967; Woodwell, Wurster, and Isaacson, 1967; Herman, Garrett, and Rudd, 1969; Anderson and Hickey, 1970; DeLong, Gilmartin, and Simpson, 1973). The analysis of this latter effect becomes a food-web, "material and information-transfer" system lending itself to computer simulation.

Most relevant studies previously undertaken ask the question, "At what exposure to a chemical will an organism die?" (see Pimentel, 1971). These studies tell nothing of populational and trophodynamic consequences. A few studies have dealt with reproductive inhibition induced by some chemicals in a few species, often extrapolating to community effects (Peakall, 1967; Bitman, Cecil, Harris, and Fries, 1969; Heath, Spann, and Kreitzer, 1969; Porter and Wiemeyer, 1969; Pimentel, 1971). A few recent studies have laid the ground work for models that can predict the kinetics of persistent residues in ecosystems (Robinson, 1967; Kapoor, Metcalf, Nystrom, and Sangha, 1970; Eberhart, Mecks, and Peterle, 1971; Metcalf, Sangha, and Kapoor, 1971).

Current environmental outcry (perhaps unreasonably) insists that total effects of chemical discharge -- industrial or agricultural -- be assessable in advance of application. Where will a given chemical end its presence and movements? At what concentration will it cease to "pollute"? When? What are the social, economic and biological costs? These are only some of the questions being asked by responsible people. We are proposing in this paper one means by which reasonable answers to such questions may be attempted.

This paper is essentially a report of work in progress based on many years of continuing investigation. Eventually we hope to apply modeling techniques to very large systems such as the San Joaquin Valley in Califoarnia in which persistent insecticides have been applied in great amounts. Similar models may then be realistically applicable to all ecosystems in which large-scale chemical discharges are proposed. Regulatory and legislative agencies have great need of such predictive capacity.

Predictive Models as Mechanisms for Understanding Biological Survival in Toxic Environments

Ecosystemic models of the "flow" of toxic chemicals can do three things. A model can give a better understanding of the problem; a model can reveal what parameters are most important to measure; and a model can assist in making predictions of future effects. If a model satisfies any one of the goals, it is successful (Patten, 1972). When preparing to construct a model that is to be used to predict natural phenomena, early decision must be made as to whether the model is to be generally applicable, realistic, or precise (Levins, 1968). To be socially useful, conceptual generality is forsaken in favor of realism and precision. Although any proposed model is an abstraction, its purpose is to represent a limited aspect of the "behavior" of a genuine system. The point of interest is only the utility of the model.

To model the long-term food-web effects of a novel substance introduced into an ecosystem, all major species present must be listed and quantified. Biological and physical activity of the chemical substance must be similarly identified. Because of the specific actions of chlorinated hydrocarbons particularly (adsorption, absorption, storage in lipids), they tend to be partitioned into specific compartments within individuals and ecosystems (Kenaga, 1972). Accumulation of a particular chemical occurs when it is selectively directed to specific cells and tissues taking in more of the chemical than they release. Trophic accumulation may follow in analogous manner in ecosystems and is well-known in chlorinated hydrocarbons and heavy metals (Hunt and Bischoff, 1960; Woodwell, 1967; Meeds, 1968). Each step of a typical food-chain may increase tissue concentrations of toxins several orders of magnitude over that of the preceeding lower trophic level.

The first models we will present will concern DDT and its lipophilic relatives and metabolites -- DDD (TDE) and DDE summed together. We refer to them as DDT-R (Kenaga, 1972). We have chosen this chemical complex for several reasons:

1. They are the most widely dispersed persistent residues in North America.
2. Their chemical characteristics are well known.
3. Analytical data are readily available.
4. They can be detected in small amounts.
5. Their chemical nature is somewhat comparable to other toxic chemicals such as PCB, BHC, toxaphene and chlorinated paraffins (Stickel, 1968).

In addition to chemical considerations, biospheric considerations must be added. There are two major biological realms -- the hydrosphere and the lithosphere, or, more familiarly, aquatic and terrestrial ecosystems. The illustrations of each we have chosen stem from ecosystems

4

highly modified by man and each will have applicability to the much larger San Joaquin Valley system we are in the process of studying.

Aquatic systems appear especially susceptible to perturbation by toxic chemicals for several reasons:

1. The medium (water) surrounding organisms contains chemical residues at all times, thereby maximizing exposure.
2. There is sustained up-take of residues by algae.
3. Aquatic systems tend to have longer food-chains, thus allowing more steps in the sequence of biological magnification of residues.
4. Avian predators (more common in the hydrosphere) are at the top of the food-chain. Many avian species have shown reproductive impairment due to accumulated residues reaching toxic threshold levels (Gress, 1970; Smith, 1971).
5. From both social and ecosystemic points of view, the most ominous consideration is that oceanic and lacustrine systems act as residue sinks. Chemical residues can be maintained in place for much longer times than that characterizing terrestrial (or, for that matter, fluvial) systems. Periodic flushing of residues is expected in the latter type of ecosystem. Unfortunately, such "cleaning" finds a more permanent station in aquatic systems.

Terrestrial systems with some exceptions may be comparably modeled:

1. The kinetics of residue movements will differ in degree and kind. We might expect as a result unforseen consequences not anticipated from studies of aquatic systems. For example, small avian predators may face a different set of food-web consequences as a result of the presence of persistent residues.
2. Small predators take in much higher concentrations of a pesticide residue because of the smaller size of their prey (Kenaga, 1972). Small prey have a much higher ratio of surface area to weight. Increased surface means more area for an aerially applied chemical to adsorb.
3. Smaller predators tend to have much higher

5

metabolic rates which results in a greater intake
of toxic food per gram of body weight.

4. Finally, insecticide resistance in many species of
   terrestrial insects may allow increases in concentrations of residues in prey species.

To begin the actual model-building, we must assume
that the transfer of DDT-R from a donor compartment within
the system to a receiving compartment is directly proportional to the amount of DDT-R contained in the donor compartment. In other words we assume the system to be linear.
Linear models have been successfully used to model the behavior of adapted systems (Lee, pers. comm.; Patten, 1971,
1972; Brylinsky, 1972; Jordan and Kline, 1972). Complex
non-linear representations have not been successfully used
to predict the behavior of natural systems and can not as
yet be applied to the problem of toxic accumulations in
ecosystems (for further discussion, see Patten, 1972).

The Clear Lake DDT-R Model

Clear Lake itself is the largest natural lake totally
within the boundaries of California. Its surface area is
17,670 hectares; its mean depth is 8 meters; and its total
water volume is 1.5 billion cubic meters. The lake is
shallow and eutrophic. The waters are very turbid and high
in inorganic dissolved material. Carp and blackfish are
harvested commercially and there is a popular sport fishery.
Clear Lake, California, has been a site of intensive
investigation for the past thirty years. During that time
the California Department of Fish and Game completed several studies on fish density and angler use. In the 1960's
the Clear Lake Algal Research Unit, directed by C. R.
Goldman, carried out many studies of physical and biological processes within the lake. The Lake County Mosquito
Abatement District has regularly collected data on bottom
fauna. The Yolo County Flood and Water Conservation Agency
has for years calculated water volumes at intake and outflow rates. In 1967 the Bureau of Sports Fisheries and
Wildlife funded a project (to Robert L. Rudd) whose purpose
was to explore the fate of pesticide residues in the lake,
especially as it concerned reproductive inhibition in an
affected avian predator, the western grebe.
With such an abundance of applicable data we concluded
that Clear Lake would be the logical site for which we

might attempt a first model of the kinetics of chlorinated hydrocarbon residues in aquatic ecosystems. We have drawn heavily from published literature to establish parameters for the model. Literature for this purpose is incorporated into Table 1. Each source is listed under the subject matter for which it was used.

Table 1. Sources used to formulate compartments and calculate state variables and fluxes for the Clear Lake DDT-R model.

Water
  Yolo County Flood Control and Water Conservation Agency.
  Herman, S. G., and R. Rudd, 1968.
Mud
  California State Department of Water Resources
  Cook, S. F., R. L. Rudd and S. G. Herman, (unpubl. data)
Plankton
  Clear Lake Algal Research Unit
  Eberhart, L. L., R. L. Meeks and T. J. Peterle, 1971.
  Horne, A. J., and C. R. Goldman, 1972.
Benthos
  Cook, S. F., Jr., R. L. Rudd and S. G. Herman (unpubl. data)
  Lake County Mosquito Abatement District
  Lindquist, A. W., A. R. Roth, 1950
  Lindquist, A. W., A. R. Roth, and J. R. Walker, 1951
Fish
    Biomass
    Anonymous, # 192 Fishery Survey Clear Lake, 1972
    Hayes, J. M., 1968
    Pucket, L. K., 1972
    Feeding
    Ahrenholz, D. W., 1973
    Bridges, W. R., B. J. Kallman and A. K. Andrews, 1963
    Brown, M. E. (ed.), 1957
    Calhoun, A., 1966
    Cook, S. F., Jr., 1962
    Cook, S. F., Jr., 1965
    Cook, S. F., Jr., and J. D. Conners, 1963
    Cook, S. F., Jr., and R. L. Moore, 1970
    Cook, S. F., Jr., R. L. Moore and J. D. Conners, 1964
    Ferguson, D. E., J. L. Ludke and G. L. Murphy, 1966

7

Table 1., continued

    Kyle, H. M., 1926
    Lagler, K. F., J. E. Bardach and R. R. Miller, 1962
Birds (other than Grebes)
    Audubon Field Notes
    Martin, A. C., H. S. Zim and A. L. Nelson, 1951
    Miller, A., 1951
Grebes
    Herman, S. G., 1973
    Herman, Rudd and Garrett, 1968
    Rudd, R. L., S. G. Herman, and S. F. Cook, Jr., 1969
Toxicities
    Heath, R. G., J. W. Spann, E. F. Hull, and J. F.
    Kreitzer, 1972
    Menzie, C. M., 1969
    Pimentel, D., 1971

_____

    Twelve thousand kg of DDD in xylene emulsion were
added to the lake in 1949 for the controlling of the Clear
Lake gnat (Lindquist, Roth, and Walker, 1951). The same
materials were added in 1954 and in 1957 excepting that 50
per cent more than the original amount was added in later
treatments. The insecticide DDD was intentionally chosen
because of its known minimal acute toxicity to lake organisms (Murphy and Chandler, 1948; Lindquist and Roth, 1950).
These conscious additions were the primary sources of
chlorinated hydrocarbons in the lake, although for several
years DDT was commonly applied to the adjacent watershed.
From samples of inflow waters we have attempted to estimate
this contribution to the lake's DDT-R load. Anaerobic conditions in parts of the lake apparently allow quick alteration of DDT to DDD (Miskus, Blair, and Casida, 1965).
    The Clear Lake ecosystem, as any system, is a collec-
tion of interacting components. Our model reflects the
appropriate interactions. Components had to be divided
into compartments to reflect the complexity of this ecosystem. The number of compartments to be used depends upon
several criteria: objectives of the model, availability of
information and degree of accuracy desired (Kowal, 1971).
Since the goal has been to trace the path of DDT-R, we have
eliminated components that have little influence on residue
pathways. We have also aggregated components (often species) whose ecological functions are similar. A non-quan-

8

tifiable but important necessity to aggregate followed from intuitive knowledge and reasoning of naturalists familiar with the ecosystem.

A final compartmentalized model might take many configurations. Our final construction is a compartment diagram representing most effectively and simplistically the Clear Lake ecosystem (see Fig. 1). The system is represented as a block diagram consisting of twelve compartments. Each compartment describes an average DDT-R content in kg. These "state" values were calculated by estimating average annual standing crop biomass for each compartment and multiplying this figure by the average concentration of DDT-R found in the whole body (wet weight) of sample organisms in that compartment. The non-biological compartments -- mud (including silt) and water (filtered) -- were calculated on a concentration times total weight basis. Obviously, most resulting values, although derived from close measures, have to be considered relative approximations in the light of the qualifications we have previously identified. The further assumption must be made that both

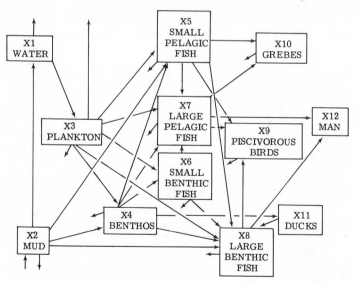

Fig. 1. Graphic compartment model of the Clear Lake ecosystem. Small arrows indicate back-flow to mud.
The small arrows from water and plankton represent
out-flow. X^n refers to labeled compartments in the
mathematical model.

the community and the individual compartments are in an energetic steady-state. In other words, the average standing-crop biomass for the various compartments has been the same year to year. This is both tenable and necessary for no better data are available.

In a flow model the assigned compartments tend to put constraints on the model that make it more realistically conform to natural flows (Patten, 1971; Caswell, Koenig, Resh and Ross, 1972). Once the variables of interest are chosen it becomes necessary to indicate paths by which DDT-R passes among the variables. This requires an intensive study of published food preferences (Table 1). The next step is to determine the proportion of DDT-R in one compartment which passes to another in a year (yearly fluxes). These transfer coefficients were arrived at from published feeding rates and physiological and toxicological information (Table 1). Table 2 shows the calculated transfer coefficients.

$\psi 02 = 16.4$,	$\psi 10 = 0.22$,	$\phi 13 = 0.155$,	$\psi 20 = 0.078$
$\phi 24 = 0.004$,	$\phi 25 = 0.00002$,	$\phi 26 = 0.000004$,	$\phi 28 = 0.00008$
$\psi 30 = 0.125$	$\phi 32 = 16.0$,	$\phi 34 = 0.442$,	$\phi 35 = 15.0$
$\phi 36 = 1.0$,	$\phi 37 = 1.0$,	$\phi 38 = 0.8$,	$\phi 42 = 0.5$
$\phi 45 = 0.5$,	$\phi 46 = 1.43$,	$\phi 47 = 0.6$,	$\phi 48 = 0.5$
$\phi 58 = 0.1$,	$\phi 411 = 0.005$,	$\phi 52 = 0.6$,	$\phi 57 = 4.0$
$\phi 67 = 5.0$,	$\phi 59 = 0.01$,	$\phi 510 = 0.002$,	$\phi 62 = 0.6$
$\phi 710 = 0.01$,	$\phi 68 = 1.8$,	$\phi 72 = 1.5$,	$\phi 79 = 0.011$
$\phi 812 = 0.16$,	$\phi 712 = 0.52$,	$\phi 82 = 0.4$,	$\phi 86 = 0.004$
$\phi 12 = 0.995*$,	$\phi 92 = 0.6$,	$\phi 102 = 0.6$,	$\phi 112 = 0.6$
$\phi 21 = 0.375*$,	$\rho 1 = 0.069$,	$\rho 2 = 0.231$	$\rho 2 (Xn) = n99$
$\phi 21 = 0.0026*$			

---

*These flows between mud and water are interchanged or set to zero as water approaches zero.

Table 2. Transfer coefficients for Clear Lake DDT-R model, units are year^{-1}.

We can then further define the system by a set of coupled first order differential equations (Brylinsky, 1972). These equations are solved simultaneously with the aid of a digital computer. The equations are based on the "income and loss" principle; all energy or substance must be accounted for (X_i = gain fluxes - loss fluxes).

Coupling is represented by shared variables; i.e., outflow from one compartment is inflow to another. Table 3 shows the mathematical model. This dynamic model is intended to be an approximate representation of the sequences actually followed by Clear Lake DDT-R residues.

$$X1 = \phi21(X2) - (\psi10 + \phi13 + \phi12)X1 \tag{1}$$

$$X2 = \psi02 + \phi32(X3) + \phi42(X4) + \phi52(X5) + \phi62(X6) + \\ \phi72(X7) + \phi82(X8) - (\psi20 + \phi21 + \phi24 + \phi25 + \phi26 + \\ \phi28 + \phi299)X2 \tag{2}$$

$$X3 = \phi13(X3) - (\psi30 + \phi34 + \phi35 + \phi36 + \phi37 + \phi38 + \\ \phi39)X3 \tag{3}$$

$$X4 = \phi24(X2) + \phi34(X3) - (\phi42 + \phi45 + \phi46 + \phi47 + \phi48 + \\ \phi411 + \phi499)X4 \tag{4}$$

$$X5 = \phi25(X2) + \phi35(X3) + \phi45(X4) - (\phi52 + \phi57 + \phi58 + \\ \phi59 + \phi510 + \phi599)X5 \tag{5}$$

$$X6 = \phi26(X2) + \phi36(X3) + \phi46(X4) - (\phi62 + \phi67 + \phi68 + \\ \phi699)X6 \tag{6}$$

$$X7 = \phi47(X4) + \phi57(X5) + \phi67(X6) - (\phi72 + \phi79 + \phi710 + \\ \phi712 + \phi799)X7 \tag{7}$$

$$X8 = \phi28(X2) + \phi38(X3) + \phi48(X4) + \phi58(X5) + \phi68(X6) - \\ (\phi82 + \phi812 + \phi899)X8 \tag{8}$$

$$X9 = \phi59(X5) + \phi79(X7) + \phi89(X8) - (\phi92 + \phi999)X9 \tag{9}$$

$$X10 = \phi510(X5) + \phi710(X7) - (\phi102 + \phi1099)X10 \tag{10}$$

$$X11 = \phi411(X4) - (\phi1102 + \phi1199)X11 \tag{11}$$

$$X12 = \phi712(X7) + \phi812(X8) \tag{12}$$

Table 3. Mathematical model of the trophodynamics of DDT-R in the Clear Lake ecosystem.

The Mathematics of the Clear Lake Model

The total amount of DDT-R in the system is the sum of DDT-R in the compartments X1 to X11 at any point in time. The compartment lebeled man (X12) is outside the system and was included only to indicate the total amount of DDT-R leaving the system in the form of fish for human consumption. DDT-R going to this compartment is an outflow.

Transfer coefficients between compartments represent either external or internal flows. External flows are flows into and out of the system calculated from data of physical processes -- i.e., average inflow rates from creeks, sedimentation rates, degradation of DDT-R to non-toxic or water-soluble products. External flows are not coupled; they appear in only one equation each. Internal flows are all coupled, based on the rate at which one compartment feeds on another, or on the rate at which one compartment degrades (e.g., excretion) to another.

The rate that compartment X_i feeds on compartment X_{i-1} is the sum of the feeding rates of species in X_i on species in X_{i-1}. Feeding rates for each species are the product of the laboratory-determined feeding rate of species S, (or similar species) in Kg/Kg/year, the biomass of S, and the proportion of S's diet made up by S_2. The flow of DDT-R back to mud completes the internal cycling of DDT-R (Eberhart, Meeks, and Peterle, 1971; Robinson, 1967). The net flux in DDT-R in all twelve compartments of the ecosystem is, as previously stated, represented by 12 simultaneous linear differential equations:

$$DX_{(t)} = \sum_{\substack{i=0 \\ i \neq j}}^{12} \phi_{ij} X_i(t) - \sum_{\substack{i=0 \\ i \neq j}}^{12} \phi_{ij} X_j(t) \qquad j = 1, 2, 3 \ldots 12,$$

where subscripts 1, 2, 3 ... 12 designate compartments of the ecosystem and 0 designates an outside compartment; X = the amount of DDT-R in a compartment at any time (t); and ϕ_{ij} = transfer coefficient. The transfer coefficients were calculated by:
where f = flux of DDT-R out of a compartment during 1968, and X = amount in the compartment averaged over the year 1968 (see Jordan, Kline and Sasscer, 1972).

$$\phi = \frac{f_{(1968)}}{X_{(1968)}}$$

Logic and mathematical models herein are similar to

those used by Robinson (1967). This model was programmed
for use by a EBDIC digital computer using the IBM CSMP/360
application-oriented language. "CSMP" is an acronym for
Continuous Systems Modeling Program and is uniquely adapted
to handle models of the type we propose (see IBM Application Program Manual H20-0367-4). The Runge-Kutta variable-
step, integration method was used to solve equations.

Transfer coefficients were originally calculated using
data collected in 1968. These data were used to experiment
with the rationality of the models' transfers. Initial
conditions of the state variables were then set at minimal
levels which might represent concentrations at the instant
of first application of DDD -- September, 1949 (here called
1950). Twelve thousand kg DDD were simulated in the water
compartment. We ran the program for 5 "years" at the end
of which another 18,000 kg DDD was infused. This value
corresponds to the amount dumped in September, 1954. This
we repeated 3 "years" hence. Figure 2 is a graph of the
computer predictions for the mud-silt compartment.

We hesitate to project conclusions too far into the
future, as subtle transfer relationships inevitable must
become more important. However, the order of magnitude and
the duration of residues seem to be reasonable projections.

Validations of the Clear Lake Model

To test the predictability of the model we must compare the model-derived data with data collected in the
field (Table 4). Graphic comparisons are presented for
several compartments. In Fig. 2 the single point in 1968
is the only available estimate for total DDT-R in mud and
silt. It is based on 15 dredge samples and one bottom core
sample. From the core sample it was found that residues in
sediment profile decline rapidly. Only the total weight of
DDT-R available to the system was considered. The high
siltation rate buries lower layers of sediment. The residues trapped in bottom strata are removed from the system.
This "burial" constitutes an outflow from the ecosystem.
Such siltation is, of course, not uniform throughout the
lake, but to deal with it more precisely would destroy the
utility of the model. We assume only DDT-R in the aerobic
zone to be available to the biotic community.

The values thus derived are obviously "ball park" estimates (Table 4). The predicted level for total DDT-R in
Figure 2 appears to be in the same ball park but to draw

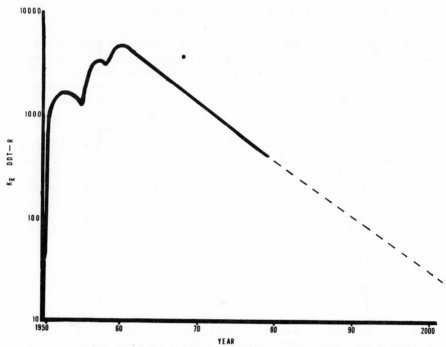

Fig. 2. Total DDT-R available from mud and silt in the Clear
Lake ecosystem. High points represent three inten-
tional applications of DDD, added amounts known.
Datum point represents estimated DDT-R in 1968 from
field-collected data.

more conclusions is unwarranted.

To graphically represent biotic compartments of middle
trophic levels, we present Figure 3, representing the DDT-R
load in large, pelagic fish (bass, crappie, etc., larger
than 2 inches). Few data are available for comparison.
Residue data are available for fish in 1958 (n = 214) and
1968 (n = 60). The computer program does not allow for die-
offs due to DDT-R, so it is unlikely that the peaks shortly
after application are realized. A significant die-off of
fish was in fact observed after each application. Other
fish compartments were similar in form although quite different in range of DDT-R load (see Table 4).

The greatest number of residue data available was for
western grebes (Aechmophorus occidentalis), a piscivorous
bird which has historically nested in large numbers at
Clear Lake. A great deal of life history data -- feeding
rates, lipid-level fluctuations, body weights and population numbers -- is available for western grebes. This compartment is therefore more precisely definable for compara-

14

Variable	Predicted	Measured
X2 - Mud 1968	1736 Kg	3820 Kg
X3 - Plankton 1968	.217 Kg	.12 Kg
X4 - Benthos 1968	2.06 Kg	4.2 Kg
X5 - Small Pelagic Fish 1968	.92 Kg	1.0 Kg
X6 - Small Benthic Fish 1968	.43 Kg	.75 Kg
X7 - Large Pelagic Fish		
1958	68 Kg	64 Kg
1968	3.43 Kg	3.5 Kg
X8 - Large Benthic Fish		
1958	38.5 Kg	92 Kg
1968	3.3 Kg	4.0 Kg
X10 - Western grebes		
1958	1.3*	.42
1959	2.6*	.59
1960	2.4*	.23
1961	1.4*	.16
1962	.85	.75
1963	.54	.3
1966	.16	.1
1967	.13	.2
1968	.092	.15
1973	.049	.07

*These predictions are for total amount of DDT-R (in Kg) in the entire population with no factor foe die-off due to DDT-R. There was in actuality a significant die-off so it would be expected that total load would actually be much lower.

Table 4. Comparison of measured values (i.e., average tissue levels x population biomass for 1968) of state variables (where data is available) with predicted values.

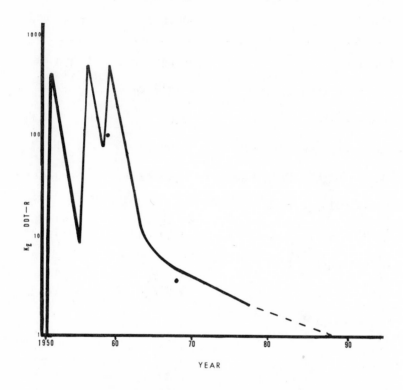

Fig. 3. Total estimated DDT-R values in large (over 2 inches
in length) pelagic fish based on residue amounts in
tissue. Data points indicate estimated total DDT-R
in this compartment in 1958 and 1968.

tive purposes.

Figure 4 is actually a composite of two graphs.
Points represent the average concentration of DDT-R in fat
of western grebes as determined from tissue analysis instead of total DDT-R in the compartment. The line represents the computer-predicted levels. The dashed area of
the line indicates concentrations that would be patholog-
ical (Heath, Spann, Hill, and Kreitzer, 1972). The computer estimate is based on an equilibrium population of adult
grebes. Our model predicts that the average bird in the
population would concentrate enough DDT-R to kill him. Indeed, most of the adult population was killed off after

16

each of the applications.

We would not expect any living grebes to be found with fat concentrations higher than 3,000 p.p.m. DDT-R, so that we would predict the decline in tissue level to begin below that point. Tissue samples tend to follow a decline that conforms to the model's prediction.

Although there is a surprisingly good fit between

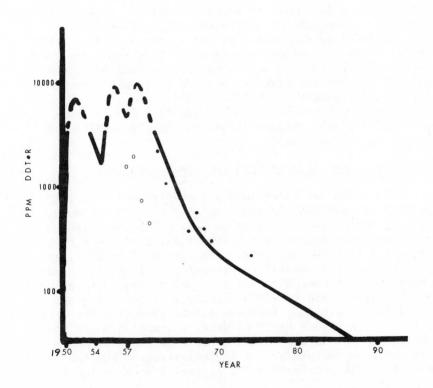

Fig. 4. Total residue concentration of DDT-R in fat of western grebes, wet weight basis. Circles and dots are averages of tissue analyses. Numbers: 1958, n = 2; 1959, n = 2; 1960, n = 5; 1961, n = 13; 1962, n = 6; 1963, n = 5; 1966, n = 12; 1967, n = 60; 1968, n = 26; 1969, n = 3; 1972, n = 5. Circles are years in which die-off due to DDT-R would significantly disrupt our predictions.

17

predicted and field samples, we must remember that precision is not the purpose of the model; rather the purpose is to indicate general trends of consequences.

Comments on Sensitivity Analysis

Because all compartments of the system are related to each other and since it is possible to alter any single parameter and determine its effect on any other parameter, it is important to test, by successive runs, which components of the model have the greatest effect. If some parameter of one compartment is changed, the system will respond by changing the values of its state variables. How sensitive are the various compartments to changes in other components? There is a multitude of such analyses which could be run and mathematical methods to compare the various sensitivities (Brylinsky, 1972).

We will not discuss here the relative and absolute sensitivity of the various flows, but merely point out the utility of such analysis.

General Conclusions from the Clear Lake Model

This model has heightened our comprehension of the kinetics of toxicants in food-chains. We feel a most significant conclusion from this work is proof that results usable by environmental and agricultural decision-makers may be had from the application of simple, linear, first-order mathematical models to natural history data. Clearly, knowledge of natural history, geophysical and chemical data must be synthesized to yield descriptions of ecological functions. Monitoring agencies should recognize the need both to collect such kinds of data contemporaneously and the need to be systematic and uniform in such data collections. Approximations of ecological functions and dependent social conclusions can logically only derive from such sources.

Physical elements are not given sufficient emphasis in current ecological investigations. Nor do chemists and toxicologists give sufficient attention to physical and ecological information. Union of all elements is necessary before effective social conclusions can be reached. Eventually, following the pattern described in this model, we may reach the "cook-book" whereby planners and decision-makers, however removed from the scientific disciplines, may be

able to utilize such predictive models for beneficial risk
judgements.

The Terrestrial Model in Man-Simplified Ecosystems

Practical productivity in forestry and agriculture requires simplification of ecological sequences. The intrusion of chemical controlling substances or the further
effects of the "wastes" of such chemical introductions become major components of reduced ecosystems.

We have currently in progress an investigation whose
purpose is two-fold. It is first an attempt to model terrestrial ecosystems in a fashion comparable to that we have
described at length for the Clear Lake ecosystem. Given
the simplified nature of agricultural ecosystems, we can
effectively reduce compartmentalization for modular systems
from 12 for Clear Lake to 8 for the farm land. Were we
dealing with undisturbed terrestrial environments, or were
we perhaps dealing with tropical productivities, we would
be unable to make such reductions. These reductions do
however fit most mid-latitude agriculture.

Our second goal is related to a simplified system of
large dimension. It is the analysis of chemical intrusion
(using the DDT-R approach) in the San Joaquin Valley,
California. We have in progress investigations which are
both general for that region (hence have lesser predictability) and a close study of a limited area near Davis,
chosen as a sample of an ecosystem reduced in complexity by
agricultural activities. Our efforts are currently directed at determining relationships of all involved biotic and
physical relationships. DDT has been deliberately applied
with the view as well of determining by residue analysis
the kinetics of residue flow in a terrestrial ecosystem of
great productive importance.

To date we have succeeded in concluding only preliminary phases. Figure 5 is a graphic model indicating food-
chain relationships commonly found throughout the central
valleys of California. Full analysis will enable us to
create an even more precise description of ecological ener-
getics in systems containing intruded chemicals than was
possible for Clear Lake. The precision we expect to obtain
may not be as much as desired, but even with margins of
error disturbing to a scientist, these margins are much
narrower than those traditionally forced on decision-makers
of any capacity. These studies, moreover, have one

19

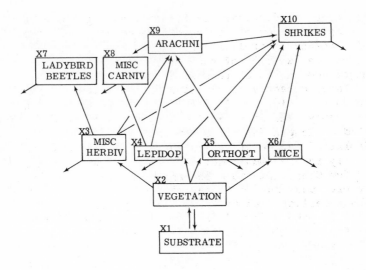

Fig. 5. Graphic compartment model of a simplified terrestrial system, based on conditions obtaining in the San Joaquin Valley, California.

important further value. Although we employ DDT-R as our basis for chemical ecokinetics, we fully recognize the transferability of this modular patterning to all groups of persistent chemicals which have the capacity to intrude into ecological sequences.

References

Ahrenholz, D. W. 1973. "Hunger and digestive response in largemouth black bass (Micropterus salmoides) under laboratory conditions." Unpubl. Ph.D. Thesis. Univ. Calif., Davis. 130 p.
Allison, D., B. J. Kallman and O. B. Cope. 1963. Science 42: 958-961.

Anderson, D. W., and J. J. Hickey. 1970. Wilson Bull. 83: 14-28.

Anonymous. 1972. Fishery survey - Clear Lake, Lake County, California. Calif. Dept. of Fish and Game memorandum. 10 p.

Bitman, J., H. C. Cecil, S. J. Harris and G. F. Fries. 1969. Nature 224:44-66.

Bridges, W. R., B. J. Kallman and A. K. Andrews. 1963. Trans. Amer. Fish. Soc. 92:421-427.

Brown, M. E. (ed.) 1957. "The Physiology of Fishes." Vol. I, II. Academic Press Inc., New York.

Brylinsky, M. 1972. "Systems Analysis and Simulation in Ecology," B. C. Patten (ed.). Academic Press, New York, pp. 81-101.

Calhoun, A. (ed.) 1966. Inland Fisheries Management. State of Calif. Dept. of Fish and Game. 546 p.

Caswell, H., H. E. Koenig, J. A. Resh, and Q. E. Ross. 1972. "Systems Analysis and Simulation in Ecology." B. C. Patten (ed.). Academic Press, New York, pp. 3-78.

Cook, S. F., Jr., 1962. J. Econ. Entomol. 55:155-157.

Cook, S. F., Jr., 1965. California Vector Views 12:43-48.

Cook, S. F., Jr., and J. D. Conners. 1963. Ann. Entomol. Soc. Amer. 57:701-707.

Cook, S. F., Jr., and R. L. Moore. 1970. Amer. Fish. Soc. Trans. 99(1):70-73.

DeLong, R. L., W. G. Gilmartin and J. G. Simpson. 1973. Science 181:1168-1169.

Diamond, J. B., and J. A. Sherburne. 1969. Nature 221:486-487.

Eberhart, L. L., R. L. Meeks and T. J. Peterle. 1971. Nature 230:60-62.

Ferguson, D. E., J. L. Ludke and G. C. Murphy. 1966. Trans. Amer. Fish. Soc. 95:335-344.

Gress, F. 1970. Reproductive status of the California brown pelican in 1970 with notes on breeding biology and natural history. State of California Dept. of Fish and Game Report no. 70-6. 18 p.

Hayes, J. M. 1968. Biological survey of Clear Lake, Lake County, California. Calif. Fish and Game contract services report. 5 p.

Heath, R. G., J. W. Spann and J. F. Kreitzer. 1969. Nature 224:47-48.

Heath, R. G., J. W. Spann, E. F. Hill and J. F. Kreitzer. 1972. Comparative dietary toxicities of pesticides to birds. USDI Special Scientific Report -- Wildlife no.

152. 57 p.

Herman, S. G. 1973. "Cyclic fluctuations in feeding rates and body weight in captive western grebes Aechmophorous occidentalis." Unpubl. Ph.D. Thesis. Univ. Calif., Davis. 56 p.

Herman, S. G., R. L. Garrett and R. L. Rudd. 1969. "Chemical Fallout." M. W. Miller and G. G. Berg (eds.) Charles C. Thomas, Publisher. Springfield, IL, pp. 24-53.

Horne, A. J., and C. R. Goldman. 1972. Limnol. and Oceanog. 17(5):628-692.

Hunt, E. G., and A. I. Bischoff. 1960. Cal. Fish and Game. 46(1):91-106.

Hurtig, H. 1972. "Environmental toxicology of pesticides." F. Matsumura, G. M. Boush and T. Misato (eds.). Academic Press, New York, pp. 257-276.

Jordan, C. F., and J. R. Kline. 1972. "Annual Review of Ecology and Systematics." R. F. Johnston (ed.) Annual Reviews, Inc., Palo Alto, pp. 33-50.

Jordan, C. F., J. R. Kline, and D. S. Sasscer. 1972. Am. Nat. 106(948):237-253.

Kapoor, I. P., R. L. Metcalf, R. F. Mystrom and G. K. Sangha. 1970. J. Agr. Food Chem. 18(6):1145-1152.

Kenaga, E. E. 1972. "Environmental Toxicology of Pesticides." F. Matsumura, G. M. Boush and T. Misato (eds.). Academic Press, New York, pp. 193-228.

Kowal, N. E. 1971. "Systems Analysis and Simulation in Ecology." B. C. Patten (ed.). Academic Press, New York, pp. 123-194.

Kyle, H. M. 1926. "The Biology of Fishes." Sidgwick and Jackson, Ltd. London. 396 p.

Lagler, K. F., J. E. Bardach and R. R. Miller. 1962. "Icthyology." John Wiley and Sons, Inc. New York. 545 p.

Levins, R. 1968. "Evolution in Changing Environments." Princeton Univ. Press. 120 p.

Lindquist, A. W., and A. R. Roth. 1950. J. Econ. Entomol. 43(3):328-332.

Lindquist, A. W., A. R. Roth and J.d J. R. Walker. 1951. J. Econ. Entomol. 44(4):572-577.

Martin, A. C., H. S. Zim and A. L. Nelson. 1951. "American Wildlife and Plants: a Guide to Wildlife Food Habits." Dover Publ., Inc. New York. 500 p.

Meeks, R. L. 1968. Jour. Wildl. Mgt. 32(2):376-398.

Menzie, C. M. 1969. Metabolism of Pesticides. Bureau of Sport Fish. and Wildl. Special Scientific Report -- Wildlife No. 127. Washington, D. C.

Metcalf, R. L., G. K. Sangha, and I. P. Kapoor. 1971.
Environ.Sci. Technol., 5:709-713.

Miller, A. H. 1951. An analysis of the distribution of the
birds of California. Univ. of Calif. Publ. Zool. U. C.
Press, Berkeley, Vol 50(6):531-644.

Miskus, R. P., D. p. Blair and J. E. Casida. 1965. J. Agr.
Food Chem. 13(5):481-483.

Moore, N. W. 1967. "Adv. in Ecological Res." Vol. 4. J. B.
Cragg (ed.). Academic Press. New York, pp. 75-129.

Murphy, G. I., and H. P. Chandler. 1948. The effects of TDE
on fish and on the plankton and littoral fauna in lower
Blue Lake, Lake County, California. Calif. Fish and Game,
Inland Fisheries Admin. No. 48-14. 10 p.

Patten, B. C. 1971. "Systems Analysis and Simulation in
Ecology." Vol. I. B. C. Patten (ed.). Academic Press,
New York, pp. 3-121.

Patten, B. C., (ed.) 1972. "Systems Analysis and Simulation
in Ecology." Academic Press, New York. 592 p.

Peakall, D. B. 1967. Nature 216:505-506.

Pimentel, D. 1961. J. Econ. Entomol. 54(1):108-114.

Pimentel, D. 1971. Ecological effects of pesticides on non-
target species. Exec. Office of the President. Office of
Science and Technology. 220 p.

Porter, R. D., and S. N. Wiemeyer. 1969. Science 165:199-
200.

Puckett, L. K. 1972. Estimated angler use and success at
Clear Lake, Lake County, California. Calif. Fish and
Game Report No. 72-1.

Ratcliffe, D. A. 1967. Nature 215:208-210.

Risebrough, R. W., D. B. Menzel, D. J. Martin and H. S.
Olcott. 1967. Nature 216:589-591.

Robinson, J. 1967. Nature 215:33-35.

Rudd, R. L. 1964. "Pesticides and the Living Lanscape."
Univ. of Wisconsin Press. 320 p.

Rudd, R. L., S. G. Herman and S. F. Cook, Jr. 1969. Studies
of pesticide kinetics and western grebes at Clear Lake,
Lake County, California. U. S. Fish and Wildlife Service
Report No. 14-008-881. 19 p.

Rudd, R. L., and S. G. Herman. 1972. "Environmental Toxicology of Pesticides." F. Matsumura, G. M. Boush and T.
Misato (eds.). Academic Press, New York, pp. 471-485.

Smith, J. J. 1972. "Global pollutants and avian population
decline." Unpubl. Master's Thesis. Calif. State Univ.,
San Jose. 32 p.

Stickel, L. F. 1968. Organochlorine pesticides in the

environment. U. S. Bureau of Sport Fisheries and Wildlife, Special Scientific Report -- Wildlife No. 119.
32 p.

Woodwell, G. M. 1967. Sci. Amer. 216(3):24-31.

Woodwell, G. M., C. F. Wurster, Jr., and P. A. Isaacson.
1967. Science 156:821-824.

Acknowledgements

We would like to thank Dr. Jeffery Lee for his help in
the construction of the Clear Lake model and to thank also
W. S. Williams, G. Suter, K. Riese, A. MacIntyre, P.
McMahan and P. Adams for their assistance in data search and
the analysis of aggregations. Many individuals and organizations have helped to acquire the data reported here.
Their assistance ranges over several years. We gratefully
acknowledge their contributions, but particularly thank
Drs. S. F. Cook, Jr., R. L. Garrett, and S. G. Herman.

ENVIRONMENTAL IMPACT OF PESTICIDES

David Pimentel and Nancy Goodman

Department of Entomology and
Section of Ecology and Systematics
Cornell University

Abstract

The effects of pesticides (insecticides, herbicides, nematocides, and fungicides) were analyzed and an assessment made of their ecological impact. Some pesticides have influenced the structure and function of ecosystems and communities; reduced species population numbers in certain regions; altered the natural habitat under some conditions; changed the normal behavioral patterns in animals; stimulated or suppressed growth in animals and plants; increased or decreased the reproductive capacity of animals; altered the nutritional content of foods; increased the susceptibility of certain plants and animals to diseases and predators; and changed the natural evolution of species populations in some regions.

All available evidence suggests that certain current pesticide usage methods have caused measurable damage to many species of birds, fishes, and beneficial insects. The full extent of damage is impossible to assess accurately because only a few (less than 1,000) species of the estimated total of 200,000 species of plants and animals in the United States have been studied. Although the data on the detrimental effects of pesticides on the life system are limited, there is ample evidence to encourage real concern about pesticide use.

Introduction

An estimated 200,000 species of plants and animals exist in the United States. These species are vital to our survival, for we can not survive with only our crop

25

plants and livestock. No one knows how many species of plants and animals can be exterminated or how far the ecosystem can be altered before man himself is in serious jeopardy.

In 1971 more than 1.2 billion pounds of pesticides were produced (USDA, 1973) (about 6 pounds per person) and more than 1 billion pounds were probably applied to our environment to control about 2,000 pest species. If these poisons hit only the target species, there would be no pollution problem, however, little pesticide (probably less than 1%) ever hits the target pests (PSAC, 1965). Often as little as 25% to 50% of the pesticide formulation ever lands in the crop area, when pesticides are applied by aircraft (Hindin, et. al., 1966; Ware, et. al., 1970; Buroyne and Akesson, 1971; Akesson, et. al., 1971). The significance of aircraft applications contributing to pesticide pollution is clear when evidence shows that about 65% of all agricultural insecticides are applied by aircraft (USDA, 1973).

Some pesticides, like the chlorinated insecticides, even after killing the target pest may still remain in the environment as pollutants. The main reasons for serious ecological problems with pesticides are: (1) pesticides are biological poisons (toxicants); (2) large quantities (about 1 billion pounds) are applied to the ecosystem annually; and (3) poor application technology (especially by aircraft) is used which results in large amounts of pesticides being widely spread in non-target areas.

A direct toxic effect on a species is frequently thought of when the effects of pesticides are discussed. Although direct toxicity is important, many other diverse effects are equally significant. Based on ecological impact, the numerous diverse other effects may be of greater danger to the ecosystem because of their number and because their action is more subtle and therefore may go undetected for long periods. In this paper we plan to summarize the evidence concerning the diverse ecological effects of pesticides (insecticides, herbicides, nematocides, and fungicides) on the life system. Particular attention will be given to direct and indirect ecological effects and we will consider the wide range of ecological effects that pesticides may have on nature.

Ecosystem Effects

Mention was made of our dependence upon the 200,000

26

species which make up the life system in the United States.
We depend upon this great variety of species for the maintenance of a quality atmosphere, for adequate food, for the
biological degradation of wastes, and for other necessities
for man's survival. In the presence of sunlight, plants
take in carbon dioxide and water and release oxygen which
is needed by man and other animals. The oxygen (as both
oxygen and ozone) also screens lethal solar ultraviolet
rays, keeping them from reaching the earth's surface. In
addition, the plants are food for many animals, passing
their life-making elements (carbon, oxygen, hydrogen, nitrogen, phosphorus, and so forth) to the animals in the
food chain. Eventually, microorganisms feeding on the dead
and other wastes release vital elements for reuse by plants.
In this way, species of the life system interact and
function to keep the life-making elements recycling in the
environment.

     With quantities of pesticides and other pollutants in-
creasing, some species populations of the life system may
serve another valuable role -- that of "indicator". Thus,
they will "tell us" when pollutant dosages may be reaching
dangerous levels in the environment.

     Pesticides and other pollutants generally have a dis-
rupting and deleterious impact on ecosystems by causing
changes in the species composition and population numbers
which make up the life system (PSAC, 1965; Pimentel, 1971).
First, if there is a sufficiently high concentration of
pesticides or other chemical pollutants in the environment,
the number of species in the particular ecosystem is reduced. Second, if the reduction in number of species is
sufficient, this may lead to instability within the ecosystem and subsequently to population outbreaks of some
species. Outbreaks result from a breakdown in the normal
check-balance structure of the system, as when a species
of predator (parasite or competitor), which limits the increase of its prey or competitor, is severely reduced in
numbers or exterminated. Third, after the pesticide or
chemical pollutant disappears from the affected ecosystem,
species in the lower part of the food chain, for example,
herbivorous animals, usually increase to outbreak levels.
This also may result in a serious disruption of the ecosystem. Fourth, predators and parasites existing at the top
of the food chain are quite susceptible to the loss of a
species and to intense population fluctuations of species
low in the food chain upon which they depend. Thus, when a

27

species low in the chain in an ecosystem is affected, many dependent species also suffer, and the entire check-balance structure may be inoperative.

Pesticides have altered certain natural habitats, thus causing significant reductions in numbers of some non-target species of plants and animals. For example, dimethoate applied at 0.56 kg/ha to a red clover field reduced the numbers of certain insect prey (Orthoptera, Hemiptera, and others) on which mice (Mus musculus) feed. The result was an 80% decline in the dependent mouse predator population (Barrett and Darnell, 1967).

Reducing some species of stream insects on which fish feed may have a striking influence on the diets and perhaps the survival of the fish. For example, crayfish were not in the diet of brook trout before treatment of a forest with 2.8 kg/ha of DDT. Immediately after treatment crayfish accounted for 99% of the trout diet (Adams, et. al., 1949). How this change in food affected the survival of the trout population was not investigated.

Herbicide destruction of plants upon which animals depend for food may cause significant reductions in animal numbers. Thus, 2,4-D applied to a gopher habitat reduced the green forbs by 83%, eventually resulting in an 87% reduction in the dependent gopher population (Keith, et. al., 1959).

Altering the structure of an ecosystem by changing the producer species with herbicides may have indirect effects upon species members of that ecosystem. For instance, the decline in numbers of Grey Partridge in England is reportedly due to decreased chick survival which, in turn, was linked to changes in the abundance of their food arthropods in cereal crops (Potts, 1970). Small arthropods are an important source of nutrients for partridge chicks, but under "favorable conditions herbicides can temporarily reduce the number of arthropods" in cereal crops by about 70% compared to untreated crops. The cause of the general arthropod reduction is both the "clean culture" and more frequent aphid outbreaks in the crops (Potts, 1970).

These examples illustrate the influence of pesticide pollutants on ecosystems and the interdependence of all species in the earth's biological system. Plants, humans, and other animals are all part of the same system or "establishment" -- if the life system is lost, the ecosystem and humankind will suffer!

Toleration and Toxic Action

Although all species are constructed of practically the same elements (C, H, N, O, P, etc.), they don't respond exactly alike because their structures are different. Of course, not only do species differ in their responses, but, also individuals differ in their responses to toxicants for similar reasons. It is these individual differences that result in different LD_{50}'s (administered dosage of pesticide that kills 50% of a test population) and LC_{50}'s (lethal concentration) when test populations are exposed to pesticide poisons.

Because of individual and species differences and the numerous modes of toxic action of pesticides, the toxicity of pesticides may vary greatly from one species population to another. For example, DDE (a highly stable metabolite of DDT) is practically non-toxic to insects, but predaceous bird species such as the American sparrow hawk are highly sensitive to DDE (Wiemeyer and Porter, 1970). This chemical affects raptorial birds' reproductive physiology causing them to produce eggs with shells significantly thinner (up to 34% in pelicans) than normal (Keith, et. al., 1970), thereby decreasing successful reproduction. A recent examination of peregrine falcon eggs showed that a mean reduction in eggshell thickness of 21.7% was correlated with a mean of 889 ppm DDE in the eggs (lipid basis) (Cade, et. al., 1971). DDT in combination with dieldrin also caused eggshell thinning in sparrow hawks (Porter and Wiemeyer, 1969), and DDT alone fed to mallard ducks induced eggshell thinning (Heath, et. al., 1969). Interestingly, seed-eating birds such as ring-necked pheasants are relatively resistant to the effects of DDT (Azevedo, et. al., 1965). DDT stimulated Bengalese finches to produce lighter-weight eggs with significantly heavier shells (Jefferies, 1969). However, ovulation times in these finches were delayed nearly twice normal by the daily administration of a dosage of 270 ug of DDT and thereby reproduction decreased (Jefferies, 1967).

Differences in mode of action and toleration in various species can be documented further by the following example: DDT in earthworms breaks down to DDE, whereas in slugs DDT breaks down mainly to TDE (Davis and French, 1969). DDE, although non-toxic to earthworms and insects, is highly toxic to predatory birds as mentioned. Clearly much more needs to be known about the toxicity and diverse modes of action of the pesticides we use.

Pesticide interaction may influence the toxic effects of pesticides upon species resulting in either decreased toxicity or increased toxicity. For example, when rainbow trout were dosed with 5 mg DDT in combination with either 0.04 mg or 0.20 mg of dieldrin, the presence of the dieldrin increased the time to death after the appearance of toxic sign from less than an hour with DDT alone up to a maximum of 48 hr. (Mayer, et. al., 1972). Houseflies exposed to the polychlorinated biphenyl (Aroclor[R]1248) and 5 organophosphorus insecticides were found to be significantly more susceptible to the combination than to the insecticides alone (Fuhremann and Lichtenstein, 1972). A similar synergism in toxicity occurred when Drosophila, houseflies, and mosquitoes (Aedes aegypti) were exposed to combinations of herbicides and insecticides (Lichtenstein, et. al., 1973). For example exposure of these insect species to carbofuran (0.5 mg), DDT (4 mg), parathion (0.35 mg), and diazinon (0.2 mg) alone resulted in mortalities of 7.5, 9.5, 8, and 10.5%, respectively. Twenty-three, 40, 6, and 10 mg of atrazine added to the above insecticide dosages, increased mortalities of the insect populations to 50%.

Environmental stresses can also alter the susceptibility of animals to pollutants. For instance, adult hen pheasants that received 16 capsules each containing 50 mg of PCB (Aroclor[R]1254) once per week and those receiving 7 capsules each containing 50 mg of PCB at 3.5 day intervals were alternately starved for 2 or 3 days and then fed for 2 days. Control hens similarly starved lived an average of 44 days whereas the PCB treated birds lived for only 27 days.

Degradation of Pollutants

The wastes produced by our livestock annually is staggering -- a total of 1.7 billion tons of manure (Miner, 1971). Each person produces about 1,200 pounds annually and one cow produces 20,000 pounds. If it were not for various microorganisms and invertebrates, these wastes would pile up and the vital elements would not be recycled for reuse by the ecosystem. Few people appreciate the tremendous numbers of microorganisms and invertebrates present per acre. A human averages only about 14 lbs. of biomass per acre in the U.S., but earthworms are estimated at about 500 lbs/A (based on Raw's [1962] data) and microorganisms might total 8,000 lbs/A (Clark, 1967). Not only do micro-organisms play a vital role in degrading organic wastes, they play a significant role in degrading pesticide pollutants (PSAC, 1965). Bacteria, for example, have been cultured which can obtain some of their carbon and other needs directly from pesticides such as 2,4-D (Alexander, 1967).

On the other hand microorganisms which cause or contribute to the breakdown of cellulose, nitrification, turnover of organic materials, and other biological activities may be adversely influenced by pesticides. For example, EPTC (herbicide) at normal use dosages impaired cellulose decomposition in soil (Sobieszczanski, 1969). Another herbicide (TCA) reduced soil nitrification (Otten, et. al., 1957). Earthworms and soil arthropods have been severely reduced by insecticides and herbicides. For example, the herbicide simazine at normal dosages (2 to 4 lb/A in WSA, 1967) caused a reduction in the numbers of soil invertebrates by 33 to 50% (Edwards, 1964). Predatory mites, hemeidaphic Collembola, and particularly the Isotomidae, were most affected by simazine. Earthworms, enchytraeid worms, dipterous and coleopterus larvae, and populations of other mites and springtails also decreased, and significant differences between numbers of those in treated and untreated soil were still obvious 3 to 4 months after simazine had been applied.

Biotic Communities

Although pesticides are aimed at one or a few species in biotic communities, usually these toxicants have some impact either directly or indirectly on most species. Pesticides may influence the structure and/or functioning of biotic communities. For example, when the animal community associated with Brassica oleracea (cole plant) was exposed to either DDT (0.25 lb/A) or parathion and endrin (0.20 and 0.18 lb, respectively) significant changes in the community were observed (Pimentel, 1961a). Initially, there was little difference in the number of herbivorous taxa present in the untreated and both treated plots (23, 20, and 19 taxa, respectively). Although the parasitic and predaceous taxa were similar in both the untreated and DDT communities (13 and 11, respectively), the parasitic and predaceous taxa in the parathion communities were practically extinct (only 2 remained). The loss of natural enemies in the

parathion community was due to two factors: (1) direct
destruction of many natural enemies and (2) indirect
destruction by reducing their food host and prey populations to such low levels that the parasite and predator
populations were unable to persist.

Densities of the various taxa per week in the three
communities varies significantly (Table 1). Note that an
aphid outbreak occurred in the DDT community and that a
large number of parasites were present. These were
attracted by the aphid outbreak. The parathion community
had been severely reduced in kinds of taxa.

TAXON	CONTROL	DDT	PARATHION
Aphids	162.7	1,106.3	20.3
Lepidoptera	12.0	4.4	1.0
Flea beetles	1,107.1	3.5	1.5
Herbivores	643.5	3.4	1.0
Parasites	27.8	481.7	0.4
Predators	8.9	7.6	0.7

Table 1. The average taxa density per week recorded in
three experimental communities.

Note that the ratios of parasites to hosts and
predators to aphid prey were quite different in the three
communities (Table 2). Aphid-parasite numbers were up but
lepidoptera parasite numbers were down in the DDT community
compared to the untreated community. Both, however, were
higher than in the parathion community. Predator to aphid
prey ratios were low in both the DDT and parathion communities.

TAXON	EXPERIMENTAL COMMUNITY		
	CONTROL	DDT	PARATHION
		Parasites	
Aphids	9	34	1
Lepidoptera	57	22	8
		Predators	
Aphids	4.4	0.6	1.2

Table 2. The ratio of parasites to hosts and of predators
to aphids in various experimental communities.

Recognizing the complexity of interactions in the B. oleracea community (Figure 1) and the different degrees of susceptibility that the various species have in the community (Pimentel, 1961b), it is at times impossible to predict exactly how any community will respond to the impact of a pesticide. Generally this community responded to pesticides similarly to the four effects on ecosystems mentioned earlier and they are: (1) reduction in species; (2) population outbreaks; (3) species low in the food chain exploded in numbers without enemies; (4) predators and parasites high in the food chain were more severely affected than those species low in the food chain.

A reduction in species diversity occurred in a fescue meadow when it was exposed to 3,9, and 27 lbs/A of the herbicide, sodium cacodylate (Malone, 1972). Recovery of species diversity of the plants was relatively rapid but was not complete at the end of the growing season. Simplification of community structure resulted in significant reductions in biomass throughout the growing season. For example, there was an 80-100% reduction in total biomass of all species except fescue within two weeks of herbicide application.

The marine diatom (Thalassiosira pseudonata) and green alga (Dunaliella tertiolecta) that were resistant and sensitive to DDT and PCB, respectively, were experimentally exposed in mixed cultures to DDT (10, 25, 50, and 100 ppb) and PCB (1, 10, and 25 ppb) (Mosser, et. al., 1972). In untreated cultures the diatom grew faster and was the dominant species. However, in the DDT and PCB treated cultures its dominance was reduced. This effect was recorded in cultures even at DDT and PCB concentrations that had no apparent effect on single species cultures. Mosser, et. al., (1972) pointed out that long lasting pollutants such as DDT and PCB could, based on their results, "disrupt the species composition of phytoplankton communities".

Other diverse effects that pesticides may have on a community are well illustrated in rice fields. Organophosphatic nematocide compounds were applied at 10 to 100 times usual rates (0.5 - 2 lb/A) (Hollis, 1972). Nematode control resulted but rice yields did not increase in spite of excellent nematode control. The reason given by Hollis was that the nematocide treatments stimulated the grassy weeds and these more effectively competed with rice. Hence, although there were fewer nematodes, the increased weed growth more than offset the expected effect of nema-

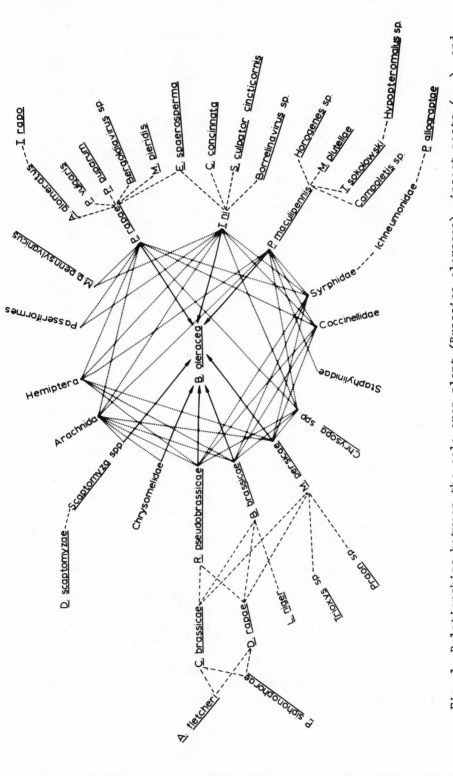

Fig. 1. Relationships between the cole crop-plant (Brassica oleracea), insect pests (——), and parasitic (---) and predaceous (•••) enemies of the pests (Pimentel, 1961b).

tode population reduction.

Populations

The application of pesticides directly to crop lands, forests, and other habitats may reduce and sometimes temporarily exterminate not only the pest, but also some non-target species in the treated region. This is not surprising for pesticides are chemically highly effective poisons applied specifically to destroy animal and plant pests. Although the direct effects of applications are relatively easily observed, the indirect effects are difficult to detect. For example, how do we discern whether numbers of a non-target species are declining because of the indirect effects of pesticides or because of the many other environmental factors which affect natural populations? In studying the indirect effects, the mode of dispersion through the environment and what dosage reaches the non-target species are difficult to determine.

Investigations of why some raptorial bird species were declining in habitats where chlorinated insecticide residues were present illustrate the complexity of the problem. Wildlife biologists suspected that DDT and other insecticide residues were having an adverse effect, but recognized that urbanization was also contributing to bird mortality. Proof that DDT and other insecticides contributed to the observed decline of some raptorial birds required the exposure of predaceous bird species to known amounts of pesticides under controlled conditions. To accomplish this, a predator species first had to be bred successfully in the laboratory (in this case the first species to be bred was the American sparrow hawk) and then fed measured amounts of either DDT and dieldrin or DDE to get body levels as occur naturally (Porter and Wiemeyer, 1969; Wiemeyer and Porter, 1970). Feeding the sparrow hawk these chemicals did cause the birds to produce eggs with significantly thinner shells and contributed to greater loss of eggs than the untreated controls. This evidence substantiated the field observations, leading to the conclusion that in these areas DDT and DDE were contributing to population declines.

The decline of lake trout in Lake George and other nearby lakes also illustrates the complexity of measuring indirect effects. For several years previous to and during the decline in the lake trout populations, about 4,535,900 kilograms of DDT had been applied yearly for pest control

35

in the Lake George watershed. A portion of the DDT found its way into the lake, but the amount was probably small. Although both adult lake trout (8 to 835 ppm of DDT in fat) and their eggs contained DDT, (3 to 355 p.p.m.) the mature lake trout appeared unaffected, and their eggs hatched normally. The cause for the decline in the lake trout population remained a mystery until it was discovered that the young fry were highly sensitive to certain levels of DDT in the eggs (Burdick, et. al., 1964). Fry died at the time of final absorption of the yolk, just when the young were ready to feed. Mortality in the fry was significant at 3 ppm and, at levels of 5 ppm or more, mortality was 100%. The reason for the observed decline in the lake trout population in Lake George was then obvious.

On the California Channel Islands there appears to be an association between premature pupping of the California sea lion and organochlorine pollutant residues (DeLong, et. al., 1973). Premature births have been occurring with increasing frequency and starting as early as January. The early premature pups are not furred and apparently die soon after birth. The later premature pups lacked motor coordination, breathing was short, and only parts of the lungs were inflated. DDT and PCB residues in blubber fat of females having premature pups averaged 824 ppm and 112 ppm, respectively; whereas residues in females producing full-term pups averaged only 103 ppm (DDT) and 17 ppm (PCB) (DeLong, et. al., 1973).

Beneficial predaceous and parasitic insect populations have been reduced and even eliminated in some regions after insecticide usage. The results are outbreaks of particular insect and mite species previously controlled by these populations. For example, when predaceous coccinellid beetles and other predator and parasite populations were unintentionally eliminated in areas treated with DDT, chlordane, and other chemicals, outbreaks of mites (Helle, 1965), aphids (Pimentel, 1961a), and scale insects (DeBach, 1947) occurred. Sometimes the densities of these plant pests increased 20-fold above the control level usually achieved by their natural enemies.

Reduced seed production may occur in plants influenced by pesticides. For example, when 2,4-DB herbicide was applied at 0.56, 1.12, and 1.68 kg/ha at three stages of growth (vegetative, bud, and flowering), there was a 10 to 50% reduction in seed production that occurred primarily at the vegetative and bud stage applications (Lee, 1972). The reductions were more severe at the higher dosages.

Insecticides may also suppress the growth of bacterial (Staphylococcus aureus) populations (Langlois and Sides, 1972). The generation time for this bacterium on a trypticase soy broth at 37°C was about 32 min. However, when 10 ug/ml of heptachlor in 99.8% absolute alcohol was applied, the generation time was reported to be increased to about 211 min and purified chlordane at the same dosage increased the generation time to about 357 min (Langlois and Sides, 1972).

Food and Energy

Elton (1927) pointed out that the whole structure and function of biotic communities is dominated by the interrelationships of species seeking food (energy). The prime input of energy is from the sun via plant photosynthesis. Herbivores, carnivores, and decomposers all seek to obtain their share of food and energy resources from the plants. Pesticides may influence the energy dynamics of species and communities by affecting the physiology of the organism so that its metabolism, growth and reproduction are changed and by altering the quality of food consumed by the animals.

Pesticides have been found to either depress growth in some species or stimulate growth in others. For example, female whitetailed deer, when fed either 5 ppm or 25 ppm of dieldrin for 3 years grew much more slowly than untreated females (Korschgen and Murphy, 1969). An herbicide (2,4-D), sprayed at 0.56 kg/ha, increased the time for growth and development of predaceous coccinellid beetle larvae by nearly 60% (Adams, 1960). Extending the growth period and thus altering their life cycle could significantly reduce the effectiveness of these animals in biological control of aphids and other pest insects. Caterpillars of the rice stemborer pest grew 45% larger on rice plants treated with 2,4-D than on untreated rice (Ishii and Hirano, 1963). They suggested the increased growth was due to changes in the rice plant caused by the 2,4-D which made the plant more nutritious to the rice stemborer. The larger borers also probably ate more. Herbicides at sublethal concentrations are known to affect the growth of plants, but insecticides may also directly affect plant growth. Corn grown in soil treated with DDT at the rate of 100 ppm weighed nearly 40% more after 4 weeks than corn grown in untreated soil (Cole, et. al., 1968). Beans, however, weighed significantly less

37

(30%) at the end of 8 weeks when grown in soil with 10 ppm of DDT.

Reproduction

Altering the reproductive physiology of animals changes the efficiency of the species and its ability to utilize food and leave offspring. Species populations are in rather delicate balance with the energy they obtain for maintenance and reproduction. Any alteration of reproduction may seriously influence the survival of a species. For example, pesticides appear to have a deleterious effect on the reproduction of some raptorial as well as other bird species. Eggshell thinning, as mentioned, was one such effect for predaceous birds. Aquatic fish-eating birds have been more severely affected than terrestrial-bird predators because the aquatic birds obtain more pesticides via their food chain than do terrestrial birds. In some natural habitats the brown pelican has been exposed to DDT and DDE. Keith et al. (1970) reported that this exposure caused egg breakage and complete reproductive failure in one area investigated. The effects of pesticides on reproduction in birds are more varied than just eggshell thinning. Ovulation times in Bengalese finches, as mentioned, were delayed (twice normal) when the birds were fed DDT at a daily dosage of 270 ug DDT (Jefferies, 1969), thus significantly increasing the time for a generation and possibly putting the breeding cycle out of phase with foods produced in the environment. When mallard ducks were fed 40 ppm DDE in their diet, embryo mortality during egg incubation ranged from 30% to 50% (Porter and Wiemeyer, 1969). Total duckling production per hen was reduced by as much as 75% when the ducks received this level of DDE. Also, ringdoves fed 10 ppm DDT showed a decrease in estradiol in the blood early in the breeding cycle, and, egg production was delayed (Peakall, 1970).

Dieldrin, DDT, and DDE were not the only chemicals to affect reproduction in birds. Herbicides 2,4-D (32% acid) and 2,4,5-T (15% active agent, 19.52 ml/liter water) sprayed on grass daily for 14 days led to reduced egg production in exposed chickens (Dobson, 1954). For 2,4-D the reduction was 8% and for 2,4,5-T, 18%. In one test, 2,4-D was also found to depress reproduction of mallard ducks fed daily levels of 1,250 and 2,500 ppm in their diet. In another test at the same dosages, reproduction was

38

reduced about 80% (USDI, 1970).

The fungicide thiram, when included in the diets of chickens at 10 to 200 ppm, caused them to produce soft-shelled and abnormally-shaped eggs (Waibel, et. al., 1955; Antoine, 1966).

Female mosquito fish aborted their young after exposure to sublethal dosages of DDT, TDE, methoxychlor, aldrin, endrin, toxaphene, heptachlor or lindane (Boyd, 1964).

Pesticides may also increase the rate of reproduction in some animals. The exposure of bean plants, for example, to sublethal dosages of 2,4-D increased aphid progeny production during a 10-day period from 139 to 764 per aphid (Maxwell and Harwood, 1960). Also 2,4-D amine caused a more rapid increase of aphids on treated corn than on un-treated barley (Oka, 1973).

Sublethal doses of DDT (1 ug/female), dieldrin (0.5 ug/female) and parathion (2 ug/female) increased egg production by the Colorado potato beetle during the second week by 50%, 33%, and 65%, respectively (Abdallah, 1968).

Chemical Composition of Plants

Pesticides also may alter the chemical makeup of plants and this may in turn affect the animals dependent upon them for food. The changes which do occur appear to be specific for both the plants and pesticides involved. Certain chlorinated insecticides increased the amounts of some macro- and micro-element constituents in corn and beans, and decreased the amounts of others (Cole, et. al., 1968). For instance, heptachlor in soil at dosages of 1, 10, and 100 ppm caused significant changes in the elements N, P, K, Ca, Mg, Mn, Fe, Cu, B, Al, Sr, and Zn measured in the aboveground portions of corn and bean plants. Zinc was significantly higher (89 ppm, dry weight) in bean plants treated with 100 ppm of heptachlor than in untreated con-trols (55 ppm); however, nitrogen levels were significantly lower (4.99%) in the treated plants than in the unexposed controls (7.25%).

Protein content increased from 10.9% to 15.5% when wheat was exposed to 2,4-D (Erickson, et. al., 1948), whereas beans grown in soil containing a low level of 2,4-D had a lower level of protein than the untreated controls (Anderson and Baker, 1950).

The potassium nitrate content of sugar beet plants

exposed to a sublethal dosage of 2,4-D increased from a normal of 0.22% (dry weight) to 4.5% (Stahler and Whitehead, 1950). This nitrate level was highly toxic to cattle. 2,4-D and other herbicides have been found both to increase and to depress the level of nitrate in various other plants (Frank and Grigsby, 1957).

Another chemical change is the sugar content of plants exposed to pesticides. When exposed to sublethal doses of 2,4-D, ragwort, a weed naturally toxic to many animals including cattle, has an increased level of sugar (Willard, 1950). The high sugar content in the weed makes it attractive to cattle and sheep, with disastrous results because the toxicity of the plant remains high.

Swanson and Shaw (1954) demonstrated that the hydrocyanic acid content of sudan grass increased by 69% when exposed to 1.12 kg/ha of 2,4,5-T. The sudan grass in the untreated control contained 36 mg/100 g of HCN (fresh weight), compared with 61 mg/100 g in the 2,4,5-T treated sudan grass. Note that 2,4,5-T is not recommended for weed control in sudan grass.

DDT, aldrin, endrin, and lindane each applied at rates of 10, 20, and 30 ppm were found to stimulate synthesis in corn of arginine, histidine, leucine, lysine, proline, and tyrosine but decreased the content of tryptophan (Thakre and Saxena, 1972). They also found that synthesis of methionine was stimulated by the application of aldrin, endrin, and lindane only, however, the synthesis of valine was suppressed by aldrin, endrin, and DDT only.

Behavior

Patterns of behavior in animals determine their survival in the habitat in which the animal lives. Each animal responds to environmental cues to help it select its food and shelter, avoid natural enemies, select a mate, and so forth. Hence, any change in an animal's normal behavioral patterns may significantly influence the survival of the population.

Pesticides have been found to alter the normal behavior of various animal species. For example, sublethal dosages of dieldrin (15 mg/kg/day) fed to sheep increased the number of trials required by the animals to relearn a visual discrimination test (Van Gelder, et. al., 1969). Also the Swedish robin, Erithacus rubecula, generally a migratory bird that moves at night, is affected by low

levels of pesticides. Ulfstrand, et. al., (1971) found that
robins given PCB (Clophen A50) so that their breast muscle
contained 164 to 467 ppb of PCB had significantly longer
than normal activity periods compared with the control
birds that contained PCB at only 51 to 120 ppb. What this
change in behavior means to actual survival of these migratory robins has not been determined.

Sublethal doses of DDT (20 ppb) caused brook trout to
lose most of their learned avoidance responses (Anderson
and Peterson, 1969). Further, Jackson, et. al., (1970)
reported that sublethal dosages of DDT altered speckled
trouts' natural repertoire of unconditioned response
patterns to a given set of conditioning procedures.

Ogilvie and Anderson (1965) found that New Brunswick
salmon from a DDT-sprayed region were unusually sensitive
to low temperatures and selected water of higher temperatures than normal for spawning. With this type of
behavior, the salmon might place their eggs in areas where
their fry could not survive. Mosquito fish exposed to low
concentrations of DDT (0.1 to 20 ppb) preferred waters of a
higher salinity level than normal for the species (Hansen,
1969). The effect of this was not studied.

Atlantic salmon parr had their ability to learn and
retain a simple conditioned response suppressed when exposed to sumithion (1 ppm), abate (5 ppm), and DDT (0.7 ppm)
(Hatfield and Johansen, 1972). With a sumithion exposure
for 24 hrs, the fish had their learning ability completely
inhibited and also appeared less active than untreated
fish. Although abate-exposed fish eventually learned the
response pattern, they had significant difficulty in the
learning process. Interestingly, salmon exposed to DDT
learned faster than controls, but the fish appeared hypersensitive to external stimuli. No effects were noted in
salmon exposed to 0.09 ppm of methoxychlor (Hatfield and
Johansen, 1972). Exposing Atlantic salmon parr to 1 ppm of
sumithion for 24 hrs made the fish more vulnerable to pred-
ation by large brook trout (Salvelinus fontinalis) than
untreated fish (Hatfield and Anderson, 1972). In an
experimental pond in which 50% of the salmon had been exposed to 1 ppm sumithion more treated salmon were eaten
(95%) by the brook trout than untreated (58%).

Goldfish (Carassius auratus) exposed to 10 ppb of DDT
for 4 days had their locomotor activity significantly suppressed (Davy, et. al., 1972). The exposure of young
Atlantic salmon to 1 ppm of fenitrothion for 15 to 16 hrs

caused a decrease (50%) in the "number of holding ter-
ritories" 6 days after treatment (Symons, 1973). Some of
the affected fish also swam stiffly and ceased feeding.

Concerning insects, the herbicide 2,4-D at 1.68 kg/ha
caused predaceous coccinellid beetles to become sluggish in
their behavior (Adams and Drew, 1965). When this happens,
they are less successful as predators than unaffected
beetles and some of their prey escape capture.

Predators, Parasites, and Herbivores

Perhaps 90% of all animals live as predators
(including parasites and herbivores) and feed on living
matter and only a few live as true saprophytes (Pimentel,
1968). These predators feeding on prey populations may
control the numbers of their food population. However, if
the prey population is to persist, the predator population
must live only on surplus prey (energy) produced by their
prey population (Pimentel, 1961a and 1968). Through what
has been termed the feedback mechanism, predator and prey
populations evolve a balanced supply-demand economy. This
balanced economy is in dynamic equilibrium and therefore
any alteration in the normal ecology of either predator or
prey species may result in serious changes in this
equilibrium. Pesticides may alter the equilibrium and
economy in several ways. For example, the exposure of
mallard ducklings to PCB (Arochlor) increased their
susceptibility to disease (duck hepatitis virus) (Friend
and Trainer, 1970). Also, the exposure of fish to carbaryl
and 2,4-D seemed to reduce their natural resistance to a
microsporidian parasite (Butler, 1969). Oka (1973) has
demonstrated that corn plants exposed to about 20 ppm of
2,4-D sprayed on plants are about twice as susceptible to
corn leaf aphid. Oka (1973) also found corn smut gall
weights on plants treated with 20 ppm of 2,4-D were twice
the weights on untreated plants.

Other plant-related instances of pesticides increasing
disease susceptibility in hosts include the following:
2,4-D (4.5×10^{-4} and 4.5×10^{-3} M) increased the size of
tobacco mosaic virus lesions on hypersensitive tobacco
(Simons and Ross, 1965); pyrazon ($6\frac{1}{2}$ lb/A) increased the
incidence of damping off in sugar beet seedlings (Altman
and Ross, 1967); trifluralin (3/4 lb/A) also predisposed
cotton seedlings to damping off (Pinckard and Standifer,
1966); several nematocides including 1,3-D (20 gal/A) in-

creased the incidence of weather fleck tobacco (Miller and
Taylor, 1970); 2,4-D, picloram + 2,4-D, or cacodylic acid +
arsenic (injected to the heartwood) increased oak wilt
fungal infections and bark beetle infestations (Rexrode, et.
al., 1971); and the number of root-knot larvae and ring nematodes in the soil at harvest was increased with azide
applied at 10 and 15 lb/A (Rodriguez-Kabana, et. al., 1972).

Another interesting pesticide phenomenon that may have
significant impact on the dynamic equilibria that exist
between predators and prey is bioaccumulation. Both
animals and plants have the ability to concentrate many
types of pesticides in their body tissues and this appears
to be a common physiological phenomenon. The chlorinated
insecticides have the greatest tendency for biological concentration, but other pesticides exhibiting biological
concentration are: diazinon (Miller, et. al., 1966), mirex
(Cope, 1966), dichlobenil (Cope, 1965), diquat (Cope,
1965), paraquat (Cope, 1965), silvex (Cope, 1965), sodium
arsenite (Cope, 1966), and 2,4-D (Smith and Isom, 1967).
The tremendous capacity for concentrating pesticides is
best illustrated with fishes, oysters, and waterfleas.
Fish (golden shiners) were reported to take DDT at 0.265
ppb in water and concentrate it 100,000 times in their
bodies (Reed, 1969); oysters took DDT at 1 ppb in seawater
and concentrated it 70,000 times (Butler, 1964); and waterfleas were similarly adulterated, taking DDT at 0.5 ppb in
water and concentrating it 100,000 times in their bodies
(Priester, 1965).

The capacity for biological concentration is usually
not as great as this, but when the procedure is repeated at
each successive link in the food chain, extremely high concentrations of toxicant can occur in the species at the top
of the food chain especially predators and parasites. This
was documented in the food chain involving soil, earthworms, and robins. Starting with DDT at a level of 9.9 ppm
in soil, it reached a level of 141 ppm in the earthworms
and 444 ppm in the brains of adult robins (Hunt, 1965).
This high concentration in the robins was toxic to some
birds.

It is obvious that if the prey species, as with the
earthworms, become toxic to their predator, the numbers of
predators may decline. The released predator pressure then
may result in an explosive increase in the prey. This has
been well illustrated when there is a differential susceptibility between predator and prey to a particular

pesticide. Earlier we mentioned the example of coccinellid beetles being more susceptible than their aphid prey resulting in an outbreak of aphids (Pimentel, 1961a). A great many examples of this have been reported by Ripper (1956) and Van den Bosch (1973).

Evolution

Under intense selective pressure from pesticide poisons many species have evolved a degree of pesticide tolerance. The effect of this pesticide resistance on the ecosystem is varied. Species with large amounts of genetic variability can evolve a high degree of tolerance and become the dominant species in the pesticide-stressed ecosystem. Such changes in dominance by some species can alter the dynamic equilibrium of the whole biotic community. This type of change in biotic communities has not been documented, but the degree of resistance (tolerance) in natural species populations has.

A wide variety of animals and plants have evolved significant levels of tolerance. For example, a house mouse population selected for resistance to DDT increased its tolerance to DDT 2-fold over 10 generations of exposure (Ozburn and Morrison, 1964). Also, a pine mouse population investigated in the field evolved a level of tolerance to endrin 12-fold above the usual levels (Webb and Horsfall, 67). Although most of this resistance was believed to be genetic, a certain amount of tolerance might be conferred by feeding the mice sublethal dosages of endrin over time as a result of enzyme induction (see p.128).

No bird species is known to have evolved resistance to the pesticides. Unfortunately, this aspect has not been well investigated in bird populations. One would expect some of the species such as robins, which have experienced high mortalities due to insecticides, to evolve some level of resistance to these chemical toxicants.

Amphibians (cricket frogs) from heavily treated cotton field areas have evolved resistance to DDT (Boyd, et. al., 1963). Also, mosquito fish populations inhabiting streams in the cotton belt had significant levels of resistance to the following insecticides: DDT (4-fold above control), strobane (300-fold), toxaphene (40-fold), chlordane (20-fold), aldrin (20-fold), heptachlor (18-fold), dieldrin (30-fold), endrin (120-fold), and dursban (2-fold) (Vinson, et. al., 1963; Boyd and Ferguson, 1964; and Ferguson, et.

44

al., 1965a). Other fish from the same region exhibiting resistance were the golden shiner, bluegill, green sunfish, and black bullhead (Ferguson, et. al., 1965a; Ferguson, et. al., 1965b).

As expected, insect and mite populations with high levels of resistance to pesticides have been found in many parts of the world. Of about 2,000 pest insect and mite species, a total of 225 species has been reported resistant to pesticides (Brown, 1969). Of this group, 121 were crop pests, 97 man and animal pests, 6 stored-produce pests and 1 forest pest. In at least one instance the level of increased resistance was 25,000-fold.

Although the evidence is inconclusive, resistance to 2,4-D may have developed in some weed plants (Abel, 1954; Hanson, 1956).

Environmental Persistence and Movement

Persistent pesticides remain in the environment for long periods and thereby have the advantage of being effective pest controls over long periods of time with fewer applications needed. An obvious disadvantage is that the longer the chemical poisons persist in the environment, the greater the likelihood that they will move out of the treated area via either soil, water, air, or organisms and injure non-target organisms. Another disadvantage is the more prolonged exposure of pests to selection, and thereby the increased chance of pesticide resistance developing.

The chlorinated insecticides may persist for long periods, ranging from 6 months to 30 years, depending on the chemical, its dosage, and characteristics of the environment. DDT, for instance, at only 1.12 kg/ha persisted in a forest environment for 9 years with little decline in the residual level (Diamond et al., 1970). Based on this rate of disappearance, the investigators estimated that DDT even at this low dosage would endure for 30 years. In contrast, residues of some economic poisons, like malathion, may persist for only a few days, lowering the chances of the chemicals becoming persistent pollutants.

Pesticides are generally widespread in the environment, and their movement throughout the environment is related in large measure to their persistence. Antarctic seals and penguins, far distant from the application of any pesticides, were found to be contaminated with DDT (Sladen, et al., 1966; Brewerton, 1969). In the Arctic region,

45

seals, caribou, and polar bears contain DDT (Holden and Marsden, 1967; Keith, 1969). Also many kinds of non-target mammals, birds, fishes, and insects are known to contain residues of numerous kinds of pesticides. In some non-target species accumulations of pesticides have become sufficiently high to be lethal to individuals of the species itself and to predators which prey on them.

With time, pesticide residues decline in living populations if use of the pesticide is halted. For example, heptachlor residues in woodcock (<u>Philohela</u> <u>minor</u>) averaged about 2.4 ppm soon after the area had been treated with heptachlor from 1956 to 1962 (McLane, et. al., 1971). About 3 years later with no further treatment heptachlor residues had declined to an average of 0.42 ppm.

Some pesticide residues are found at low levels in water throughout the United States. However, in the southeast and west, pesticide residues were present at fairly high levels (Nicholson, et. al., 1964; Butler, 1969; Modin, 1969). A surprising find was the fairly high levels of pesticides detected in the atmosphere. Concentrations of DDT far distant from any treated area, for example, ranged from below detectable levels to 23 ng/m^3 (Tabor, 1965).

Movement through the atmosphere seems to provide an effective means for transport of some pesticides to widely dispersed habitats. The quantity of pesticide released into the atmosphere over the crop, but never reaching the treated crop, is well illustrated with aircraft spraying. For example, in treating corn only 26% of DDT sprayed from the aircraft reached the corn when measured at tassel height (Hindin, et. al., 1966). Off-tract waste of insecticide is generally 50 to 60% (Brooks, 1947).

Accumulated pesticides in living organisms may also travel long distances via the organism itself. For example, DDT and other pesticides are carried by migrating robins and woodcocks. The impact of this type of pesticide movement through the environment probably has been underestimated.

Herbicides are generally less persistent than insecticides, but materials such as picloram and monuron have been found to persist for 2 to 3 years in the soil (Hamaker, et. al., 1963; Birk, 1955). Fungicides break down fairly rapidly, but some, like the mercury compounds, may leave various stable forms which could move in the biosphere for at least 45 years (Jernelov, 1972).

References

Abdallah, M. D. 1968. Bull. Entomol. Soc. Egypt Econ. Ser. 2: 211–217.

Abel, A. L. 1954. Brit. Weed Con. Conf. Proc. 2: 249–253.

Adams, J. B. 1960. Can. J. Zool. 38: 285–288.

Adams, J. B. and M. E. Drew. 1965. Can. J. Zool. 43: 789–794.

Adams, L., M. G. Hanavan, N. W. Hosley, and D. W. Johnston. 1949. J. Wildl. Manag 13: 245–254.

Akesson, N. B., S. E. Wilce and W. E. Yates. 1971. Annual Meeting Amer. Soc. of Agr. Engineers. Chicago, Ill. Dec. 7–10, 1971. Paper 71–662.

Alexander, M. 1967. "Agriculture and the Quality of the Environment," N. C. Brady (ed.). Amer. Assoc. Advan. Sci., Washington, D. C., pp. 331–342.

Altman, J. and M. Ross. 1967. Plant Disease Reporter 5: 86–88.

Anderson, G. R. and C. O. Baker. 1950. Agron. J. 42: 456–458.

Anderson, J. M. and M. R. Peterson. 1969. Science 164: 440–441.

Antoine, O. 1966. Parasitica (Gembloux) 22: 107–114.

Azevedo, J. A., E. G. Hunt, and L. A. Woods. 1965. Calif. Fish Game 51: 276–293.

Balicka, N. 1969. Report derived from PL-480 Project Ewl-CR-30 (FG-Po-172).

Barrett, G. W. and R. M. Darnell. 1967. Amer. Midland Natur. 77: 164–175.

Birk, L. A. 1955. Can. J. Agr. Sci. 35: 377–387.

Boyd, C. E. 1964. Progr. Fish-Cult. 26: 138.

Boyd, C. E., S. B. Vinson, and D. E. Ferguson. 1963. Copeia 2: 426–429.

Brewerton, H. V. 1969. New Zealand J. Sci. 12: 194–199.

Brooks, A. F. 1947. Agr. Engin. 28(6): 233–239.

Brown, A. W. A. 1969. Can. Med. Assoc. J. 100: 216–221.

Burdick, G. E., E. J. Harris, H. J. Dean, T. M. Walker, J. Skea, and D. Colby. 1964. Trans. Amer. Fish. Soc. 93: 127–136.

Buroyne, W. E. and N. B. Akesson. 1971. Agr. Aviation 13: 12–23.

Butler, P. A. 1964. "The Effects of Pesticides on Fish and Wildlife." U. S. Fish Wildl. Serv. Circ. 226, pp. 65–77.

Butler, P. A. 1969. M. W. Miller and G. G. Berg (eds.), "Chemical Fallout." C. C. Thomas, Springfield, Illinois, pp. 205-220.

Cade, T. J., J. C. Lincer, C. M. White, D. G. Roseneau, and L. G. Swartz. 1971. Science 172: 955-957.

Clark, F. E. 1967. A. Burges and F. Raw (eds.), "Soil biology." Academic Press, London, pp. 15-49.

Cohen, J. M. and C. Pinkerton. 1966. Adv. Chem. Ser. No. 60: 163-176.

Cole, H., D. MacKenzie, C. B. Smith, and E. L. Bergman. 1968. Bull. Environ. Contam. Toxicol. 3: 141-154.

Cope, O. B. 1965. S. Weed Conf. Proc. 8: 439-445.

Cope, O. B. 1966. J. Appl. Ecol. 3)supplement on pesticides in the environment and their effects on wildlife): 33-34.

Davis, B. N. K. and M. C. French. 1969. Soil Biol. Biochem. 1: 45-55.

Davy, F. B., H. Kleerekoker and P. Gensler. 1972. J. Fish. Res. Bd. Can. 29: 1333-1336.

DeBach, P. 1947. Calif. Citrograph 32: 406-407.

DeLong, R. L., W. G. Gilmartin and J. G. Simpson. 1973. Science 181: 1168-1170.

Diamond, J. B., G. Y. Belyea, R. E. Kadunce, A. S. Getchell, and J. A. Blease. 1970. Can. Entomol. 102: 1122-1130.

Dobson, N. 1954. J. Ministry Agr. (Brit.) 110: 415-418.

Edwards, C. A. 1964. Brit. Ecol. Soc. Symp. 5: 239-261.

Elton, Charles. 1927. "Animal ecology." MacMillan Company, New York, p. 56.

Erickson, L. C., C. I. Seely, and K. H. Klagas. 1948. J. Amer. Soc. Agron. 40: 659-660.

Ferguson, D. E., W. D. Cotton, D. T. Gardner, and D. D. Culley. 1965a. J. Miss. Acad. Sci. 11: 239-245.

Ferguson, D. E., D. D. Culley, W. D. Cotton, and R. P. Dodds. 1965b. BioScience 14: 43-44.

Frank, P. A. and B. H. Grigsby. 1957. Weeds 5: 206-217.

Friend, M. and D. O. Trainer. 1970. Science 170: 1314-1316.

Fuhremann, T. W. and E. P. Lichtenstein. 1972. Toxicol. Appl. Pharamacol. 22(4): 628.

Hamaker, J. W., H. Johnston, R. T. Martin, and C. T. Redemann. 1963. Science 141: 363.

Hansen, D. J. 1969. Quarterly Report, July 1969 to September 1969. Cen. Estuarine and Menhaden Research. U. S. Fish Wildl. Ser., Bur. Com. Fish.

Hanson, N. S. 1956. Down to Earth 12(2): 2-5.
Hatfield, C. T. and J. M. Anderson. 1972. J. Fish. Res. Bd. Can. 29: 27-29.
Hatfield, C. T. and P. H. Johansen. 1972. J. Fish. Res. Bd. Can. 29: 315-321.
Heath, R. G., J. W. Spann, and J. F. Kreitzer. 1969. Nature 224: 47-48.
Helle, W. 1965. Advan. Acarol. 2: 71-93.
Hindin, E., D. S. May, and G. H. Dunstan. 1966. "Organic Pesticides in the Environment." Amer. Chem. Soc. Publ., pp. 132-145.
Holden, A. V. and K. Marsden. 1967. Nature 216: 1274-1276.
Hollis, J. B. 1972. Plant Disease Reporter 56: 420.
Hunt, L. B. 1965. "The Effects of Pesticides on Fish and Wildlife." U. S. Fish Wildl. Ser. Circ. 226, pp. 12-13.
Ishii, S. and C. Hirano. 1963. Entomol. Exp. Appl. 6: 257-262.
Jackson, D. A., J. M. Anderson, and D. T. Gardner. 1970. Can. J. Zool. 48: 577-580.
Jefferies, D. J. 1967. Ibis. 109: 266-272.
Jefferies, D. J. 1969. Nature 222: 578-579.
Jernelov, A. 1972. R. Hartung and B. D. Dinman (eds.), "Environmental mercury contamination." Ann Arbor Science Publ. Inc., Michigan, pp. 176-201.
Keith, J. A. 1969. Presented at the 33rd Federal Provincial Wildlife Conf., Edmonton, 8 July 1969. Mimeo. 6 p.
Keith, J. O., R. M. Hanse, and A. L. Ward. 1959. J. Wildl. Manag. 23: 137-145.
Keith, J. O., L. A. Woods, and E. C. Hunt. 1970. Presented at the 35th N. Amer. Wildl. Natur. Res. Conf. Mimeo. 15 p.
Korschgen, L. J. and D. A. Murphy. 1969. Missouri Federal Aid Project No. 13-R-21 (1969) Work Plan No. 8, Job No. 1, Progress Report. 55 p.
Langlois, B. E. and K. G. Sides. 1972. Bull. Environ. Contam. Toxicol. 8: 158-164.
Lee, W. O. 1972. Weed Sci. 20: 330-331.
Lichtenstein, E. P., T. T. Liang and B. N. Anderegg. 1973. Science 181: 847-849.
Malone, C. R. 1972. Ecology 53: 507.
Maxwell, R. C. and R. F. Harwood. 1960. Ann. Entomol. Soc. Amer. 53: 199-205.
Mayer, F. L., Jr., J. C. Street and J. M. Neuhold. 1972.

Toxicol. Appl. Pharmacol. 22(3): 347-354.
McLane, M. A. R., L. F. Stickel and J. D. Newsom. 1971.
Pest. Monit. J. 5: 248-250.
Miller, C. W., I. E. Demoranville, and A. J. Charig. 1966.
Weeds 14: 296-298.
Miller, P. M. and G. S. Taylor. 1970. Plant Disease
Reporter 54: 672.
Miner, J. R. (ed.). 1971. N. Cent. Reg. Res. Publ. 206.
Iowa Agr. Exp. Sta. Spec. Rep. 67. 44 p.
Modin, J. C. 1969. Pest. Monit. J. 3: 1-7.
Mosser, J. L., N. S. Fisher and C. F. Wurster. 1972.
Science 176: 533-535.
Nicholson, H. P., A. R. Grzenda, G. J. Lauer, W. S. Cox,
and J. I. Teasley. 1964. Limnol. Oceanogr. 9: 310-317.
Ogilvie, D. M. and J. M. Anderson. 1965. J. Fish Res. Bd.
Can. 22: 503-512.
Oka, I. N. 1973. Personal communication. Dept. of Entom-
ology, Cornell University.
Otten, R. J., J. E. Dawson, and M. M. Schreiber. 1957.
N.E. Weed Control Conf. Proc. 11: 120-127.
Ozburn, G. W. and F. O. Morrison. 1964. Can. J. Zool. 42:
519-526.
Peakall, D. B. 1970. Science 168: 594-595.
Pimentel, D. 1961a. J. Econ. Entomol. 54: 108-114.
Pimentel, D. 1961b. Ann. Entomol. Soc. Amer. 54: 323-333.
Pimentel, D. 1968. Science 159: 1432-1437.
Pimentel, D. 1971. U. S. Govt. Printing Office. 220 p.
Pinckard, J. A. and L. C. Standifer. 1966. Plant Disease
Reporter 50: 172-174.
Porter, R. D. and S. N. Wiemeyer. 1969. Science 165:
199-200.
Potts, G. R. 1970. Proc. 10th Br. Weed Control Conf.:
299-302.
Priester, L. E. 1965. Ph.D. Thesis, Clemson University.
74 p.
PSAC. 1965. Pres. Sci. Adv. Comm., The White House.
317 p.
Randell, R. 1971. Coop. Ext. Serv. Univ. of Ill. and Ill.
Nat. Hist. Survey, pp. 104-105.
Raw, F. 1962. Ann. Appl. Biol. 50: 389-404.
Reed, J. K. 1969. Completion Rept. No. 13 OWRR Project
No. A-013-SC, Clemson University. 11 p.
Rexrode, C. O., R. P. True and R. R. Jones. 1971. Plant
Disease Reporter 55: 1106-1107.
Ripper, W. E. 1956. Ann. Rev. Ent. 1: 403-438.

Rodriguez-Kabana, R., P. A. Backman, H. Ivey and
L. L. Farrar. 1972. Plant Disease Reporter 56: 362.
Simons, T. J. and A. F. Ross. 1965. Phytopath. 55:
1076-1077.
Sladen, W. J. L., C. M. Menzie, and W. L. Reichel. 1966.
Nature 210: 670-673.
Smith, G. E. and B. G. Isom. 1967. Pest. Monit. J. 1:
16-21.
Sobieszczanski, J. 1969. 1st Nat. Congr. Soil Sci. Soc.
Sofia, N. Balicka.
Stahler, L. M. and E. K. Whitehead. 1950. Science 112:
749-751.
Swanson, C. R. and W. C. Shaw. 1954. Agron J. 46:
418-421.
Symons, P. E. K. 1973. J. Fish. Res. Bd. Can. 30:
651-655.
Tabor, E. C. 1965. 58th Annual Meeting of the Air Pol-
lution Control Assoc., Toronto, Canada, June 20-24. In
J. M. Cohen and C. Pinkerton, (eds.), Adv. Chem. Ser.
No. 60, 1966. p
Thakre, S. K. and S. N. Saxena. 1972. Plant and Soil 37:
415-418.
Ulfstrand, S., A. Sodergren and J. Rabol. 1971. Nature
231: 467-468.
USDA. 1973. The Pesticide Review 1972. Agr. Stab. and
Cons. Ser., 58 pp.
USDI. 1970. Personal communication. Patuxent Wildl. Res.
Center. U. S. Department of the Interior.
Van den Bosch, R. and P. S. Messenger. 1973. "Biological
control." Intext Educational Publishers, New York,
180 p.
Van Gelder, G. A., W. B. Buck, R. Sandler, J. Maland, G.
Karas, and D. Elsberry. 1969. "The Biological Impact
of Pesticides in the Environment." Environ. Health Ser.
1, Oregon State University, pp. 125-133.
Vinson, S. B., C. E. Boyd, and D. E. Ferguson. 1963.
Science 139: 217-218.
Waibel, P. E., B. S. Pomeroy, and E. L. Johnson. 1955.
Science 121: 401-402.
Ware, G. W., W. P. Cahill, P. D. Gerhardt, and J. M. Witt.
1970. J. Econ. Entomol. 63: 1982-1983.
Webb, R. E. and F. Horsfall, Jr. 1967. Science 156: 1762.
Wiemeyer, S. M. and R. D. Porter. 1970. Nature 227:
737-738.
Willard, C. J. 1950. Proc. N. Central Weed Cont. Conf. 7:

110-112.

WSA.   1967.   "Herbicide handbook of the Weed Society of
America."   Humphrey Press, Inc., Geneva, N. Y.   293 p.

Acknowledgments

This study was supported in part by grants from the
Ford Foundation (Ecology of Pest Management) and the
National Science Foundation grant No. GB19239.

ENVIRONMENTAL POLLUTION IN RELATION TO ESTUARINE BIRDS

Harry M. Ohlendorf, Erwin E. Klaas, and T. Earl Kaiser

U. S. Bureau of Sport Fisheries and Wildlife
Patuxent Wildlife Research Center

Abstract

Eggs of anhingas, herons, and ibises were collected during the 1972 nesting season at coastal and inland localities from Florida to New Jersey. Eggshell thinning was not detected among those species for which adequate samples were available for pre-1946 and post-1945 eras. Measurable residues of DDE occurred in all 209 eggs. The highest mean value (4.0 p p m , wet weight) was found in great egrets from New Jersey. Among the coastal localities, levels of DDE as well as total DDT progressively declined toward the south. PCBs occurred second most frequently and also reached their highest mean level (4.2 p p m) in the great egret eggs from New Jersey. However, the pattern of occurrence of PCBs was not like that of the DDT compounds. Higher levels of PCBs were also found in eggs from eastern Florida (anhinga, 2.0 p p m). Other pollutants occurred less frequently and at lower levels. Geographic differences in occurrence and concentration were more apparent than species differences with these less frequently occurring chemicals. Wherever judgments can be made concerning species differences that are independent of geographic differences relative to total DDT residues, it seems that great egrets carry higher residues. Glossy ibises, snowy egrets, and little blue herons have residues at intermediate levels, and other species have residues at lower levels.

Introduction

Changes in eggshell characteristics (thickness, weight, and thickness index) of a number of avian species have been associated with the advent of widespread use of persistent organochlorine pesticides (Ratcliffe, 1967, 1970; Hickey and Anderson, 1968; Anderson et al., 1969; Anderson and Hickey, 1970, 1972; Blus, 1970). The affected species are terminal consumers, generally those feeding on aquatic organisms (primarily fish) or birds.

Experimentation has established that changes in eggshell characteristics can be caused by ingestion of certain organochlorine pesticides. American kestrels, Falco sparverius, fed diets containing dieldrin and DDT in combination produced thinner-shelled eggs and destroyed more of their eggs than did controls (Porter and Wiemeyer, 1969). (Chemical names of compounds referred to in the text are indicated in Appendix A, p.74). Eggshell thinning was also induced when DDE was administered in the diets of kestrels (Wiemeyer and Porter, 1970). In other studies, DDE has caused eggshell thinning in mallards, Anas platyrhynchos, black ducks, A. rubripes, and screech owls, Otus asio (Heath et al., 1969; Longcore et al., 1971; McLane and Hall, 1972).

The soils of estuaries may act as reservoirs for pollutants. Biologic magnification of these chemicals in higher trophic levels may result in a relatively high exposure for secondary and tertiary consumers in these habitats (Woodwell et al., 1967). Herons and ibises are abundant in marsh and estuarine habitats and are important consumers of fish and other small organisms in these ecosystems. Thus, they are an appropriate group of animals for investigations of pollutant occurrence and effect.

Certain herons have been included in general surveys of organochlorine residues in piscivorous birds in the United States and Canada (Keith, 1966; Vermeer and Reynolds, 1970; Anderson and Hickey, 1972; Baetcke et al., 1972). Such residues and their possible effects in herons and related wading birds have also been studied at more restricted localities (Causey and Graves, 1969; Greenberg and Heye, 1971; Faber et al., 1972; Flickinger and Meeker, 1972). The most comprehensive study of a heron species was made on the grey heron, Ardea cinerea, in Great Britain (Prestt, 1969).

This is a preliminary report of our studies of the anhinga (Anhingidae), herons (Ardeidae), and ibises (Threskiornithidae) in the eastern United States. We attempt to discern geographic and species differences in the occurrence and concentration of the residues of organochlorine pesticides and other organochlorine pollutants. We collected eggs from a wide range of localities for shell thick-

ness measurements and chemical analysis of contents. The
eggshell thicknesses of these and other modern eggs in
museum collections were compared to those of archival
shells from the same areas.

Methods

Eggs were collected at coastal (estuarine) and inland
(freshwater) localities from Florida to New Jersey in 1972.
Data from different localities were consolidated when proximity and similarity of habitat, chemical residues, and
eggshell thickness indicated that this was valid.

Entire clutches were collected. In the field, one egg
was selected randomly from each clutch and wrapped in aluminum foil to prevent contamination from the plastic con-
tainer into which it was placed to retard moisture loss.
These eggs were refrigerated until the contents could be
removed, placed into chemically cleaned jars, and frozen
pending analysis.

Egg volumes were measured to the nearest 1.0 ml by
water displacement prior to removing the contents. Residues were adjusted to fresh wet weight, assuming specific
gravity of 1.0 as suggested by Stickel et al., (1973).

Eggshell thickness was measured to the nearest 0.01 mm
using a modified Starrett micrometer. Thickness was measured after the shells had dried at room temperatures for at
least one month. After one year, eggshell thickness was
measured again on a sample of 40 of these eggs and was
found not to have changed. Three measurements were taken
at the "equator" of each egg and included the shell and
shell membranes. Measurements were averaged to yield a
single value for each egg in the clutch. Statistical testing (two-way, non-random model, analysis of variance) was
based on clutch mean thickness.

In this report we considered only those localities
from which we had three or more clutches for one or more of
the following species: anhinga, Anhinga anhinga; green
heron, Butorides virescens; little blue heron, Florida
caerulea; cattle egret, Bubulcus ibis; great egret, Casmer-
odius albus; snowy egret, Egretta thula; Louisiana heron,
Hydranassa tricolor; glossy ibis, Plegadis falcinellus; and
white ibis, Eudocimus albus. Nomenclature for common and
scientific names follows the A. O. U. check-list of North
American birds (1957) and the recent supplement (1973).

A 5- or 10-g subsample of the egg homogenate was

blended with sodium sulfate and extracted 7 to 8 hours with
hexane in a Soxhlet apparatus. Cleanup of the extract, and
separation and quantitation of pesticides and polychlorinated biphenyls (PCBs) was similar to the procedure used for
the analysis of pelican carcasses (Blus et al., in press).
In summary, an aliquot of hexane extract equivalent to 5 g
of subsample was passed through a Florisil column to remove
lipids. An aliquot of this eluate was column chromato-
graphed on silicic acid to separate the pesticides and PCBs.
The organochlorines separated into three silicic-acid
eluates were identified and quantitated by gas chromatography on a 1.83-m glass column packed with 4% SE-30/6% QF-1
on 100-120 mesh Supelcoport. Residues in 10% of the samples were confirmed with a combined gas chromatograph-mass
spectrometer.

Recoveries of pesticides and PCBs from spiked egg tissue ranged from 83% to 104%. Residues in this report were
not adjusted on the basis of these recoveries. Sensitivity
of detection for the gas chromatograph was 0.1 p p m for
pesticides and 0.5 p p m for PCBs. When PCBs were detected in trace amounts (<0.5 p p m), they were considered as
0.25 p p m for purposes of this report.

Differences in mean chemical residues were not tested
statistically because of the small sample sizes for each
species at individual localities. Geometric means were
calculated as a measure of central tendency because of the
logarithmic distribution of data.

Collecting Localities

Collecting localities referred to in the text are
coded alphanumerically and indicated in Table 1. We collected most of the eggs on or near National Wildlife Refuges because of logistical considerations and because of
the occurrence there of favorable nesting habitat. Samples
from refuges are considered to be representative of the
general area, because herons and ibises often travel several miles from the nesting area to feed (Dusi et al.,
1971). These birds also disperse widely during the non-
breeding season.

Localities referred to as "inland" are freshwater,
whereas those referred to as "coastal" are essentially estuarine. The latter, however, included several areas where
the birds were nesting at freshwater pools within a few
miles of tidal waters. The Potomac River (Maryland)

Table 1. Collection Localities[1]

General	Specific
Florida; west coast (A)	Wakulla Co., St. Marks National
Florida; east coast (B)	Wildlife Refuge (1)
Florida; inland (C)	Levy Co., Cedar Keys National
Georgia; coast (D)	Wildlife Refuge (2)
Georgia; inland (E)	Brevard Co., Merritt Island Nat-
South Carolina; inland (F)	ional Wildlife Refuge (3)
South Carolina; coast (G)	Alachua Co., Orange Lake (4) and
North Carolina; coast (H)	vicinity of Gainesville (5)
Maryland-Virginia;	McIntosh Co., Blackbeard Island
coast (I)	National Wildlife Refuge (6)
Maryland; Potomac River (J)	Chatham Co., Wassaw National
New Jersey; coast (K)	Wildlife Refuge (7) and Savan-
	nah National Wildlife Refuge
	(8-part of which is in South
	Carolina: Jasper Co.)
	Ware Co., Okefenokee National
	Wildlife Refuge (9)
	Berkeley Co., Lake Marion (10)
	Charleston Co., Cape Romain Nat-
	ional Wildlife Refuge and vic-
	inity (11)
	Dare Co., Pea Island National
	Wildlife Refuge (12)
	Hyde Co., Mattamuskeet National
	Wildlife Refuge (13)
	Virginia: Accomac Co., Shelly
	Bay (14-contiguous with
	Chincoteague Bay)
	Maryland: Worcester Co.,
	Chincoteague Bay, South Point
	(15)
	St. Marys Co., St. Catherine
	Island (16)
	Atlantic Co., Reeds Bay (17)
	Cape May Co., Great Egg Harbor
	Bay (18)

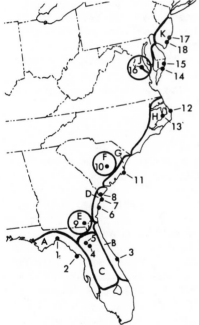

Fig. 1. Approximate location of general (coded alphabetically) and specific (numerically) collecting localities referred to in text. See Table 1 for identification.

[1]Alphanumeric coding was used to indicate these localities in Fig. 1.

locality is in the tidal portion of that river, but 80
miles from Chincoteague Bay (Virginia). The inclusion of
eggs from different habitats allows comparison of the
freshwater and estuarine environments where they were sampled within a relatively small geographic area.

Chemical Residues

All 209 eggs had measurable amounts of DDE; DDT occurred in 24.4% of the eggs (Table 2). DDT residues were
associated with levels of DDE that almost always exceeded 1
p p m (wet weight). Eggs with DDE levels lower than 1
p p m seldom contained measurable amounts of DDT. DDD was
found in only 5.3% of the eggs. PCBs occurred second most
frequently, appearing in 76.1% of the eggs. Dieldrin was
measured in 25.8% of the eggs and mirex in 17.7%. Alpha
chlordane occurred in only 2.9% of the samples and oxychlordane in 1.4%. Hexachlorobenzene was not detected.

These data depict the relative occurrence of the various chemicals. However, it is more meaningful to examine
geographic and species differences because chemical residues are probably not uniformly distributed in the environment and the species studied have dissimilar feeding habits.

Geographic differences

We analyzed three to seven samples of each species
from two or more localities. The species had different
distributional patterns and habitat requirements (Bent,
1922, 1926; Palmer, 1962) and did not all nest at any one
locality. Patterns of chemical residue distribution are
especially difficult to interpret because migratory birds
that nest in a particular locality may have over-wintered
in dissimilar areas. Different migratory routes also could
contribute to different exposures. Nevertheless, we are
able to discern certain patterns in the distribution of
chemical residues. In this preliminary report we did not
attempt to evaluate all possible contributing factors, but
report the residues measured and the patterns observed.

When data for all localities and species are graphed
and arranged by locality (Figs. 2 and 3) geographic residue
differences transcend differences attributable to species.
The numbers of samples for each locality and species, numbers of samples with measurable residue, geometric means of
residues, and extreme values of residues are presented in

Table 2. Frequency of Occurrence of Measurable Chemical Residues [Per cent of eggs in which residues were measured (Number of eggs in which residues were measured)]

Species (no. of eggs)	DDE	DDD	DDT	Dieldrin	Mirex	Chlordanes Alpha	Chlordanes Oxy	PCB
Anhinga (10)	100.0 (10)				20.0 (2)			100.0 (10)
Green heron (27)	100.0 (27)		3.7 (1)	18.5 (5)	18.5 (5)			44.4 (12)
Little blue heron (36)	100.0 (36)	2.8 (1)	27.8 (10)	27.8 (10)	13.9 (5)	5.6 (2)	2.8 (1)	66.7 (24)
Cattle egret (26)	100.0 (26)		38.5 (10)	38.5 (10)	42.3 (11)	3.8 (1)	3.8 (1)	100.0 (26)
Great egret (20)	100.0 (20)	20.0 (4)	45.0 (9)	35.0 (7)	35.0 (7)	5.0 (1)	5.0 (1)	95.0 (19)
Snowy egret (30)	100.0 (30)	13.3 (4)	23.3 (7)	33.3 (10)	6.7 (2)	6.7 (2)		60.0 (18)
Louisiana heron (30)	100.0 (30)	3.3 (1)	10.0 (3)	6.7 (2)	10.0 (3)			100.0 (30)
Glossy ibis (21)	100.0 (21)	4.8 (1)	52.4 (11)	47.6 (10)				52.4 (11)
White ibis (9)	100.0 (9)				22.2 (2)			100.0 (9)
TOTALS % (no.)	100.0 (209)	5.3 (11)	24.4 (51)	25.8 (54)	17.7 (37)	2.9 (6)	1.4 (3)	76.1 (159)

59

Appendix B (pp.75-81).

DDT did not exceed 1 p p m in most eggs. It occurred
more frequently and at higher concentration in samples from
inland South Carolina, coastal Maryland, Virginia, and New
Jersey than in samples from most other collection sites.
Eggs from New Jersey had the highest incidence of DDD and
the highest levels of DDE. Total DDT residues (DDT plus
metabolites) were found in an apparent clinal pattern among
coastal localities (Fig. 2); low levels occurred in Florida
samples and high levels in New Jersey samples. Whereas the
samples from inland South Carolina contained high residues
of several chemicals, those from inland Florida and Georgia,
particularly those from the Okefenokee Swamp, contained
much lower concentrations.

Dieldrin occurred in a greater proportion of the samples from South Carolina northward (38 of 106) than in samples from Florida and Georgia (16 of 103), although residue
concentrations were generally less than 1 p p m   Mirex was
measured at highest levels in samples from coastal Georgia
(principally Savannah), and most frequently in samples from
this locality, inland South Carolina, and inland Florida.
Alpha chlordane and oxychlordane were not found in any
clearly defined pattern, although there was some indication
of greater incidence in samples from eastern Florida.

The highest levels of PCBs were in samples from New
Jersey. No PCBs were measured in samples from inland
Georgia where the birds probably feed primarily in the
Okefenokee Swamp. Samples from eastern Florida contained
higher mean levels of PCBs than those from other areas
south of Virginia.

Species differences

The species studied have different feeding behaviors
and consume different prey (Bent, 1922, 1926; Palmer, 1962).
The occurrence of various levels of organochlorine residues
is shown in Figures 2 and 3 and Appendix B. Species differences are apparent when all samples from a particular
locality are considered.

Of the species examined, great egret eggs had the
highest mean residues of DDE (4.0 p p m , New Jersey).
This species also had the highest mean values (1.9 p p m
or greater) at the three other localities where eggs were
collected. Glossy ibis eggs had relatively uniform mean
DDE residues (1.4 and 1.5 p p m) and extreme values

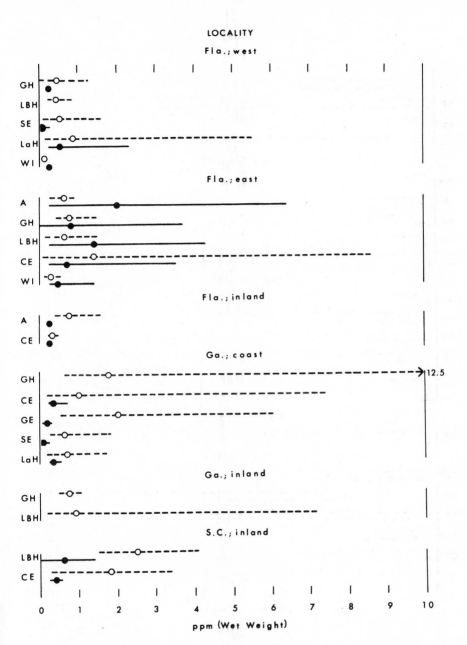

Fig. 2. Extreme values and geometric means for residues of total DDT (— O —) and of PCBs (— ● —) in eggs of estuarine birds (ppm wet weight). Localities are further identified in Fig. 1 and Table 1.

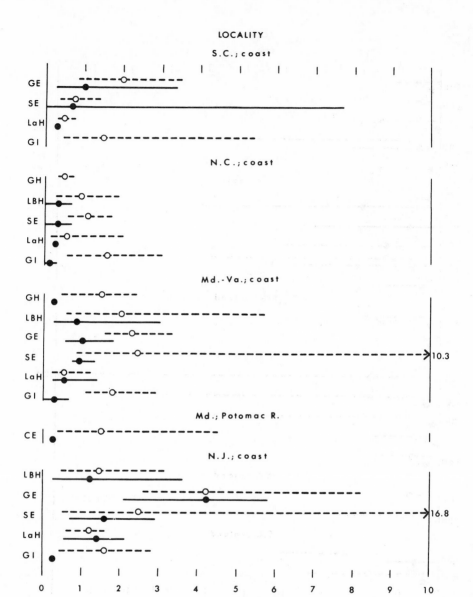

Fig. 2 cont'd. Species are coded as follows: anhinga (A), green heron (GH), little blue heron (LBH), cattle egret (CE), great egret (GE), snowy egret (SE), Louisiana heron (LaH), glossy ibis (GI), and white ibis (WI).

(Appendix B) at each of the four localities where they were collected. Little blue heron, snowy egret, and cattle egret samples had mean values of 1 p p m or greater at three localities. Eggs of other species generally had lower levels of DDE. One green heron egg from coastal Georgia and one snowy egret egg from New Jersey each contained 12 p p m of DDE, the highest individual levels detected.

Species differences for DDT and DDD are difficult to interpret because these residues occurred in fewer samples. There is no clearly defined pattern of species differences for these chemicals. A snowy egret sample (the same one with 12 p p m DDE) had the highest levels of DDT (3.6 p p m) and DDD (0.94).

Dieldrin and mirex residues were more intimately related to geographic location than to species. Nevertheless, incidence of measurable dieldrin residues tended to be higher in cattle egret and glossy ibis. The highest dieldrin concentration in a single sample was in a snowy egret (3.8 p p m). The highest individual value for mirex was in cattle egret (2.9 p p m) and the highest mean (0.74 p p m) in green heron samples from coastal Georgia.

New Jersey great egret eggs had the highest mean level of PCBs (4.2 p p m). Other mean levels greater than 1.5 p p m include the anhinga samples from eastern Florida (2.0 p p m) and snowy egrets from New Jersey (1.6 p p m). A snowy egret egg from South Carolina had the highest individual level (7.7 p p m). Green heron, cattle egret, Louisiana heron, glossy ibis, and white ibis samples had low levels of PCBs (i.e., usually < 1 p p m).

Eggshell Characteristics

Significant geographic variation in eggshell thickness is known to occur in some species (Anderson and Hickey, 1970, 1972). It is therefore necessary to compare recent eggs with archival eggs from the same general locality to appropriately determine whether any change has occurred. We tested for differences in clutch mean shell thickness, by species and locality, in 859 clutches (3,045 eggs) to determine whether changes in eggshell thickness have occurred since 1945 (Table 3). We found no statistically significant differences between pre-1946 and post-1945 shell thicknesses.

Numbers of eggs collected were few for any one species at a locality, even fewer eggs per locality were chemically

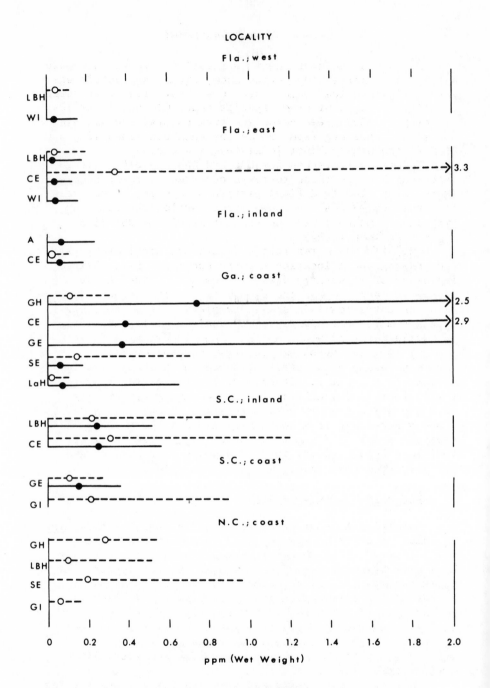

Fig. 3. Please see legend on following page.

Fig. 3, continued.

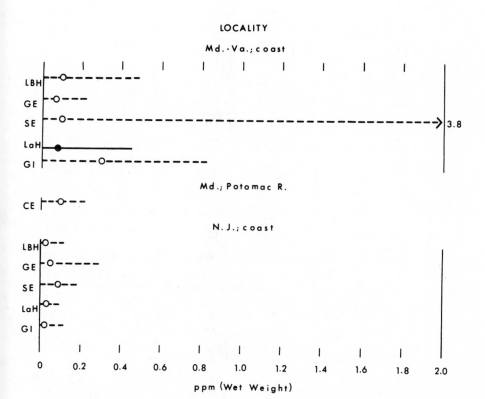

Fig. 3. Extreme values and geometric means for residues of dieldrin (—O—) and Mirex (—●—) in eggs of estuarine birds. Localities and species are identified as in Figure 2. Species (and one locality) with no measurable residues are not shown (Appendix B).

analyzed and no changes in shell thickness were found.

Species	Pre–1946		Post–1945	
Locality	no.	$\bar{x} \pm 95\%$ C.L.	no.	$\bar{x} \pm 95\%$ C.L.
Anhinga				
Fla.; east	18	0.336 ± 0.010	13	0.352 ± 0.011
Fla.; inland	31	0.355 ± 0.009	7	0.348 ± 0.015
Green heron				
Fla.; west	8	0.185 ± 0.009	8	0.187 ± 0.005
Fla.; east	34	0.184 ± 0.004	21	0.186 ± 0.004
Ga.-S.C.; coast	43	0.181 ± 0.002	8	0.177 ± 0.008
Va., Md., N.J.; coast	66	0.184 ± 0.002	9	0.180 ± 0.007
Little blue heron				
Fla.; west	81	0.237 ± 0.003	5	0.239 ± 0.019
Fla.; east	35	0.240 ± 0.004	9	0.236 ± 0.014
S.C.	11	0.234 ± 0.008	12	0.232 ± 0.005
Great egret				
Ga.-S.C.; coast	20	0.298 ± 0.006	16	0.291 ± 0.011
Snowy egret				
Fla.; west	16	0.227 ± 0.009	12	0.219 ± 0.005
Ga.-S.C.; coast	42	0.233 ± 0.004	15	0.234 ± 0.007
Louisiana heron				
Fla.; west	54	0.227 ± 0.003	13	0.225 ± 0.007
Ga.-S.C.; coast	17	0.230 ± 0.006	15	0.237 ± 0.006
White ibis				
Fla.; west	79	0.346 ± 0.005	10	0.339 ± 0.010
Fla.; east	86	0.350 ± 0.004	45	0.346 ± 0.005

Table 3. Mean shell thicknesses (mm) of clutches of eggs collected prior to 1946 and those collected after 1945 (no. = no. of clutches). Localities are further identified in Table 1. No significant differences ($P < 0.05$) were detected.

Discussion and Conclusions

Our study was oriented toward determining whether egg-shell thickness had changed since the advent of widespread use of persistent organochlorine pesticides in the mid-1940s. We further hypothesized a priori that there would be geographic differences in the occurrence of these pesticides and other organochlorine pollutants related to differences in application. It also follows that species differences in levels of contamination would exist because of differences in prey selection. We have interpreted our data in relation to these three subject areas.

a. Eggshell thickness

We did not detect significant decreases in shell thickness in any species at sampling localities included in this report. Additional eggs were collected in 1973, for these as well as other species and localities, and are in the process of analysis.

Eggshell thinning is known to vary interspecifically in response to the degree of exposure to DDE (Anderson and Hickey, 1972; Keith and Gruchy, 1972). Certain herons have exhibited shell thinning at some localities, but they apparently are not as susceptible as some other species. Our report does not include data on the great blue heron, Ardea herodias, nor the black-crowned night heron, Nycticorax nycticorax, in both of which thinning has been reported in some regions (Vermer and Reynolds, 1970; Anderson and Hickey, 1972). Our data on these species are presently incomplete but will be included in later reports.

Great egret eggshells in California have shown significant thinning, but the associated DDE residues were higher than those we measured (Faber et al., 1972). As much as a 20% reduction in shell thickness has been reported in the gray heron, A. cinerea, in England (Prestt, 1969). Residue levels of DDE and dieldrin also exceeded those we observed. Mean DDE residue levels of 4-5 p p m were found only in the great egret eggs from New Jersey, but the paucity of archival eggshell samples from that area precluded statistical comparisons of shell thickness. A 15% reduction in shell thickness in eggs of the brown pelican, Pelecanus occidentalis, in South Carolina was associated with 4-5 p p m DDE (Blus et al., 1972). Our samples of heron and ibis eggs from the same locality had lower levels of this pollutant.

We may speculate that DDE residues did not reach sufficient levels in 1972 at the localities considered in this report to cause eggshell thinning in the species we sampled. It is also possible that these species (except the great egret) are more resistant to shell thinning by organochlorines, or that our sample size was too small.

b. Geographic differences in residue levels and occurrence

Interpretation of differences in the geographic distribution of persistent pollutants in the environment is difficult. Usage patterns of these chemicals are not well known, and they change widely in space and time. Certain chemicals found in biologic samples are the result of agricultural or silvicultural applications, whereas others may originate from industrial uses. Species and individual differences in feeding habits, biologic magnification in higher trophic levels, and migration of individual birds to different localities may further complicate interpretation.

However, certain patterns of geographic distribution are evident. In our study, the most clear-cut patterns occurred with mirex and DDT (and its metabolites). Mirex appeared almost exclusively in samples from the South and was absent in nearly all samples north of North Carolina. This coincides with the widespread use of mirex in the South for "attempted" control of the imported fire ant, Solenopsis saevissima. Unfortunately, samples containing mirex are insufficient in numbers to adequately compare estuarine with freshwater ecosystems. The widespread occurrence of DDT and its metabolites, particularly DDE, is well known; this study confirms their continued presence in the environment. All samples contained measurable amounts of DDE. Quantitatively, the samples from New Jersey for each species usually contained the highest levels of total DDT and of DDE. Among the coastal localities, these residues generally declined toward the South.

Mallards, Anas platyrhynchos, and black ducks, A. rubripes, also show their highest levels of DDE in the northeastern states (Heath, 1969; Heath and Hill, in press). Fish analyzed as part of the National Pesticide Monitoring Program from the states in our study had the highest mean residues of total DDT in New Jersey (Henderson et al., 1969, 1971). This suggests that there may be a relationship between the residue levels in fish and the levels found in the eggs because all of these herons are primarily fish-eaters.

In a recent survey of organochlorines in estuarine mollusks, DDT was found in all New Jersey samples (Butler, 1973). However, the mean level for that state was exceeded by several other states. The samples from New Jersey (as well as Alabama, the only other state of the 15 in the survey in which DDT was found in all samples) were from a single drainage basin, whereas samples of mollusks from other states were from several distinct drainage basins. The incidence of DDT or metabolites was not correlated with the magnitude of residues. DDT residues in mollusks reached a peak in 1968 and have declined markedly since 1970 (Butler, 1973).

When states are ranked on the basis of the percentage of mollusk samples in which DDT and metabolites were detected at levels exceeding 5 p p b (Butler, 1973), the geographic distribution approximates that in which we found these chemicals in our egg samples. It is also important that the high levels (as high as 5.39 p p m) found in mollusks on the west coast of Florida were obtained considerably south of our collecting localities. Those samples from near our localities had comparatively lower levels (0.02-0.07 p p m).

Starlings, Sturnus vulgaris, the avian species monitored in terrestrial environments by the National Pesticide Monitoring Program, have higher DDE residues in the South (Martin, 1969; Martin and Nickerson, 1972). Starlings from the northeastern states were low in DDE. Woodcocks, Philohela minor, have also been analyzed as representatives of the terrestrial environment (Clark and McLane, unpublished manuscript; McLane et al., in press). The pattern of chemical residue concentration is similar to that in the starlings. Residue levels of six chlorinated hydrocarbons in whole carcasses of woodcocks from 23 eastern states were negatively correlated with latitude of the collection site. This correlation was strongest in residues of DDE. Woodcock wings from Georgia, South Carolina, and North Carolina had significantly higher concentrations of total DDT than those from other states.

Perhaps the observed difference between terrestrial and the aquatic species is related to chemical usage. In the Northeast, DDT has been used extensively for mosquito control in marshes whereas in the South it has been applied extensively to agricultural crops.

Our results indicate higher residues of dieldrin north of Georgia, although dieldrin did not occur in many samples. We also found more dieldrin in eggs from inland South Carolina than in eggs from coastal areas. In the National Pesticide Monitoring Program, dieldrin was reported in a greater proportion of starling samples (Martin, 1969; Martin and Nickerson, 1972) than in duck samples (Heath, 1969; Heath and Hill, in press). These observations indicate that this toxicant is more widely dispersed in terrestrial than in estuarine habitats. In the duck survey, dieldrin was either absent or present at low levels in samples from Georgia and Florida. However, of the states in common with our study, starlings had highest levels in the Southeast, as did the woodcock samples (Clark and McLane, unpublished manuscript; McLane et al., in press)

Fish from New Jersey had the highest mean residues of dieldrin, among states in common with our study (Henderson et al., 1969, 1971). Relatively high dieldrin levels were also reported in fish from Savannah. Dieldrin was the second most common organochlorine (after DDT) found in estuarine mollusks (Butler, 1973). The pattern of distribution is not very clearly defined. Georgia had greater incidence (higher percentage with levels exceeding 5 p p b) than neighboring states. However, with this exception the samples from northern states had a greater percentage exceeding 5 p p b.

PCBs were the second most prevalent group of chemicals in our samples, in frequency of occurrence and mean concentrations. Higher mean levels tended to occur in the northern states except for the eastern coastal locality in Florida. These results generally agree with the distribution of PCBs in duck wings (Heath and Hill, in press). In contrast, PCB residue levels in woodcocks were higher in samples from the South (Clark and McLane, unpublished manuscript; McLane et al., in press).

c. Species differences in residue levels and occurrence

The occurrence of different organochlorine residues in different species may be partly due to dissimilar food preferences. For example, great egrets feed on larger fish of different species than do the other bird species studied (Bent, 1922, 1926; Palmer, 1962). Cattle egrets and the ibises feed more extensively on invertebrate primary consumers. Cattle egrets are essentially terrestrial in feeding, whereas ibises feed extensively in mud flats. The other species of our study feed primarily in aquatic areas on fish of various sizes and on other organisms.

Cattle egret and glossy ibis eggs contained more DDT (in relation to metabolites) and dieldrin, but less PCBs, than did the eggs of most of the other species. Apparently the DDT had not yet been metabolized in the food chain before it was acquired by the birds. The larger fish taken by great egrets may contain higher residue levels and cause

70

the eggs of this species to contain higher levels than
those of the other aquatic-feeding herons. The anhinga
also feeds on larger fish and had higher PCB residue levels
in eastern Florida than did the herons from that locality.
We were unable to obtain great egret eggs from eastern
Florida in 1972.

Some data indicate that certain fish species contain
higher levels of chemical residues but large variations in
residues within species overshadow the species differences
(Henderson et al., 1969, 1971). No statistical correlation was found between residue levels in the different
fish species. However, these authors did find that some
species are consistently among those having highest residues whereas others are usually among those having lowest
residues.

We found considerable individual differences within
species, most noticeably among the snowy egrets. This variability is possibly related to differences in metabolism
and migratory patterns or dietary preferences.

Summary

Eggshell thinning is one of the more easily determined
manifestations of the adverse effects of organochlorines in
birds, but it may not be the only significant one. Population declines and reproductive failures may be associated
with other less well understood effects of these toxicants.
Intensive, long-term studies of reproductive success and
population dynamics in various species are needed, both in
areas having high and those having low residue levels. Our
report may assist in the selection of localities and
species for such studies.

References

American Ornithologists' Union Committee. 1957. "Check-list
    of North American birds," 5th ed. Baltimore, Amer.
    Ornithol. Union.
American Ornithologists' Union Committee. 1973. Auk, 90:
    411-419.
Anderson, D. W., and J. J. Hickey. 1970. Wilson Bull. 82:
    14-28.
Anderson, D. W., and J. J. Hickey. 1972. Proc. XV Int.
    Ornithol. Cong.:514-540.
Anderson, D. W., J. J. Hickey, R. W. Risebrough, D. F.

Hughes, and R. E. Christensen. 1969. Canadian Field-Nat. 83:91-112.

Baetcke, K. P., J. D. Cain, and W. E. Poe. 1972. Pest. Monit. J. 6:14-22.

Bent, A. C. 1922. Bull. U. S. Nat. Mus., 121.

Bent, A. C. 1926. Bull. U. S. Nat. Mus., 135.

Blus, L. J. 1970. BioScience 20:867-869.

Blus, L. J., C. D. Gish, A. A. Belisle, and R. M. Prouty. 1972. Nature 235:376-377.

Blus, L. J., A. A. Belisle, and R. M. Prouty. Pest. Monit. J. (In press).

Butler, P. A. 1973. Pest. Monit. J. 6:238-362.

Causey, M. K., and J. B. Graves. 1969. Wilson Bull.. 81:340-341.

Dusi, J. L., R. T. Dusi, D. L. Bateman, C. A. McDonald, J. J. Stuart, and J. F. Dismukes. 1971. Res. Inst. Bull., 5.

Faber, R. A., R. W. Risebrough, and H. M. Pratt. 1972. Environ. Pollut. 3:111-122.

Flickinger, E. L., and D. L. Meeker. 1972. Bull. Environ. Contam. Toxicol. 8:165-168.

Greenberg, R. E., and P. L. Heye. 1971. Wilson Bull. 83:95-97.

Heath, R. G. 1969. Pest. Monit. J. 3:115-123.

Heath, R. G., and S. A. Hill. Pest. Monit. J. (In press).

Heath, R. G., J. W. Spann, and J. F. Kreitzer. 1969. Nature 224:47-48.

Henderson, C., W. L. Johnson, and A. Inglis. 1969. Pest. Monit. J. 3:145-171.

Henderson, C., A. Inglis, and W. L. Johnson. 1971. Pest. Monit. J. 5:1-11.

Hickey, J. J., and D. W. Anderson. 1968. Science 162:271-273.

Keith, J. A., and I. M. Gruchy. 1972. Proc. XV Int. Ornithol. Cong.:437-454.

Keith, J. O. 1966. J. Appl. Ecol. 3:71-85.

Longcore, J. R., F. B. Samson, and T. W. Whittendale, Jr. 1971. Bull. Environ. Contam. Toxicol. 6:485-490.

Martin, W. E. 1969. Pest. Monit. J. 3:102-114.

Martin, W. E., and P. R. Nickerson. 1972. Pest. Monit. J. 6:33-40.

McLane, M. A. R., and L. C. Hall. 1972. Bull. Environ. Contam. Toxicol. 8:65-68.

McLane, M. A. R., L. F. Stickel, E. R. Clark, and D. L. Hughes. Pest. Monit. J. (In press).

Palmer, R. S. 1962. "Handbook of North American birds," vol.

1. Yale University Press, New Haven and London.
Porter, R. D., and S. N. Wiemeyer. 1969. Science 165:199–200.
Prestt, I. 1969. IUCN Eleventh Technical Meeting I:95–102.
Ratcliffe, D. A. 1967. Nature 215:208–210.
Ratcliffe, D. A. 1970. J. Appl. Ecol. 7:67–115.
Stickel, L. F., S. N. Wiemeyer, and L. J. Blus. 1973. Bull. Environ. Contam. Toxicol. 9:193–196.
Vermeer, K., and L. M. Reynolds. 1970. Canadian Field-Nat. 84:117–130.
Wiemeyer, S. N., and R. D. Porter. 1970. Nature 227:737–738.
Woodwell, G. M., C. F. Wurster, Jr., and P. A. Isaacson. 1967. Science 156:821–824.

Acknowledgments

Many persons in addition to those mentioned here contributed to our study. We were granted collecting permits by the several states involved in the survey. Assistance was received from numerous personnel of National Wildlife Refuges (listed in text) where eggs were collected, and from Stephen A. Nesbitt for the inland Florida locality.

We acknowledge the cooperation of curatorial personnel in the following museums where oological collections were examined: American Museum of Natural History, Carnegie Museum, Clemson University, Delaware Museum of Natural History, Florida State Museum, Louisiana State University, Museum of Comparative Zoology, Ohio State University, Peabody Museum of Natural History, Philadelphia Academy of Natural Sciences, University of Kansas, University of Massachusetts, and U. S. National Museum.

Although only one of us (T. E. K.) represents the Section of Chemistry, Patuxent Wildlife Research Center, most of the individuals of that unit took part in the chemical analyses.

Kenneth P. Burnham wrote the computer program and provided useful suggestions relative to statistical treatment and interpretation of data.

We appreciate critical reviews of the manuscript by Lawrence J. Blus, Donald R. Clark, Jr., William L. Reichel, and Lucille F. Stickel. The manuscript was typed by T. Madaline Schumacher.

Appendix A. Chemical names of compounds mentioned

Compound	Chemical Name
Alpha (cis) chlordane	1-exo,2-exo,4,5,6,7,8,8-octachloro-2,3,3a,4,7,7a-hexahydro-4,7-methanoindene
DDD	1,1-dichloro-2,2-bis(p-chlorophenyl)ethane
DDE	1,1-dichloro-2,2-bis(p-chlorophenyl)ethylene
DDT	1,1,1-trichloro-2,2-bis(p-chlorophenyl)ethane
Dieldrin	1,2,3,4,10,10-hexachloro-6,7-expoxy-1,4,4a,5,6,7,8,8a-octahydro-1,4-endo-exo-5,8-dimethanonaphthalene
Mirex	dodecachlorooctahydro-1,3,4-metheno-1H-cyclobuta[cd]-pentalene
Oxychlordane	1-exo,2-endo,4,5,6,7,8,8-octacloro-2,3-epoxy-2,3,3a,4,7,7a-hexahydro-4,7-methanoindene
PCB	Mixtures of chlorinated biphenyl compounds having various percentages of chlorination

Appendix B. Chemical residues measured in eggs of estuarine birds. Localities are further identified in Figure 1 and Table 1.

| Species: Locality (no.) | Residues in ppm (wet weight)[1] | | | | | Chlordanes | | PCB |
	DDE	DDD	DDT	Dieldrin	Mirex	Alpha	Oxy	
Anhinga:								
Fla.; east (5)	(5) 0.64 (0.29–0.93)							(5) 2.0 (0.25–6.4)
Fla.; inland (5)	(5) 0.76 (0.39–1.6)				(2) 0.07 (0–0.24)[2]			(5) 0.25 (0.25)
Green heron:								
Fla.; west (5)	(5) 0.47 (0.19–1.3)							(5) 0.25 (0.25)
Fla.; east (5)	(5) 0.78 (0.43–1.5)							(4) 0.81 (0–3.7)
Ga.; coast (6)	(6) 1.7 (0.62–12)		(1) 0.02 (0–0.16)	(3) 0.11 (0–0.31)	(5) 0.74 (0–2.5)			
Ga.; inland (5)	(5) 0.71 (0.48–1.1)							

Appendix B – (cont'd, page 2)

Species: Locality (no.)	Residues in ppm (wet weight)[1]							
	DDE	DDD	DDT	Dieldrin	Mirex	Chlordanes Alpha	Chlordanes Oxy	PCB
N.C.; coast (3)	(3) 0.47 (0.33–0.70)			(2) 0.28 (0–0.53)				
Md.-Va.; coast (3)	(3) 1.5 (0.42–2.4)						(0.25)	(3) 0.25
Little blue heron:								
Fla.; west (5)	(5) 0.44 (0.27–0.84)			(2) 0.04 (0–0.11)				
Fla.; east (5)	(5) 0.64 (0.15–1.5)			(1) 0.04 (0–0.20)	(1) 0.03 (0–0.18)	(1) 0.02 (0–0.097)	(1) 0.03 (0–0.16)	(5) 1.4 (0.25–4.3)
Ga.; inland (5)	(5) 0.85 (0.18–6.1)		(1) 0.13 (0–0.85)					
S.C.; inland (5)	(5) 2.2 (1.4–3.3)		(5) 0.35 (0.09–0.72)	(3) 0.22 (0–0.98)	(4) 0.24 (0–0.52)	(1) 0.02 (0–0.10)		(4) 0.61 (0–1.4)
N.C.; coast (5)	(5) 0.92 (0.28–1.7)		(1) 0.03 (0–0.15)	(1) 0.09 (0–0.51)				(4) 0.33 (0–0.68)

Appendix B – (cont'd, page 3)

Species Locality (no.)	Residues in ppm (wet weight)[1]					Chlordanes		
	DDE	DDD	DDT	Dieldrin	Mirex	Alpha	Oxy	PCB
Md.-Va.; coast (5)	(5) 1.9 (0.57-5.5)		(3) 0.09 (0-0.23)	(2) 0.10 (0-0.48)				(5) 0.84 (0.25-3.0)
N.J.; coast (6)	(6) 1.4 (0.45-3.1)	(1) 0.02 (0-0.094)		(1) 0.02 (0-0.12)				(6) 1.2 (0.25-3.6)
Cattle egret: Fla.; east (6)	(6) 1.4 (0.18-8.3)		(2) 0.08 (0-0.37)	(3) 0.34 (0-3.3)	(2) 0.04 (0-0.13)	(1) 0.02 (0-0.11)	(1) 0.02 (0-0.12)	(6) 0.70 (0.25-3.5)
Fla.; inland (5)	(5) 0.30 (0.22-0.41)			(1) 0.02 (0-0.10)	(2) 0.06 (0-0.18)			(5) 0.25 (0.25)
Ga.; coast (5)	(5) 0.96 (0.18-7.0)		(1) 0.06 (0-0.36)		(3) 0.39 (0-2.9)			(5) 0.33 (0.25-0.70)
S.C.; inland (5)	(5) 1.6 (0.27-3.2)		(3) 0.24 (0-0.92)	(3) 0.31 (0-1.2)	(4) 0.25 (0-0.57)			(5) 0.42 (0.25-0.57)
Md.; Potomac R (5)	(5) 1.4 (0.24-4.3)		(4) 0.12 (0-0.22)	(3) 0.10 (0-0.22)				(5) 0.25 (0.25)

77

Appendix B – (cont'd, page 4)

Species: Locality (no.)	DDE	DDD	DDT	Dieldrin	Mirex	Chlordanes Alpha	Oxy	PCB
Residues in ppm (wet weight)[1]								
Great egret:								
Ga.; coast (4)	(4) 1.9 (0.54–4.6)	(1) 0.03 (0–0.14)	(1) 0.23 (0–1.3)		(2) 0.37 (0–2.0)			(3) 0.18 (0–0.25)
S.C.; coast (6)	(6) 1.9 (0.82–2.9)	(1) 0.03 (0–0.16)	(3) 0.10 (0–0.36)	(4) 0.10 (0–0.27)	(5) 0.15 (0–0.36)	(1) 0.02 (0–0.11)		(6) 1.0 (0.25–3.4)
Md.–Va.; coast (5)	(5) 2.3 (1.6–3.1)		(2) 0.07 (0–0.21)	(2) 0.07 (0–0.22)				(5) 1.0 (0.57–1.8)
N.J.; coast (5)	(5) 4.0 (2.5–7.4)	(2) 0.04 (0–0.11)	(3) 0.18 (0–0.83)	(1) 0.05 (0–0.29)			(1) 0.02 (0–0.11)	(5) 4.2 (2.1–5.8)
Snowy egret:								
Fla.; west (5)	(5) 0.54 (0.098–1.6)					(1) 0.03 (0–0.16)		(2) 0.09 (0–0.25)
Ga.; coast (5)	(5) 0.60 (0.25–1.8)			(2) 0.15 (0–0.71)	(2) 0.06 (0–0.18)			(1) 0.05 (0–0.25)
S.C.; coast (5)	(5) 0.73 (0.36–1.3)	(1) 0.02 (0–0.098)	(1) 0.02 (0–0.10)			(1) 0.03 (0–0.15)		(2) 0.67 (0–7.7)

Appendix B – (cont'd, page 5)

Species: Locality (no.)	Residues in ppm (wet weight)[1]							
	DDE	DDD	DDT	Dieldrin	Mirex	Chlordanes Alpha	Oxy	PCB
N.C.; coast (5)	(5) 1.0 (0.61–1.6)		(2) 0.05 (0–0.15)	(3) 0.19 (0–0.96)				(3) 0.29 (0–0.65)
Md.-Va.; coast (5)	(5) 2.2 (0.79–9.2)		(3) 0.23 (0–1.2)	(2) 0.10 (0–3.8)				(5) 0.88 (0.73–1.3)
N.J.; coast (5)	(5) 2.2 (0.50–12)	(3) 0.21 (0–0.94)	(1) 0.36 (0–3.6)	(3) 0.09 (0–0.18)				(5) 1.6 (0.72–2.9)
Louisiana heron:								
Fla.; west (6)	(6) 0.69 (0–15–5.4)		(1) 0.02 (0–0.13)					(6) 0.53 (0.25–2.3)
Ga.; coast (7)	(7) 0.64 (0.17–1.7)		(1) 0.03 (0–0.26)	(1) 0.01 (0–0.10)	(2) 0.09 (0–0.65)			(7) 0.32 (0.25–0.51)
S.C.; coast (5)	(5) 0.44 (0.29–0.73)							(5) 0.25 (0.25)
N.C.; coast (4)	(4) 0.55 (0.11–2.0)							(4) 0.25 (0.25)

Appendix B – (cont'd, page 6)

			Residues in ppm (wet weight)[1]					
Species:	DDE	DDD	DDT	Dieldrin	Mirex	Chlordanes		PCB
Locality (no.)						Alpha	Oxy	
Md.-Va.; coast (5)	(5) 0.52 (0.23-1.2)				(1) 0.08 (0-0.45)			(5) 0.53 (0.25-1.4)
N.J.; coast (3)	(3) 1.1 (0.63-1.6)	(1) 0.03 (0-0.091)	(1) 0.06 (0-0.18)	(1) 0.03 (0-0.096)				(3) 1.4 (0.53-2.1)
Glossy ibis:								
S.C.; coast (5)	(5) 1.5 (0.46-5.4)			(3) 0.21 (0-0.89)				
N.C.; coast (5)	(5) 1.4 (0.53-2.7)		(3) 0.20 (0-0.71)	(2) 0.05 (0-0.16)				(1) 0.05 (0-0.25)
Md.-Va.; coast (6)	(6) 1.5 (0.57-2.8)	(1) 0.02 (0-0.13)	(5) 0.26 (0-0.73)	(4) 0.30 (0-0.83)				(5) 0.27 (0-0.66)
N.J.; coast (5)	(5) 1.4 (0.42-2.7)		(3) 0.17 (0-0.46)	(1) 0.02 (0-0.12)				(5) 0.25 (0.25)

80

Appendix B — (cont'd, page 7)

Species: Locality (no.)	Residues in ppm (wet weight)[1]					Chlordanes		
	DDE	DDD	DDT	Dieldrin	Mirex	Alpha	Oxy	PCB
White ibis: Fla.; west (5)	(5) 0.13 (0.10–0.16)				(1) 0.03 (0–0.15)			(5) 0.25 (0.25)
Fla.; east (4)	(4) 0.32 (0.12–0.54)				(1) 0.04 (0–0.16)			(4) 0.47 (0.25–1.4)

[1]Values are indicated in the following sequence:
(no. with residues)   Means were computed by first coding all values (as X + 1) to
geometric mean   resolve the problem of "0" values, computing the geometric mean,
(extreme values)   and then decoding.

[2]Lower extreme values of "0" indicate that none was detected at sensitivity level of 0.1 ppm
for pesticides and 0.5 ppm for PCBs.

81

SUBLETHAL EFFECTS OF OIL, HEAVY METALS AND PCBs ON MARINE ORGANISMS

J.W. Anderson, J.M. Neff and S.R. Petrocelli

Department of Biology
Texas A&M University

Introduction

The increased utilization of the near-shore areas of bays and estuaries as sites of industrial development as well as the continued rise in effluent inputs from inland activities has resulted in a rapid increase in the level of contamination of these areas. While individual effluents have in some cases been reduced due to recent regulations, there is still much concern about the effects of an increasing pollution load on marine organisms and on the marine environment as a whole (Darnell, 1971).

In order to evaluate the impacts on the marine environment of the influx of a multitude of contaminants, biologists, oceanographers, engineers and chemists for several years have been involved in the measurement of pollutant levels in the water and biota and in the evaluation of the physiological and toxicological effects of specific contaminants on a variety of marine organisms. Considerable information is now available on the baseline concentrations of many contaminants in the water and biota and on the relative toxicities of these contaminants to several species of marine organisms. For reviews of this background information, the reader is referred to Moore et al. (1973), Nelson-Smith (1973) and Anderson et al. (1974) for oil data, Doudoroff and Katz (1953) and Saha (1972) for reviews on heavy metals in general and mercury in particular, and Peakall (1972) and Risebrough and de Lappe (1972) for the polychlorinated biphenyls (PCBs).

Because of the mass of toxicity data compiled to date, several problems arise in attempting to estimate the present and future impacts of different pollution loads on marine organisms and on the marine environment. Results of bio-

assays and studies of sublethal effects of various pollutants performed in different laboratories are not always
comparable. This is due in part to:
1. Variations in experimental techniques
2. Variations between species
3. A general lack of information on the qualitative
    and quantitative nature of the test solutions after
    preparation and after aeration
4. Lack of correlation between exposure concentration
    of a pollutant and its content in tissues
5. Lack of information on recovery rates and/or con-
    taminant release rates following exposure

To clarify the significance of the toxicity data and
to provide a more realistic means of evaluating damage to
the marine ecosystem, recent emphasis has been placed on
the determination of the sublethal effects of pollutants.
Since a wide range of biological investigations can and
should be included under this broad heading, an outline of
several of these may be helpful (Table 1).

Table 1. Possible means of determining sublethal effects of
         pollutants.

   I. Accumulation and release
      A. Measurement of the extent of accumulation
      B. Measurement of the rates of uptake and release
      C. Measurement of the specific composition of accumu-
         lated and depurated substances
      D. Identification of the sites of exchange with the
         environment and storage within the organism
      E. Correlation of tissue content with toxicity data
      F. Food web accumulation

  II. Physiological studies
      A. Metabolism
         1. Whole organism respiration
         2. Tissue respiration
         3. Homogenate respiration
         4. Enzyme activity
      B. Osmoregulation
         1. Decrease in rate and extent of regulation
         2. Change in ionic composition
      C. Feeding and nutrition
      D. Chemical analyses
         1. Change in relative composition of carbo-

Table 1, (cont'd.)

               hydrates, proteins and lipids
      2. Change in concentration of specific amino acids
          and metabolic intermediates
      3. Increase in mucous production
      4. Alteration in blood proteins

III. Behavioral studies
    A. Loss of equilibrium
    B. Modification in locomotor patterns
    C. Modification of threshold for detection of nutritive
       or reproductive chemical stimuli

IV. Reproduction
    A. Alteration in breeding behavior
    B. Interference with spawning
    C. Decrease in gamete production
    D. Decrease in success of fertilization
    E. Decrease in survival of larval and juvenile stages
    F. Decrease in capacity of breeding by second
       generation

V. Growth
    A. Decrease in rate of cell production
    B. Decrease in the rate of growth
    C. Modification of the number of larval stages or
       adult molts
    D. Modification of correlation between various
       allometric relationships

VI. Histological studies
    A. Development of abnormal growths
    B. Damage to respiratory or sensory membranes
    C. Damage to reproductive organs

VII. Interactions
    A. Temperature – pollutant combinations
    B. Salinity – pollutant combinations
    C. Temperature – salinity – pollutant combinations
    D. Dissolved oxygen – pollutant combinations
    E. Multiple pollutant combinations

Although most sublethal studies conducted thus far
could be placed under one or more of the headings in Table 1,

this list is only presented for convenience and is not exhaustive. For additional comments on methods for evaluating sublethal effects of pollutants, the reader is referred to Sprague (1971) and Waldichuk (1973). Where possible, field studies should be combined with controlled laboratory investigations, as both are needed to reach a definitive conclusion about the impact of a pollutant on the marine environment. Under field conditions, interactions among pollutants and between pollutants and natural physical parameters may greatly modify the response of an organism to any single factor. Interactions may be classified as simple additive, synergistic, supplemental synergistic or antagonistic. A simple additive effect is one in which the effect of the interaction is equal to the sum of effects of the individual components. If the observed effect is greater than the simple sum of each component, the interaction is termed synergistic or supplemental synergistic, depending on degree. If the observed effect is less than the sum, the interaction is termed antagonistic. Before examining the physiological response of an organism to interactions, thorough knowledge of its physiology must be obtained under controlled conditions. In essence, any biological parameter which can be quantitated and which provides a reproducible response is suitable for the evaluation of sublethal effects of pollutants on organisms. Frequently the response to a pollutant may provide new insight or pose new questions regarding the nature of the basic parameter under investigation. With Table 1 as a guide, this paper will compare experimental results which enhance our knowledge of the response of marine organisms to petroleum hydrocarbons, heavy metals and PCBs.

It may be assumed that benthic intertidal marine organisms exposed to pollutants as a result of accidental spills or effluents from industrial operations become contaminated to some extent by these compounds. The questions regarding contamination by any pollutant include: (1) are the substances accumulated in the tissues and what mechanisms are involved , (2) what tissue levels can the organism tolerate and survive , (3) how long are the contaminants retained in the tissues and what is the mechanism of their eventual release, if this is possible? Each of these general questions should bring to mind several related problems, which are too numerous to discuss at this time. Since the second question concerns toxicity and we are limiting our comments to sublethal effects,

86

this discussion will be confined to the accumulation and release of pollutants.

Accumulation and Release:

Heavy metals

The accumulation of heavy metals from dilute sea water solution by marine and estuarine animals has been well demonstrated. Among the more recent studies, Eisler et al. (1972) have shown that mummichogs or common killifish Fundulus heteroclitus, scallops Aquipecten irradians, oysters Crassostrea virginica and northern lobsters Homarus americanus, exposed for 21 days to flowing sea water containing 10 ug/l (ppb) of cadmium accumulated the metal to levels equivalent to 45, 114, 352 and 41 percent, respectively, higher per unit wet weight than baseline levels of cadmium in the controls. Pentreath (1973) determined that exposure of the estuarine mussel, Mytilus edulis to zinc, manganese, iron and cobalt in sea water solution for 49 days resulted in maximum concentration factors of approximately 500, 250, 5000, 1000 respectively. Vernberg and O'Hara (1972) studied the effects of temperature-salinity stress on mercury uptake and accumulation in the gill and hepatopancreas tissues of the fiddler crab Uca pugilator and found significant uptake over 72 hours of exposure, with gill tissue accumulating greater amounts than hepatopancreas under all conditions. While very few data are available regarding the retention times for heavy metals, there are indications that metals accumulated in animal tissues are retained at significant concentrations for several months. The effect of the various temperature-salinity regimes on mercury toxicity will be discussed in a later section.

Polychlorinated Biphenyls (PCBs)

PCBs have been shown to be accumulated to an even greater extent than heavy metals by marine animals. Hansen et al. (1971) measured uptake and retention of Aroclor 1254 by the estuarine pinfish Lagodon rhomboides and spot Leiostomus xanthurus. Exposure of pinfish for 35 days and spot for 45 days to 5 ppb of Aroclor 1254 resulted in tissue concentrations which were $2X10^4$ and $3X10^4$ times greater than ambient. When PCB-exposed spot were transferred to

clean water, the accumulated PCBs were lost relatively
slowly, 84 days being required for the depuration of 61%.
Sanders and Chandler (1972) found that exposure of aquatic insects and crustaceans to Aroclor 1254 at concentrations of the order of 1 ppb resulted in magnification factors as large as 2.7×10^4. Goldfish exposed to Clophen A50
at concentrations of 0.01, 0.05 and 0.1 ppm for 18 days
and 0.5 ppm for 6 days contained residues of approximately
10, 60, 265 and 410 ppm, respectively (Hattula and Karlog,
1973). There was a 70% decrease in Clophen A50 residues
in the tissues after 70 days of depuration.

Petroleum Hydrocarbons

Blumer et al. (1970) have indicated that bivalves exposed to oil may retain aromatic hydrocarbons for a period
of months or perhaps indefinitely. However, Lee et al.
(1972a) demonstrated that the mussel Mytilus edulis accumulated several different petroleum hydrocarbons but released
approximately 95% of these in a period of 2 weeks. Lee et
al. (1972b) showed that polycyclic aromatic hydrocarbons
taken up by several species of marine fish were metabolized
and the products discharged in the urine. Lee and Benson
(1973) stated that petroleum hydrocarbons resulting from a
distant small spill were accumulated by Mytilus but members
of the same population showed no contamination three weeks
after the spill. Stegeman and Teal (1973) exposed oysters
to 106 ug/liter of a #2 fuel oil for periods up to 50 days.
They found that short term accumulation was correlated with
total body weight and long term accumulation was correlated
with the fat content of the oysters. The maximum levels
of hydrocarbons detected in oyster tissues were 334 and 161
ug/g wet weight for high and low fat oysters, respectively.
After one month in their post-exposure "cleaner" sea water
system the oysters still retained approximately 34 ug/g
total petroleum hydrocarbons, but since there was a small
amount of contamination in this system (11 ug/liter), continued low level accumulation could not be ruled out.

During the past two years we have been studying the
comparative effects of 4 test oils on several species of
marine and estuarine fish and invertebrates. These studies
have included: (1) toxicity of different oils and specific
petroleum hydrocarbons, (2) effects of exposure to sublethal
concentrations of oil on various physiological parameters,
and (3) uptake and release of petroleum hydrocarbons. The

four test oils were provided by the American Petroleum Institute and include two crude oils (Kuwait and South Louisiana), and two refined oils; a high aromatic (40%) #2 oil and a heavy residual oil, Venezuelan bunker C. Our studies include work with oil-water dispersions (OWD) of 3 oils and water soluble fractions (WSF) of all 4 oils.

The OWDs were prepared by adding a specific volume of oil to Instant Ocean and shaking the mixture vigorously for 5 minutes at approximately 200 cycles per minute on a shaker platform. In most cases the dispersions were prepared in 1 quart glass jars which were sealed with Teflon-lined caps during mixing. The oil and water layers were allowed to separate for 30 to 60 minutes before test animals were added or the aqueous layer was sampled for hydrocarbon analysis. The WSFs were prepared by mixing with a magnetic stirrer an oil-water solution containing 1 part oil (1.5 liters) to 9 parts Instant Ocean (13.5 liters) for 20 hours in a 5-gallon Pyrex bottle. The mixing speed was adjusted such that the vortex did not extend more than one-quarter of the distance to the bottom. The water phase was carefully siphoned from beneath the oil and this solution (100% WSF) was diluted with synthetic sea water for use in the various experiments. Detailed analyses of the specific hydrocarbons found in the 4 WSFs and 3 OWDs are described elsewhere (Anderson et al. 1974).

Characteristics of the test oils and their WSFs are shown in Table 2. It should be noted that the two refined oils and the WSFs prepared from them contain significantly higher relative concentrations of aromatic hydrocarbons than do the 2 crude oils and their WSFs. Bivalve molluscs exposed to rather high concentrations of these oils have been shown to accumulate many of the oil derived hydrocarbons in their tissues (Tables 3 and 4). The estuarine clam, Rangia cuneata, accumulated both saturated and aromatic hydrocarbons from the OWD of #2 fuel oil (Table 3). Similar results were obtained when oysters were exposed to OWDs of the 4 test oils (Table 4). The hydrocarbon type accumulated to the greatest extent by both species, regardless of the exposure oil, was the "naphthalenes". In general, the dimethylnaphthalenes were the members of this class accumulated to the greatest extent by both species and for all 4 oils. It should be noted that in additional studies with Rangia and oysters (to be described below), the tissue content of naphthalenes decreased to levels below detection (0.1 ppm) during periods in clean water of between 14 and

Table 2. The total concentration of soluble hydrocarbons
in the water soluble fractions (WSF) of four
test oils, and the relative proportion of aromatics
in the oils and soluble fractions. (Quantities of
the various components in water and tissue samples
were determined by gas liquid chromatography by
Dr. Warner of Battelle Laboratories, Columbus,
Ohio (see also Anderson et al. 1974).)

OIL	Total hydrocarbons WSF (ppm)	Aromatics n-paraffins WSF (ratio)	Aromatics n-paraffins Oil (ratio)
South Louisiana crude	19.8	3.43	0.24
Kuwait crude	10.4	18.75	0.15
#2 fuel oil	8.7	42.60	1.24
bunker C	6.3	77.92	3.42

Table 3. Oil-derived hydrocarbons in the tissues of the
clam, Rangia cuneata, following 24 hours of exposure to a 1000 ppm (ug/ml) oil-water dispersion
of #2 fuel oil. Totals include the unresolved
petroleum hydrocarbon "envelope" for the two major
hydrocarbon fractions.

Hydrocarbon	Tissue content (ppm)	Hydrocarbon	Tissue content (ppm)
n-paraffins		aromatics	
C_{13}	0.1	tetralin	9.2
C_{14}	0.3	naphthalene	22.4
C_{15}	0.1	2-methylnaphthalene	37.2
C_{16}	0.2	1-methylnaphthalene	20.8
C_{17}	0.3	dimethylnaphthalenes	44.0
C_{18}	0.2	trimethylnaphthalenes	5.2
C_{19}	0.1	misc. di- and triaromatics	6.1
Total n-paraffins	3.0	Total aromatics	158

Hydrocarbon	#2 fuel oil	Total	S.La. crude	Total	bunker C	Total	Kuwait crude	Total
C_{16} n-paraffin	0.7		2.2		0.3		5.3	
C_{17} n-paraffin	0.6		1.7		0.4		4.5	
Total C_{12}–C_{25} n-paraffins	3.1	3.1	13.8	13.8	1.1	1.1	46.0	46.0
naphthalene	6.3		1.8		1.3		4.3	
2-methylnaphthalene	15.4		5.5		8.5		5.7	
1-methylnaphthalene	9.4		4.2		7.0		4.8	
dimethylnaphthalenes	35.6		19.8		18.8		23.2	
trimethylnaphthalenes	17.4	84.1	12.7	44.0	5.7	41.3	17.1	55.1
biphenyl	0.2		0.5		0.1		0.3	
methyl-biphenyl	1.0		0.6		0.2		0.3	
fluorene	1.2		0.5		0.4		0.4	
dimethylbiphenyl	0.7		0.5		0.1		0.1	
methylfluorene	1.7		1.7		0.7		1.1	
dibenzo-thiophene	0.6		0.1		0.1		0.6	
phenanthrene	1.7		0.9		1.3		0.4	
dimethyl-fluorene	0.5		1.0		0.4		0.8	
methylphenanthrene	1.7		1.7		1.7		1.5	
dimethyl-phenanthrene	0.2	9.5	0.5	8.0	0.5	5.0	0.5	6.0
Total oil-derived hydrocarbons		96.7		65.8		47.4		107.1

Table 4. Oil-derived hydrocarbons in tissues of oysters
Crassostrea virginica following exposure to 1% oil-
water dispersions for 4 days. All concentrations are
in ppm (ug/g wet weight of tissue).

52 days.

In the depuration tests, oysters were exposed in a
similar fashion to OWDs of South Louisiana crude oil and #2
fuel oil. Following exposure, a portion of each group was
placed in a flowing sea water system on Galveston Island
for depuration studies. Table 5 shows the depuration of all
classes of hydrocarbons by the contaminated oysters. Oysters held in a "clean" environment for periods of 24 to 52
days were found to contain less than 0.1 ppm of all classes
of oil derived hydrocarbons. In other experiments, R. D.
Anderson (1973) has shown that oysters exposed to 1%

(10,000 ppm) OWDs of each of the 4 oils for 96 hours accumulated 10 to 83 ppm of mono- and di-aromatic hydrocarbons, but within 52 days in clean sea water they had depurated to background levels (below 0.1 ppm total oil derived hydrocarbons).

The results of numerous experiments with bivalves (Anderson, 1973), crustaceans and fish (Anderson et al., unpublished data), have indicated that naphthalenes are the oil-derived hydrocarbons most highly accumulated in animal tissues exposed to oils or their water-soluble extracts. While these aromatics appear to be retained longer than the n-paraffins and other detectable aromatics, their association with the tissues is reversible. Since it seems likely that there will be a relationship between the degree of tissue contamination by a given pollutant and its toxic and sublethal effects on the organism, the role of naphthalenes in petroleum toxicity should be investigated further.

Respiration:

There is a vast amount of information on the effects of endogenous and exogenous factors on the respiratory rate of estuarine, marine and intertidal animals. For recent reviews, the reader is referred to Newell (1970, 1973) and for specific effects on crustaceans and fish to McFarland and Pickens (1965) and Fry (1971) respectively. Much fewer data are available on the respiratory response of marine organisms to the stress of a man made pollutant.

Heavy Metals

Recently, respiratory rates of a bivalve mollusc and a crustacean have been measured while the animals were exposed to heavy metals. Brown and Newell (1972) reported a series of experiments in which the mussel, Mytilus edulis, was exposed to copper and zinc in the form of their sodium citrate salts. It was determined that copper sodium citrate at a concentration of 500 ppm caused a 50% depression in respiratory rate of the whole animal as compared to unexposed controls and sodium citrate-exposed controls. The copper salts depressed gill tissue respiration and ciliary activity but had no effect on the respiration of the digestive gland. Zinc apparently did not affect either of these parameters. From these data it was concluded that copper decreases the respiratory rate of whole organisms by inhibiting the

Oil (%)	Exposure (Days)	Depuration (Days)	Saturated hydrocarbon (ppm)	Mono- and diaromatic hydrocarbon (ppm)	"Triaromatic" hydrocarbon (ppm)
South Louisiana crude (5%)	4		0.3	37.4	5.2
		27	0.1	—(a)	—
South Louisiana crude (5%)	7		—	10.2	2.6
		24	—	—	—
		35	—	—	—
#2 Fuel Oil (1%)	4		1.8	11.8	0.7
		7	0.2	2.6	0.9
		13	0.1	2.2	1.0
		52	—	—	—
Control			—	—	—

(a) Where no value is given the amount was less than 0.1 ppm.

Table 5. Hydrocarbon content of oyster tissues exposed to South Louisiana crude oil and #2 fuel oil and subsequent levels after various periods of depuration.

energy-consuming process of ciliary activity.

Vernberg and Vernberg (1972) studied the effect of inorganic mercury ($HgCl_2$) on the oxygen consumption of fiddler crabs, Uca pugilator. After determining baseline values for respiratory rates of male and female crabs, they exposed the animals to 0.18 ppm of mercury in seawater solution and measured their oxygen consumption periodically for 28 days. A significant difference between male and female crabs was observed. The respiratory rate of the males was unchanged through day 3. However, rates had decreased to 32, 48 and 20% that of the controls on days 7, 21 and 28, respectively. The oxygen consumption of the female crabs, on the other hand, was similarly depressed at day 7 but had returned to control baseline values by day 14 and remained unchanged through day 28.

De Coursey and Vernberg (1972) determined the effects of sublethal concentrations of mercuric chloride on the respiratory rate of fiddler crab larvae. Stage I, III and V zoea were exposed to mercury concentrations of 0.18 ppm, 1.8 ppb and 18 pptr (parts per trillion) and oxygen consumption was measured. After one hour of exposure at each of the three concentrations of mercury, the respiratory rate of stage I zoea was not different from that of controls. However, after 6 hours of exposure at 0.18 ppm, there was a significant depression in oxygen consumption rates for all zoeal stages with the greatest decrease (1/3 that of controls) observed in stage V zoea. Even after 24 hours of exposure there was no effect of 18 pptr of mercury on stage I zoea but 1.8 ppb did cause a decreased rate. Twenty four hours exposure of stage III and V zoea to 1.8 ppb or 18 pptr mercury tended to increase respiratory rates, while larvae reared in mercury solutions showed a differect response. That is, the respiratory rate of stage V zoea reared in mercury was depressed while that of stage III zoea was unchanged.

Polychlorinated Biphenyls (PCBs)

To the best of our knowledge, there are no reports in the literature of studies on the effects of sublethal concentrations of PCBs on the respiratory rates of marine animals.

In our laboratory we have recently begun to perform measurements of the effects of heavy metals and PCBs on respiratory rate, as measured by oxygen probes and the Carpenter modification of the Winkler titration method. Exposures of the grass shrimp Palaemonetes pugio to 1 ppm of mercury in seawater solution increased respiration slightly but not significantly. In two experiments, the mean respiratory rates of 20 shrimp before and after exposure to mercury were 2.43 and 2.96 ml O_2/g dry weight/hour. However, exposure of this species to 100 ppb of Aroclor 1254 resulted in a respiratory rate 3.6 times higher than that of unexposed controls. The rate of consumption of the controls was 1.36 ml O_2/g dry weight/hour (n = 10) and that of the exposed shrimp was 4.96 ml O_2/g dry weight/hour (n = 30) (Petrocelli et al., unpublished data).

In another series of experiments, the respiratory rates of 25 Gulf killifish, Fundulus similus, were measured prior to and immediately after exposure to 1 ppm Aroclor 1254, each fish thus serving as its own control. The respiratory rates of the fish following exposure to the PCB (mean, 0.275 ml O_2/g dry weight/hour) were only about 20% of the rates of the same fish prior to exposure (mean, 1.413 ml O_2/g dry weight/hour). Oxygen consumption of the fish before exposure showed the characteristic inverse relationship between weight specific respiratory rate and body weight. However, this relationship was not evident after exposure to PCB (Petrocelli et al., unpublished data). Since fish respiratory rates were not determined at different times after they had been returned to clean sea water, it is not yet known if recovery will occur.

Petroleum Hydrocarbons

Steed and Copeland (1967) examined the effects of exposure to industrial effluents on the respiratory rates of the fish Cyprinodon variegatus, Lagodon rhomboides, and Micropogon undulatus and the pink and brown shrimp, Penaeus duorarum and P. aztecus. While there was considerable variation, there was a trend for low concentrations of the effluent to depress and for higher concentrations to stimulate respiration of Cyprinodon variegatus. The other two species of fish showed an even more variable respiratory response to the pollutant. Respiratory rates of the test shrimp were not significantly different from those of unexposed controls. Wohlschlag and Cameron (1967) studied the effect of exposure to diluted petrochemical waste products on the respiratory rate of the pinfish Lagodon rhomboides. Respiratory rates, particularly of the larger fish (approximately

95

100 g) at the extreme exposure temperatures (10° and 30°C) were apparently depressed by exposure to the contaminated water. Brocksen and Bailey (1973) studied the effects of exposure to benzene on the respiratory rates of juvenile salmon and striped bass. Respiratory rates of the fish were determined at various intervals during a 96-hour exposure to either 5 or 10 ppm benzene in a flowing system. At an exposure concentration of 10 ppm, juvenile salmon had respiratory rates significantly higher than those of unexposed controls. The respiratory rates of exposed salmon returned to control values within ten days after return to clean sea water. The mussels Mytilus edulis and Modiolus demissus responded to exposure to as little as 1 ppm crude oil with elevated respiratory rates and decreased net carbon balance (Gilfillan, 1973).

In extensive bioassay studies (Anderson et al., 1974), the mysid crustacean, Mysidopsis almyra, consistently demonstrated the greatest sensitivity to the various petroleum solutions. The respiratory rate of this mysid was measured, using the Carpenter modification of the Winkler titration method for dissolved oxygen determination, during or shortly after exposure to different sublethal concentrations of the OWDs and WSFs. Animals exposed to the WSFs of #2 fuel oil, bunker C and Louisiana crude oil for 2 hours before respiratory measurements were made in clean sea water did not exhibit respiratory rates which were significantly different from controls. However, exposure to the WSF of Kuwait crude oil produced respiratory rates which were significantly above control levels (solid line, Fig. 1A). The rates tended to increase gradually from control level to a high

Fig. 1. Relationship between the concentration of hydrocarbons in the exposure medium and the respiratory response of Mysidopsis almyra. Vertical bars represent standard errors; mean control and experimental values connected for convenience.
A. Measurements taken in clean water after 2 hours of exposure to WSFs of Kuwait crude oil (solid line; 10 animals/container and 5 containers/concentration). Measurements taken during exposure to WSFs of #2 fuel oil (dashed line; 5 animals/container and 5 containers/concentration).
B. Measurements taken in clean water after 2 hours exposure to OWDs of #2 fuel oil. Each point represents the mean value from 3 containers with 10 animals each. (From Cox and Anderson, unpublished data).

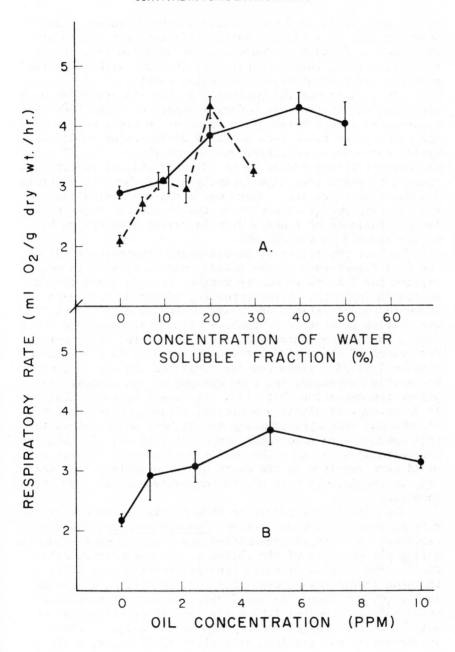

Fig. 1. See legend on previous page.

at 40% WSF, but at 60% there was a slight decrease in consumption rate (not significantly different from the 20 or
40% level). In each of these studies with the WSFs of the
test oils, there were 5 respiratory chambers with 10 mysids
each for all concentrations including controls.

Since there was the possibility that the organisms were
respiring at abnormal rates during exposure to the WSFs, but
returned to normal rates after transfer to clean water, oxygen consumption rates were measured during exposure of the
mysids to various concentrations of the WSF of #2 fuel oil.
All concentrations tested (5 to 30% WSF) induced respiratory
responses, which were significantly higher than the controls
(dashed line, Fig. 1A). There was a sharp and significant
rise in respiratory rate between the 15 and 20% exposure
levels, followed by a sharp drop in oxygen consumption by
mysids exposed to the 30% WSF.

To test the effect of an oil-water dispersion (OWD) on
the respiratory rate of the mysids, groups of animals were
exposed for 2 hours to concentrations between 1 and 10 ppm
of the #2 fuel oil. After exposure, 30 mysids from each
exposure concentration, including controls, were placed in
respiration chambers (10/chamber) with clean water and their
oxygen consumption rates measured. As before, the respiratory rates of the mysids increased gradually to a maximum of
between 1.5 and 2 times control levels as the exposure concentration increased, and then dropped at the highest exposure concentration (Fig. 1B). It should be noted that,
in an attempt to elicit a sublethal effect, concentrations
of OWDs and WSFs approximating the 24 hour LC-50 values for
this species were used (Anderson et al., 1974). The highest
concentrations to which the mysids were exposed in each test
would have resulted in the death of the organisms, and the
drop in respiratory rate may be indicative of the near lethal
condition.

The effect of exposure to WSFs of oil on the respiratory
rate of postlarval brown shrimp, Penaeus aztecus, was also
examined. All oxygen consumption measurements were conducted
during the exposure of the shrimp to the hydrocarbon solutions. The results of three separate experiments, utilizing
the same techniques as described for the mysids, are shown
in Fig. 2. It should be noted that the control respiratory
rates vary as expected from a log-log linear regression of
weight specific oxygen consumption versus weight. Those
postlarvae of the smallest size class (2.25 mg, mean dry
weight) consumed significantly greater amounts of oxygen

per unit weight under control conditions than did the larger shrimp. In each experiment, animals at the higher concentrations exhibited increased activity, an abnormal spiraling swimming pattern and some were on their backs with only the pleopods beating at the termination of the exposure.

The pattern of respiratory response was remarkably similar in each of the three experiments. It is interesting that Mysidopsis exhibited increased respiratory rates, while Penaeus postlarvae responded by depressing their oxygen consumption, particularly at the lowest exposure concentrations. The intermediate range of concentrations generally resulted in respiratory rates which were near or statistically equivalent to control levels. A greater respiratory response was exhibited by the postlarvae exposed to WSFs of #2 fuel oil than by those exposed to the South Louisiana WSFs. This may be due to the differences in the hydrocarbon composition of the two WSFs or to the smaller size of the shrimp exposed to the #2 fuel oil WSF or a combination of both factors (Fig. 2A). Based on the differences between figures 2B and 2C, it would appear that larger shrimp are more tolerant than smaller ones to the WSF of South Louisiana crude oil. However, the respiratory response may not be directly related to the long term tolerance of an organism, since bioassay data on this species indicates that sensitivity increases as size increases (Cox and Anderson, unpublished data).

In an attempt to relate the extent of respiratory response to the content of petroleum hydrocarbons in the shrimp tissues, an additional series of measurements was taken. Two groups of shrimp, from the same collection and of the same size class (5.68 mg, mean dry weight) were exposed to a 30% WSF of #2 fuel oil for four hours. Respiratory rates of the first group and of a third unexposed control group of shrimp were then determined. Each group was then placed in a separate aquarium containing oil-free sea water which was constantly recirculated through a charcoal filter. At 6 and 26 hours after exposure, the respiratory rates of the first and third (control) groups were again determined. At the same time, shrimp from the second exposure group were sacrificed and their tissues were analyzed for naphthalene and alkylnaphthalenes by the ultraviolet spectrophotometric method of Neff and Anderson (unpublished). Because the method required approximately 0.1 g of tissue, 15 to 20 postlarvae were pooled for each analysis.

99

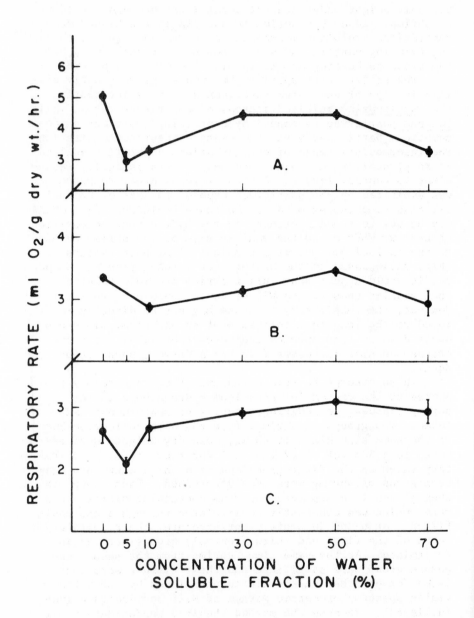

Fig. 2.   See legend on following page.

Table 6 shows the results of both respiratory and tissue content measurements taken at the various time intervals. It should be noted that the respiratory rates of the 12 postlarvae exposed to the 30% WSF were significantly higher than those of the control group at all time intervals. While the tissue content of naphthalene and alkylnaphthalenes decreased considerably during the 27-hour recovery period, approximately 10 and 12 percent, respectively, remained after 27 hours. There would appear to be a relationship between the presence of petroleum hydrocarbons in the tissue and high respiratory rate. Similar studies should be conducted utilizing longer recovery periods to determine whether or not oxygen consumption returns to the control rate when the hydrocarbons have been completely depurated.

The respiratory response of an animal may be merely indicative of its ability to regulate in some way to an irritating environment. From the results presented above, it would appear that mysids have little ability to regulate their metabolic rate when faced with an adverse environment, and as irritant concentration increases, the response is intensified. Apparently the rate is maximal at the highest sublethal concentration and beyond this point a sharp drop occurs which may be indicative of the onset of death. In these respiratory studies and earlier toxicity tests (Anderson et al., 1974), mysids exhibited a greater sensitivity to the oils and their WSFs than did the postlarval Penaeus aztecus.

Fig. 2. Relationship between the concentration of water-soluble hydrocarbons in the exposure medium and the respiratory response of Penaeus aztecus postlarvae during a 4 to 5-hour exposure. Vertical bars represent standard errors; mean control and experimental values connected for convenience.
A. Postlarvae with a mean dry weight of 2.253 mg (5 containers with 3 postlarvae each at all concentrations) during exposure to WSFs of #2 fuel oil.
B. Postlarvae with a mean dry weight of 3.464 mg (5 containers with 2 postlarvae each at all concentrations) during exposure to WSFs of South Louisiana crude oil.
C. Postlarvae with a mean dry weight of 12.079 mg (5 containers with 2 postlarvae each at all concentrations) during exposure to WSFs of South Louisiana crude oil. (From Cox and Anderson, unpublished data).

Time	Oil Exposed						Control
	Exposure water (ppm)		Tissue (ppm)		Respiratory rate		Respiratory rate
	N*	A*	N*	A*	(ml O_2/g/hr)		(ml O_2/g/hr)
Exposure Period:							
Initial	0.39	0.66					
After 4 hours	0.30	0.42	12.06	42.36	5.239 ± 0.801 **		3.139 ± 0.242
Recovery Period:							
After 6 hours			1.86	6.83	4.747 ± 0.588		3.287 ± 0.407
After 27 hours			1.17	5.07	5.516 ± 0.378		3.096 ± 0.280

* N = Naphthalene and A = Alkylnaphthalenes

** The exposed rate was taken during the 4 hours of exposure to the 30% WSF.

Table 6. Respiratory rates and tissue napthalenes content of postlarval Penaeus aztecus exposed to a 30% WSF of Fuel Oil. Respiratory chambers each contained 2 shrimp and there were 12 animals used in both control and exposure measurements.

As the concentration of the hydrocarbons in solution (irritant) increased, postlarval and juvenile brown shrimp did not show increased intensity of response. In fact, the strongest suppression in respiratory rate occurred at the lowest hydrocarbon levels. It would appear that contact with low hydrocarbon concentrations elicits a specific response which differs from the possible "regulatory response" exhibited by shrimp exposed to higher concentrations. Such differences could well be triggered by the hydrocarbon content of the tissues, and particularly the levels associated with the nervous system. There is some indication that the intensity of respiratory depression may be related to the size and therefore the age of the brown shrimp. It is possible that more mature individuals have a greater capacity for reducing the level of hydrocarbon contamination in the tissues. Since other evidence shows that mature shrimp are less resistant to acutely toxic hydrocarbon levels, differences in permeability between the size classes seem likely.

Additional evidence of the permeability and regulatory differences between postlarvae and large juvenile shrimp has been obtained from accumulation and depuration studies (Cox and Anderson, unpublished data). Large juvenile shrimp rapidly accumulated higher levels of naphthalene and alkylnaphthalenes than smaller juveniles and postlarvae but began releasing this material back to the environment sooner. From this information it would appear that the earlier stages in the life history of Penaeus aztecus are less permeable to hydrocarbons, but once the compounds have been accumulated, these immature forms have not fully developed regulatory mechanisms for reducing their internal concentration. While the experiments have not yet been conducted, it would appear that in order to demonstrate an effect on the respiratory activity of large juvenile and adult shrimp, the respiratory rate must be measured during the initial exposure to the petroleum hydrocarbons.

These data indicate that while respiratory rate may be affected by sublethal levels of various pollutants, it is virtually impossible at this stage to predict the direction or magnitude of the response. Furthermore, there is not enough known concerning recovery to normal respiratory rates upon removal of the animal from test solutions. These factors are under investigation in our laboratory.

Osmotic and Ionic Regulation:

Marine and particularly estuarine organisms have evolved a wide diversity of adaptations to cope with a changing ionic environment. Some organisms (stenohaline species) are restricted to a narrow salinity range, while other organisms (euryhaline species) are able to tolerate a wide range of environmental salinities. There are several excellent reviews (Kinne, 1967, 1973; Potts and Parry, 1964) dealing with the mechanisms and parameters of adaptation to different osmotic and ionic environments. Environmental pollutants, by inhibiting or interfering with these adaptive mechanisms, might be expected to reduce the ability of marine organisms to tolerate stressful salinities.

Chlorinated Hydrocarbons and Heavy Metals

Janicki and Kinter (1971) studied the effect of DDT on osmoregulation of excised intestine from salt water adapted eels Anguilla rostrata, and found inhibition of Na^+, K^+ and Mg^{2+} ATPases, resulting in disruption of normal osmoregulation. More recently these investigators (Kinter et al., 1972) studied effects of DDT and Aroclor 1221 (a PCB containing 21% chlorine by weight) on the osmoregulatory ability of the killifish Fundulus heteroclitus, and the eels studied previously. These two organochlorine compounds were used because of their chemical similarity. Fish were exposed to ethanol solutions of these compounds dissolved in sea water. After exposure, osmolarity and concentrations of sodium and potassium ions in the whole blood were measured. Blood of DDT-and PCB-exposed fish exhibited elevated Na^+ and K^+ levels and higher osmolarity, compared to the ethanol controls. Kinter et al. (1972) concluded that both DDT and Aroclor 1221 decreased, by about the same degree, the ability of these organisms to osmoregulate.

In our laboratory, we have studied the effects of sublethal levels (as determined by bioassay prior to physiological experimentation) of inorganic mercury ($HgCl_2$) and the PCB, Aroclor 1254, on the chloride ion levels in the blood of estuarine shrimp and crabs (Roesijadi et al., unpublished data). The effects of these compounds on two different processes were measured. In one series of experiments, animals acclimated to a given salinity were exposed to the compound under investigation and subsequent alterations in the Cl^- levels of the blood were measured. In the second series, a group of animals acclimated to 14°/oo salinity were exposed to the pollutant at the same salinity. The animals were

rapidly transferred to different salinities and the rate of
ionic adjustment of the blood was monitored and compared to
the adjustment rate of unexposed controls. The protocols
for the two experiments are outlined schematically in Fig. 3.

In the case of the porcelain crab, <u>Petrolisthes armatus</u>,
the Cl^- concentrations of the blood of both control animals
and animals exposed to 50 ppb mercury for 24 hours were
hyperchloride to the medium at salinities of 7, 14, and
$21°/oo$ and hypochloride at 28 and $35°/oo$. Except at $35°/oo$
in the 24-hour exposed group, there was no significant difference between control and exposed crabs (by student's t-
test, p = 0.05) (Fig. 4). Similarly, in the experiments involving salinity shock, after exposure to 50 ppb of mercury,
adjustment of internal Cl^- concentration to the new medium
was essentially completed within 3 hours with no significant
changes at 12 or 24 hours. Furthermore, there were no differences between the blood chloride levels reached by controls and exposed animals (Fig. 5). The ability of this animal to regulate its internal Cl^- concentration very ef-
ficiently may be related to its mode of life on oyster reefs
which are subject to extremes of salinity due to exposure,
salt-water immersion and freshwater flooding.

In similar experiments we measured the Cl^- concentration of the blood of grass shrimp <u>Palaemonetes pugio</u>, as affected by 10 ppb of Aroclor 1254. We found the Cl^- concentration of the shrimp blood to be hyperchloride to the
medium at salinities of 1, 7 and $14°/oo$ and hypochloride at
19, 25 and $31°/oo$. There was a significant difference at 1
and $7°/oo$ between the response of control and exposed animals with the latter showing somewhat lower blood chloride
levels (Fig. 6). In the salinity shock experiments, the effects of the PCB were also observed (Figs. 7-9). At the 6-
hour determination, blood Cl^- levels of exposed shrimp at
$1°/oo$ were significantly below that of the controls (Fig. 7).
At 24 hours, both groups were approaching a new steady state
level, but the PCB-exposed shrimp showed a greater lag.
There are no measurements for exposed shrimp at $1°/oo$ beyond
this point since mortalities prior to the 72-hour reading
had reduced the number of shrimp to fewer than 5, preventing
further measurements. At 7, 14 and $19°/oo$ the Cl^- concentration of both groups of shrimp were at the new acclimation
level and not significantly different from one another at the
6-hour determination. However, at the 24-hour interval the
chloride level of blood from exposed shrimp at $7°/oo$ (Fig. 8)
was slightly less than that of the controls and mortalities

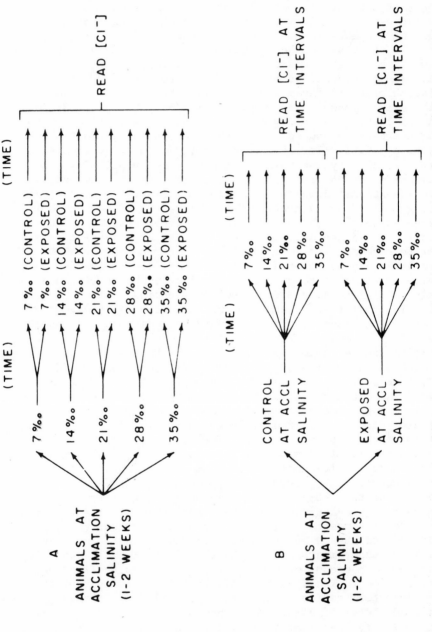

Fig. 3. Protocol for experimentation on the chloride regulation of _Petrolisthes armatus_ and _Palaemonetes pugio._

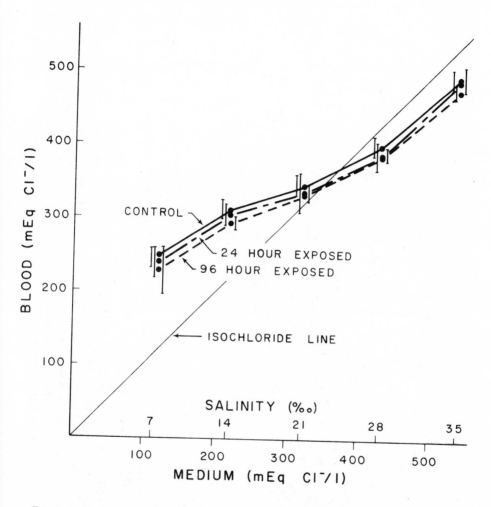

Fig. 4. Relationship between the medium chloride level and
that of the blood of specimens of Petrolisthes
armatus acclimated to various salinities as compared
to individuals similarly acclimated and exposed to
50 ppb mercury for 24 or 96 hours. Vertical bars
represent standard deviations, where n = 10 for
controls and 5 for exposed groups. (From Roesijadi
et al., unpublished data.)

107

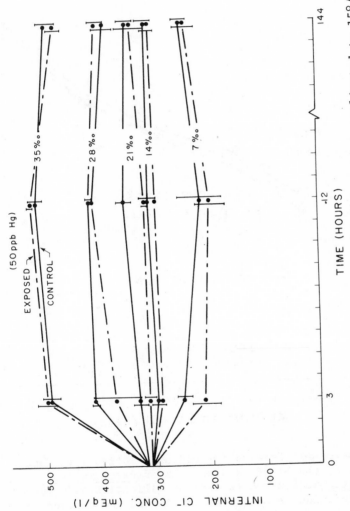

Fig. 5. The blood chloride regulation of Petrolisthes armatus acclimated to 15°/oo on transfer to various salinities after exposure to 50 ppb of mercury for 72 hours. (Values for 144-hour determinations represent data from 24-hour exposed groups presented in Fig. 4 and shown above for comparison.) Vertical bars represent standard deviations, where n = 5 for controls and 2 for exposed groups. (From Roesijadi et al., unpublished data.)

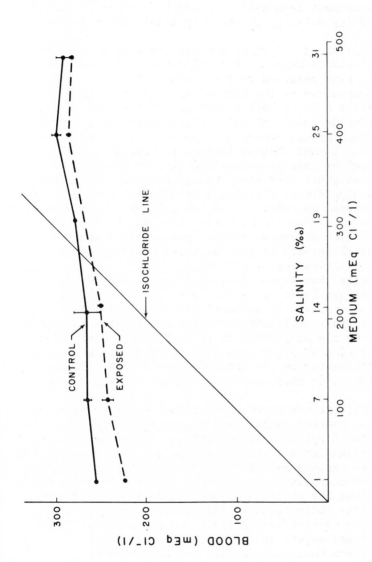

Fig. 6. Relationship between the medium chloride concentration and the blood chloride level of specimens of Palaemonetes pugio exposed to 10 ppb Aroclor 1254 for 5 days during acclimation to various salinities. Vertical bars represent standard deviations, where 2 replicates were taken from the pooled blood of 5 animals. (From Roesijadi et al., unpublished data.)

occurred. Depression in chloride level of the exposed shrimp
continued to the 72-hour reading with further mortalities,
but then the levels in both groups increased until 120 hours
when the experiment terminated. Blood Cl⁻ levels of shrimp
at 14 and 19°/ₒₒ salinity showed only slight changes thereafter.

At 25°/ₒₒ blood chloride concentrations of both control
and exposed animals were slightly elevated, and some minor
fluctuations were observed to 120 hours. Effects of the PCB
were most pronounced at the highest salinity tested (31°/ₒₒ,
Fig. 9). After 6 hours both groups had significantly over-
shot the chloride level, at which acclimation would eventually occur. Both groups showed a decrease in blood Cl⁻ concentration at the 24-and 72-hour intervals. The blood Cl⁻
levels of control animals approached the new acclimation
values at a slightly more rapid rate, and, even at 72 hours
there was a significant difference between Cl⁻ levels of controls and exposed animals. As in the case of the animals at
1°/ₒₒ, there were significant mortalities in the 31°/ₒₒ exposed group which prevented further measurements after 72
hours. Control animals at this salinity experienced no significant mortalities during this time.

One factor that should be considered is that dilution of
full strength synthetic sea water to the lowest salinity
tested (1°/ₒₒ) results in an equal dilution of all ions,
which is not truly representative of natural estuarine water.
While chloride ion proportion is probably not greatly altered, the ratios of other ions such as Ca:Na and K:Na does
change significantly in the estuarine environment (Kinne,
1973). However, in these experiments, any effects due to

Figs. 7-9. Differences between chloride regulatory abilities
of control animals and Palaemonetes pugio exposed
to 10 ppb of Aroclor 1254 for 4 days at the acclimation salinity of 14°/ₒₒ and then transferred
to various salinities. Vertical bars represent
standard deviations, where 2 replicates were taken
from the pooled blood of 5 animals. The dashed
line indicates the final acclimation level, while
the control (solid line) and experimental (broken
line) points are connected for convenience.
(From Roesijadi et al., unpublished data.)
Fig. 7. On transfer to 1°/ₒₒ salinity.
Fig. 8. On transfer to 7°/ₒₒ salinity.
Fig. 9. On transfer to 31°/ₒₒ salinity.

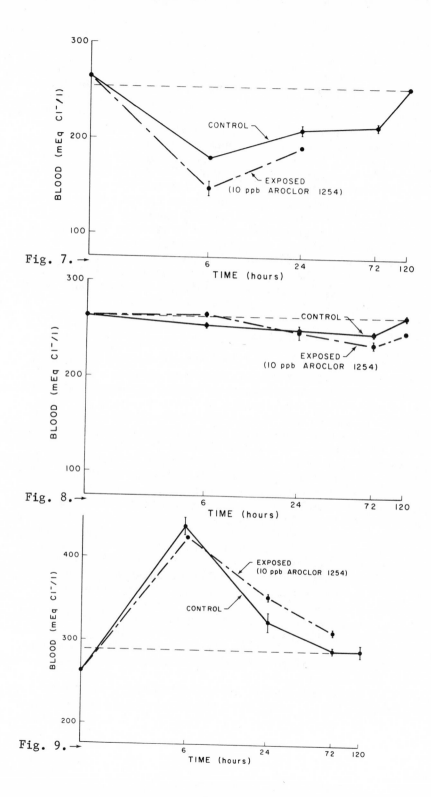

Fig. 7. →

Fig. 8. →

Fig. 9. →

dilution and changes in ionic proportions were accounted for
by the measurements made on control animals and the fact that
the blood Cl⁻ levels of control and exposed groups were significantly different at 1°/oo, but not different at the intermediate salinities of 7, 14 and 19°/oo.

From these results it appears that relatively high (50
ppb) sublethal levels of inorganic mercury do not affect the
chloride ion regulation of Petrolisthes armatus, while 10
ppb of Aroclor 1254 significantly affects the ability of
Palaemonetes pugio to adjust to rapid fluctuations in the
salinity of the environment. Thus, exposure of these
shrimp to sublethal concentrations of Aroclor 1254 during a
time of heavy rainfall with the resulting rapid decrease in
salinity could cause mortalities which would not be predicted
on the basis of the toxicity of Aroclor 1254 alone. That is,
the PCB makes this animal less able to withstand and adjust
to the normal fluctuations in its environment.

Petroleum Hydrocarbons

In our studies on the adult brown shrimp, Penaeus
aztecus, chloride levels of the blood were determined after
4 and 6 hours of acclimation to 5, 10, 14, 25 and 35°/oo
salinities. This species was shown to be an active chloride
regulator demonstrating hyperchloride regulation at levels
up to 22°/oo and hypochloride regulation at higher salinities.
The osmoregulatory abilities of penaeid shrimp were documented previously by Williams (1960) and McFarland and Lee
(1963). A large group of animals (average weight, 5 grams
per individual), was acclimated to 20°/oo salinity for 5
days. A sub-sample of this group was transferred to 20% WSF
of #2 fuel oil in 20°/oo sea water for 10 hours. At the end
of the exposure period, half of the exposed animals were
transferred to 10°/oo clean water, while the other half was
placed in 30°/oo water and the chloride concentration of the
blood was determined at several time intervals (Fig. 10).
At the time of transfer, control individuals were also
placed in 10 and 30°/oo sea water. At time intervals of 1,
6, 24, 48, 96 and 192 hours, 3 exposed and 3 control shrimp
from both salinities were sacrificed for blood chloride ion
determinations. The points shown in Figure 10 represent the
mean Cl⁻ levels of three replicate samples of the blood from
each of 3 shrimp.

Although exposure to the WSF produced a temporary loss
of equilibrium in several of the shrimp, only one death oc-

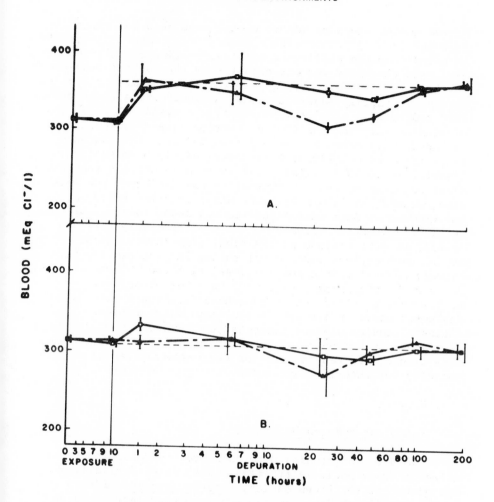

Fig. 10. Differences between the chloride regulatory ability
of control animals and <u>Penaeus</u> <u>aztecus</u> exposed to
20% WSF of #2 fuel oil in 20°/oo sea water for 10
hours. Control animals (solid line) and those exposed (broken line) were transferred from 20°/oo
water to either (A) 30°/oo or (B) 10°/oo salinity
sea water and the blood chloride levels monitored.
Each point represents the mean values from 3 replicate samples of the blood from each of 3 shrimp.
Vertical bars represent standard deviations, and the
dashed line indicates the final acclimation level.
(From Cox and Anderson, unpublished data.)

curred during exposure and no deaths were recorded after transfer from $20^\circ/_{oo}$ to either 10 or $30^\circ/_{oo}$ water. It should be noted that the ability to maintain acclimated chloride levels in the blood was not affected by the 10-hour exposure to the WSF. It would also appear that the ability of Penaeus aztecus to rapidly adjust to a new salinity was not directly affected by such exposure. However, the steady state of regulation of chloride ion during the time intervals studied was apparently upset by the exposure to oil. The fluctuations in blood chloride levels, particularly by organisms transferred to $30^\circ/_{oo}$ (Fig. 10A), were more erratic than the minor adjustments made by control organisms during the same time period. At 24 and 48 hours after transfer to $30^\circ/_{oo}$, the exposed animals were significantly lower in blood Cl^- levels than control animals. This was apparently only a transitory effect since at the final time interval (192 hours) both exposed and control shrimp had reached the previously determined acclimation level of blood chloride. The recovery of the animals after 192 hours in clean water may be due to the release of hydrocarbons from their tissues as discussed above in the section on respiratory response. Additional studies will be conducted to determine whether tissue damage or hydrocarbon accumulation, perhaps in the nervous tissue, are responsible for the temporary decreased capacity for chloride regulation.

Growth:

Petroleum hydrocarbons

Two types of studies were conducted to determine the effect of water-soluble fractions (WSF) of #2 fuel oil, on the growth of the brown shrimp, Penaeus aztecus. First, small juvenile shrimp were exposed to a near-lethal concentration (acute exposure) of the WSF (70%) for 2 hours and then placed in clean sea water. In the second experiment (chronic exposure), shrimp were exposed for 2 hours to a 30% WSF of #2 fuel oil, placed in clean water for one week, and then exposed 4 times at one week intervals for 2 hours to a 15% WSF. Over the first 25 days of this 6-week period, the molting frequency of each group was recorded. The rate of growth in length and weight was recorded at various intervals during the 6 weeks and the total increases, with standard deviations, are listed in Table 7. Neither acute nor chronic exposure to #2 fuel oil WSFs produced growth indices significantly different from those of the control animals.

The effect of exposure to WSFs of the test oils on phytoplankton growth has also been studied. Concentrations (in % of the WSF) required to decrease the growth rates of Isochrysis galbana, Cyclotella nana, and Glenodinium halli by 50% (EC_{50}) are shown in Table 8. It should be noted that there is quite good agreement between the EC_{50} values obtained by cell counts (Coulter counter) and those derived from chlorophyll a determinations. In these as in other studies (Anderson et al., 1974) the refined oils were shown to be more toxic than the two crude oils tested. The detergent dodecyl sodium sulfate (DSS) was used as a reference toxicant (LaRoche et al, 1970) to compare the tolerance of the three test species. From the data available, it would appear that all three species of phytoplankton responded to the hydrocarbon solutions in a similar manner, but Glenodinium was significantly more tolerant to DSS. As evidenced by the somewhat larger EC_{50} values at 72 hours in several cases, a good portion of the algal population survived the exposure to the WSFs and resumed normal growth during longer exposure periods. Additional tests have shown that subcultures of organisms subjected to concentrations greater than the EC_{50} values resumed normal growth rates after only 48 hours in new medium (Mills and Ray, unpublished data).

Interactions:

Heavy metals

Vernberg and Vernberg (1972) studied the interaction between the natural environmental stresses, temperature and the toxicity of mercury to the fiddler crab, Uca pugilator. It was found that mercury concentrations of 0.18 ppm were significantly more toxic to crabs acclimated at 25°C and salinity, and 30°/$_{oo}$ and then placed in a condition of stress at a temperature of 5°C and a salinity of 5°/$_{oo}$. The males appeared to be more affected by these stresses than the females. Survival times upon exposure to mercury were similarly reduced when temperature was maintained at the acclimation value and salinity alone was decreased.

Our preliminary studies on the toxicity of inorganic mercury ($HgCl_2$) to the porcelain crab, Petrolisthes armatus, indicated that salinity might be an important modifying factor in survival (G. Roesijadi et al., unpublished data). After 10 days of acclimation to each of 5 salinities,

115

Table 7. The effect of chronic and acute exposure to the WSF of #2 fuel oil on the molting frequency and growth of Penaeus aztecus.*

	Control	Acute exposure	Chronic exposure
Molting frequency (days per molt)	6.9 ± 1.9	7.4 ± 2.2	6.6 ± 1.2
Final Weight (mg dry wt)	29.2 ± 9.4**	31.4 ± 9.5	29.9 ± 10.6
Final length (cm)	2.86 ± 0.32**	2.97 ± 0.30	2.86 ± 0.35

*n = 15 for each condition in molting studies and n = 60 for each condition in growth studies. Ten shrimp were sacrificed each week under each condition for length-weight determinations.

**The overall mean and standard deviation for the initial length and weight of all test animals were 1.36 ± 0.4 mg dry weight (from Cox and Anderson, unpublished manuscript).

Table 8. Effects of the WSFs of four oils on the cell number and chlorophyll a levels in three species of marine algae. EC-50 values are per cent of WSFs. (From Mills and Ray, unpublished data.)

OIL	EC-50 values by cell density measurements				
	Isochrysis galbana		Cyclotella nana		Glenodinium halli
	48 hr.	72 hr.	48 hr.	72 hr.	72 hr.
S. La. crude	30	28	22	22	16
bunker C	5	7	-	11	10
#2 fuel oil	6	7	6	6	7
Kuwait crude	36	39	51	63	62
DSS (ppm)	-	0.65	-	0.54	1.58
OIL	EC-50 values by chlorophyll a measurements				
	Isochrysis galbana		Cyclotella nana		Glenodinium halli
	48 hr.	72 hr.	48 hr.	72 hr.	72 hr.
S. La. crude	31	19	14	18	11
bunker C	15	4	-	8	7
#2 fuel oil	6	7	3	6	5
Kuwait crude	46	27	28	39	48

subsequent tests were conducted utilizing 4 concentrations of mercury. It was found that the 96-hour LC_{50} values were not salinity dependent, but the rate at which mortality occurred did increase with decreasing salinity. Significant mortality was observed at the lowest test salinities (7 and $14^{\circ}/_{oo}$) during the initial 24 hours, and after 48 hours at 75 ppb of mercury, survival was 0, 40 and 60% at salinities of 7, 14 and $21^{\circ}/_{oo}$, respectively. This indicates that crabs exposed to excessively large drainages of pollutants introduced by rivers into the estuary or heavy pollutant input into an estuary during or immediately after a heavy rainfall would be very seriously stressed. Coupled with possible thermal stresses, these deleterious synergistic effects could be further multiplied.

Discussion

This review described what has been and is now being done in the study of the sublethal effects of three major classes of pollutants commonly found in the estuarine environment. The material presented indicates that there is still a great deal of baseline information on the "normal" responses and functions of marine and estuarine species needed before the effects of pollutants on these parameters can be assessed fully. Furthermore, physiological parameters and the effects of pollutants on them are greatly complicated by natural factors such as season of the year, condition of the animal, its sex, its life stage and countless other variables. This is especially evident in the data derived from respiration studies in which the exposed animals may significantly increase or decrease the rate of oxygen consumption, may vary the response depending on concentration of pollutant and duration of exposure or may not respond measurably at all. Therefore, in any assessment of sublethal effects of pollutants, the biology of the organism under investigation must be well understood by the researcher so that alterations in response can be directly related to the effects of that specific pollutant under the conditions of the experiment. It is also necessary that field studies be undertaken to assess these responses under natural conditions as influenced by all of the operating environmental factors. With the fluctuations of the natural environment, it is likely that organisms never attain the petroleum hydrocarbon levels which were produced in the laboratory. It is also probable that in the estuaries, periods of flushing

117

from heavy rainfall allow the organisms to release some portion of the accumulated contamination. Only by combining laboratory and field studies can the effects of pollutants be fully assessed.

While the chemical nature of the pollutants discussed and their behavior in sea water are beyond the scope of this paper, it would be appropriate to mention the fact that there are many problems associated with both exposure of animals to these compounds and subsequent analysis of residues present in sea water and tissues. Even short-term maintenance of a stable concentration of a pollutant in the exposure medium is relatively difficult. These compounds or their solvent carriers are generally highly volatile and tend to be lost from sea water solution on aeration. They also have a great affinity for physical adsorption to the surface of containers and to small particulate materials, resulting in either case, in a less-than-anticipated amount in the exposure water (i.e. nominal vs. measured concentration). Finally, the problem of analysis of exposure water and tissues of exposed and control organisms needs to be considered. Many of the techniques and procedures used for the analysis of these compounds are relatively new and some are still in the developmental or research phase. Once identification and quantitation of a pollutant is made it should be confirmed by at least one and preferably two different analytical methods. Furthermore, the detection sensitivities of present-day instruments are such that contamination of samples is a very significant problem. All of these factors combined make it difficult for an analytical laboratory to process many samples on a routine basis. This reinforces the concept that in conducting experiments of the types described above, it is desirable, if not imperative, for the biologist to coordinate with a full-time analytical chemist.

Finally, it should be noted that the concentrations of pollutants used to elicit the sublethal responses observed were significantly higher than those reported in the natural environment. By refining the studies already described and by utilizing additional, more sensitive physiological parameters, it may be possible to demonstrate sublethal effects at near environmental levels. Measurements of the effects of sublethal concentrations of pollutants on organisms, if performed and evaluated intelligently, will be a powerful and effective tool in the assessment of man's impact on the environment.

Summary

1. Virtually any biological parameter which can be quantitated and which provides a reproducible response is suitable
for the evaluation of the effects of sublethal pollutant
doses on an organism.

2. Heavy metals and chlorinated hydrocarbons are in general
accumulated to a greater extent and bound to organisms much
more firmly than petroleum hydrocarbons. Retention of petro-
leum-derived hydrocarbons by animals in clean water may vary
from several days to approximately two months, and is species
dependent.

3. The class of petroleum hydrocarbons accumulated to the
greatest extent and retained the longest is the "naphthalenes". Significant members of this group are naphthalene,
1-methylnaphthalene, 2-methylnaphthalene and dimethylnaphthalenes.

4. Utilizing concentrations well above environmentally realistic levels, inorganic mercury, Aroclor 1254 and petroleum hydrocarbons have been shown to affect the respiratory
rate and chloride ion regulation of selected marine animals.

5. There is some indication that the levels of petroleum hydrocarbons in the animal tissues may act to temporarily alter
the regulatory ability of the test individuals. This inter-
ference was shown in several instances to be transitory, presumably due to the dynamics of hydrocarbon release from the
tissues to the environment.

References

Anderson, J. W. 1973. Background paper, submitted to the
    National Academy of Sciences Workshop on Inputs, Fates
    and Effects of Petroleum in the Marine Environment,
    Airlie, Virginia, May 21-25. pp. 690-708.
Anderson, J. W., J. M. Neff, B. A. Cox, H. E. Tatem and G.
    M. Hightower. 1974. Mar. Biol. (submitted).
Anderson, R. D. 1973. Ph.D. dissertation presented to the
    Biology Department, Texas A&M University, 146 p.
Blumer, M., S. Souza and J. Sass. 1970. Mar. Biol. 5:
    195-202.
Brocksen, R. W. and H. T. Bailey. 1973. Proc. Joint Conf.

on Prevention and Control of Oil Spills. API, EPA & USCG. March 13-15, pp. 783-792.

Brown, B. E. and R. C. Newell. 1972. Mar. Biol. 16: 108-118.

Darnell, R. M. 1971. Intecol. Bull. 3: 3-20.

DeCoursey, P. J. and W. B. Vernberg. 1972. Oikos 23: 241-247.

Doudoroff, P. and M. Katz. 1953. Sewage and Ind. Wastes 25: 802-839.

Eisler, R., G. E. Zaroogian, and R. J. Hennekey. 1972. J. Fish. Res. Bd. Can. 29: 1367-1369.

Fry, F. E. J. 1971. W. S. Hoar and D. J. Randall (eds.), "Fish Physiology," Vol. VI. Academic Press, New York. pp. 1-99.

Gilfillan, E. S. 1973. Proc. Joint Conf. on Prevention and Control of Oil Spills. API, EPA & USCG. March 13-15, pp. 691-695.

Hansen, D. J., P. R. Parrish, J. I. Lowe, A. J. Wilson, Jr. and P. D. Wilson. Bull. Environ. Contam. Toxicol. 6: 113-119.

Hattula, M. L., and O. Karlog. 1973. Acta. Pharmacol. Toxicol. 32: 237-245.

Janicki, R. H. and W. B. Kinter. 1971. Science 173: 1146-1148.

Kinne, O. 1967. In: G. H. Lauff (ed.), Estuaries. AAAS, Washington, D.C. pp. 525-540.

Kinne, O. (Ed.). 1973. Marine Ecology. A Comprehensive Integrated Treatise on Life in Oceans and Coastal Waters. Vol. 1, Part 2 - Salinity. Wiley Interscience, New York. pp. 683-1083.

Kinter, W. B., L. S. Merkens, R. H. Janicki and A. M. Guarino. 1972. Environ. Health Perspect. Iss. No. 1: 169-173.

Lee, R. F. and A. A. Benson. 1973. Background paper, submitted to the National Academy of Sciences Workshop on Inputs, Fates and Effects of Petroleum in the Marine Environment, Airlie, Virginia, May 21-25. pp. 541-551.

Lee, R. F., R. Sauerheber and A. A. Benson. 1972. Science 177: 344-346.

Lee, R. R., R. Sauerheber and G. H. Dobbs. 1972. Mar. Biol. 17: 201-208.

McFarland, W. N. and B. D. Lee. 1963. Bull. Mar. Sci. Gulf. Carrib. 13: 391-417.

McFarland, W. N., and P. E. Pickens. 1965. Can. J. Zool. 43: 571-585.

Moore, S. F., R. L. Dwyer and A. M. Katz. 1973. Report No.

162, Ralph M. Parsons Lab. for Water Resources and Hydro-
dynamics. School of Engineering, MIT, Cambridge, Mass.
162 p.

Nelson-Smith, A. 1973. "Oil Pollution and Marine Ecology."
Plenum Press, New York. 260 p.

Newell, R. C. 1970. "Biology of Intertidal Animals."
American Elsevier Publ., New York. 555 p.

Newell, R. C. 1973. American Zool. 13: 513-528.

Peakall, D. B. 1972. Residue Rev. 44: 1-21.

Pentreath, R. J. 1973. J. Mar. Biol. Assoc. U. K. 53: 127-
143.

Potts, W. T. W. and G. Parry. 1964. "Osmotic and Ionic
Regulation in Animals." Pergamon Press, Oxford. 423 pp.

Risebrough, R. W. and B. DeLappe. 1972. Environ. Hlth.
Perspect., Iss. No. 1: 39-45.

Saha, J. G. 1972. Residue Rev. 42: 103-163.

Sanders, H. O. and J. H. Chandler. 1972. Bull. Environ.
Contam. Toxicol. 7: 257-263.

Sprague, J. B. 1971. Water Res. 5: 245-266.

Steed, D. L. and B. J. Copeland. 1967. Contrib. Mar. Sci.,
Univ. Texas 12: 143-159.

Stegeman, J. J. and J. M. Teal. 1973. Mar Biol. 22: 37-44.

Vernberg, W. G. and J. O'Hara. 1972. J. Fish. Res. Bd.
Can. 29: 1491-4194.

Vernberg, W. B. and F. J. Vernberg. 1972. Fishery Bull.
70: 415-420.

Waldichuk, M. 1973. CRC Critical Reviews in Environmental
Control, Chemical Rubber C. Press, Cleveland, Ohio. pp.
167-211.

Wohlschlag, D. E. and J. N. Cameron. 1967. Contrib. Mar.
Sci., Univ. Texas 12: 160-171.

Williams, A. B. 1960. Biol. Bull. 119: 560-571.

Acknowledgments

The authors gratefully acknowledge the research efforts
of Dr. Roger D. Anderson, Mr. Guri Roesijadi and Mr. Bruce A.
Cox. We are also indebted to Dr. J. Scott Warner of Battelle
Laboratories, Columbus Ohio, for the expert and unparalleled
identification of petroleum hydrocarbon in water and tissue
samples. This research was supported by Grants GX37344,
GX37347 and GX37349 from the I.D.O.E. branch of the National
Science Foundation and by contract #0S20C from the American
Petroleum Institute, which has also supported the research
of Dr. Warner.

SECTION II

DETOXICATION AS A MECHANISM

FOR SURVIVAL

R. H. Adamson, presiding

"It has been necessary for the body to call to its aid a chemical defense mechanism to guard against poison absorbed from the gastrointestinal tract. After many generations the chemical defense mechanism has been so perfected that it is now quite able to cope with many of the foreign organism compounds..."

-Sherwin 1922

An Introduction to Detoxication as a
Mechanism of Survival

R. H. Adamson[1]

This is the second section of the symposium on
mechanism of survival in toxic environments. The
first session was concerned with the effects of
pesticides and other chemical pollutants on the
environment and this section will be concerned with
the detoxication and metabolism of some of these
biocides and other foreign chemicals by microorganisms, invertebrates, fishes and other species.

The term xenobiotic is derived from the Greek
meaning "a substance foreign to living organism";
this term was introduced by Professor R. Tecwyn
Williams over two decades ago and is now internationally accepted and synonymous with foreign
compounds. Furthermore, there is now a journal
entitled Xenobiotica[2] which publishes manuscripts
concerned with the metabolism and disposition of
xenobiotics (foreign compounds) by various species
and biological systems.

The fate of a xenobiotic in an animal, after
exposure or administration, depends to a great extent on the lipid solubility of a compound for it
is the lipid solubility of a compound which determines its ability to traverse biological membranes
and this in turn determines to a large extent the
absorption, distribution, excretion, and metabolism
(detoxication) of the xenobiotic. Foreign compounds, therefore, are eliminated from the body by
excretion (renal, biliary and extrarenal), metabolism (non-microsomal or microsomal) and by a combination of these mechanisms. Without mechanisms
for the metabolism of xenobiotics some lipid
soluble drugs (e.g., thiopental or chlorpromazine)
would exert their effects for a lifetime and drug
therapy as we know it today might be impossible.

The general patterns for metabolism of xenobiotics consist of a few reactions in which the
xenobiotic is oxidized, hydrolyzed or reduced
(phase I) or conjugated (phase II) or both phase
I and phase II reactions may occur.

[1]National Cancer Inst., N. I. H., Bethesda, Md.
[2]Printed and published by Taylor and Francis Ltd.,
10-14 Macklin Street, London, England.

```
       phase I                      phase II
Xenobiotic → Oxidation, red.    Synthetic → Conjugated
             or hydrolysis      reaction    metabolite
```

The reaction of both phases is catalyzed by enzymes occuring in the plasma or various organs. These enzymes may be distributed in the microsomal sub-cellular fraction which is derived from the endo-plasmic reticulum, the mitochondria or occur in the cell sap. The microsomal oxidative enzymes are present mainly in the liver with other organs having less enzyme activity, e.g. lung.

While a xenobiotic undergoing one of the reactions usually gives rise to a more polar metabolite, the metabolite is not always less toxic or pharma-cologically inactive. This is especially true of metabolites resulting from oxidation, reduction, and hydrolysis. Examples of foreign compounds whose metabolic products are more active than the parent compound are abundant (Table 1). Conjugation reactions however are detoxication mechanisms par excellence since they nearly always yield metab-olites which are inactive and readily excreted.

TABLE 1. Metabolic activation of foreign compounds

Foreign compound	Reaction	Metabolite	Activity of metabolite
Prontosil	Reduction	Sulfanilamide	Anti-bacterial
Chloral hydrate	Reduction	Trichlo-roethanol	Hypnotic
Acetophene-tidin	Oxidation	p-Acetamido-phenol	Antipyretic, analgesic
Cyclophospha-mide	"	Aldophospha-mide	Antineo-plastic
Parathion	"	Paraoxon	Anticholines-terase
2-Acetylamino-fluorene (2AAF)	"	N-hydroxy-2AAF	Carcinogen

Removal of an unnecessary chemical is a process which is constantly occurring in all animals and there is data which indicates this may also be happening when xenobiotics are chemically altered by the body. To explain why and how this is done, several hypotheses have been formulated and these may be referred to as the:

Surface Tension Hypothesis of Berczeller
Chemical Defense Hypothesis of Sherwin
Increase Acidity Hypothesis of Quick
Special Mechanism Hypothesis of Brodie
Extended Capacity Hypothesis of Adamson

The surface tension hypothesis (Berczeller, 1917) states that during a conjugation process a change in surface tension occurs bringing the surface tension of the metabolite closer to that of water than the surface tension of the parent compound. This will result in lower toxicity since the metabolite will not accumulate at surfaces in toxic concentrations. The surface tension of a number of parent compounds and their conjugates was measured and results were obtained which supported this hypothesis. However, this hypothesis only involves conjugations as detoxication mechanisms and does not account for metabolic alterations as a result of reduction, oxidation or hydrolysis. Furthermore, the hypothesis has been criticized for stressing the quantitative aspects of toxicity and minimizing the qualitative or specific aspects of toxicity (Ross and Sherwin, 1926).

The view that detoxication processes are special defense mechanisms was developed by Sherwin (1922) who regarded the metabolism of foreign compounds as defense mechanisms against toxic compounds formed in vivo or absorbed from the gastrointestinal tract. According to Sherwin "the body has at its command a series of chemical reactions. The first method of attacking a foreign molecule seems to be an attempt to complete oxidation. This, in the majority of cases, meets with at least partial success.... In some cases reduction is used as a precursor of oxidation, and in a few

127

including steroid hormones, other hormones, fatty
acids, bile acids, and bilirubin to its glucuronide.
Adamson et al. (1965) have suggested that reducing
enzymes may have evolved before the oxidative
enzymes and have developed what might be called the
extended capacity hypothesis of xenobiotic metabolism. Stated simply, enzymes both microsomal and
non-microsomal have evolved to metabolize normal
body chemicals and in particular the microsomal
enzymes have evolved to metabolize and detoxify
lipid soluble steroids and other hormones, products
produced by bacteria and to conjugate bilirubin.
The variety of products produced by bacteria alone
allows for development of non-specific enzyme
systems for detoxication. As fish and animals
become exposed to more toxic chemicals in their
food (trimethylamine, terpenes, steroids, alkaloids)
the non-specific enzymes developed to a more extended capacity. Furthermore, development of enzyme
induction allowed this metabolic capacity to be
further extended so that a major accumulation of
toxic matter over a short time interval could be
detoxified. These mechanisms wide in scope, non-
specific in substrate specificity and readily inducible thus prepared the organism for the onslaught
of synthetic molecules produced by the organic
chemist and pharmacologist during the last century.

References

Adamson, R. H. 1967. Fed. Proc. 20:1047-1055.
Adamson, R. H., R. L. Dixon, F. L. Francis, and
    D. P. Rall 1965. Proc. Nat. Acad. Sci. 54:
    1386-1391.
Berczeller, L. 1917. Biochem. Z. 84:75-79.
Brodie, B. B. 1956. J. Pharmacy and Pharmacol.
    8:1-17.
Quick, A. J. 1932. J. Biol. Chem. 97:403-419.
Rose, A. R. and C. P. Sherwin, 1926. J. Biol. Chem.
    68:565-573.
Sherwin, C. P. 1922. Physiological Rev. 2:238-276.

MICROBIAL DEGRADATION OF PESTICIDES

Fumio Matsumura

Department of Entomology
University of Wisconsin
Madison

Introduction

Pesticides belong to the group of environmental microcontaminants. Generally they are present in such small quantities that they do not affect the physical quality of the environment. The reason these compounds could become a serious threat is that they can affect biological systems. In other words, problems of microcontamination should be studied only from the biological view.

When pesticides are introduced into the environment many physical, chemical and biological forces begin to act upon them. The key to an understanding of the behavior of pesticides in the environment lies in their high biological affinity. This is natural, since these chemicals are designed as biocidal agents and particularly true in one group of pesticides which are designed to kill insects. Insect pests generally possess lipophilic outer cuticles which are resistant to polar substances but very susceptible to attack by apolar chemicals. This means that pesticidal molecules in polar media such as soil and water tend to accumulate in organic matter, especially in biological systems.

Assuming that pesticides are applied to soil or aquatic systems, one can immediately foresee two independent reactions adsorption-binding by soil or aquatic sediment particles and that by biological material. It is known that pesticides bound to soil and sediments can eventually be transferred to biological systems, though the speed of transfer will be much slower than direct reaction to biological systems.

It has generally been said that environmentally applied pesticides disappear through processes that follow pseudo-first order kinetics. That is, if one plots the logarithm of the amount of the given pesticide remaining at the site against time, one can observe linear patterns of disappearance. More often than not, such lines follow two step reactions: i.e. the initial "fast phase" and the subsequent "slow phase." The initial fast disappearance is related to physico-chemical factors such as evaporation, leaching and mechanical removal. It is the second "slow phase" reactions that are ascribed to the biological (and some physical) alteration processes working on pesticidal molecules in nature. These are metabolic reactions of microbial, plant and animal systems as well as actions of sunlight, heat, pH and other catalytic reactions by various soil and sediment substances such as clay particles, ferrous ions, etc. Generally speaking, only the first two types of reactions (biological and sunlight) play important roles in altering stable pesticides in nature. Also it is important to stress here that pesticide which disappears through "fast phase" reactions should not be regarded as permanently eliminated. The reactions in this "fast phase" largely represent translocation in the environment, and such processes do not, therefore contribute to overall reduction of the total environmental pesticide load. Among biological reactions, microbial activities are regarded as most important in the elimination of pesticidal chemicals from the environment.

Characteristics of Microbial Metabolism

Although there have been many reports suggesting toxic actions of pesticidal chemicals on micro-

bial populations in soil, etc. the general concensus
of the scientific community is that pesticides do
not permanently alter microbial populations. Of
course, such a generalization does not include
fungicides, algicides, etc. which are intended to
control specific microorganisms. Even in these
cases, however, microorganisms are known for their
ability to develop resistant populations. It is
not unusual to find microorganisms which are highly
capable of metabolizing specific pesticides in areas
that have been heavily treated with such chemicals.
For instance we could isolate microorganisms
capable of degrading dieldrin from the loading dock
soil of a dieldrin factory (Matsumura et al., 1968)
and from the farm area known to be heavily treated
by dieldrin (Matsumura and Boush, 1967). Raghu
and MacRea (1966) observed that the second addition
of BHC to submerged soil of a paddy field increased
metabolic activity by microorganisms, suggesting
the development of microorganism populations capable
of degrading BHC during the first incubation period.
It is also probable that the other type of microbial
adaptatation, i.e. "induction" of enzyme systems
to degrade pesticidal molecules, takes place when
microorganisms are under heavy pressure by pesticidal chemicals. We have, for instance, subjected
microorganisms to heavy dieldrin pressure, and
found that a strain of Trichoderma koningi can grow
in a carbon deficient medium with colossal levels
of dieldrin (Bixby et al., 1971). This strain was
found to produce CO_2 from dieldrin, indicating that
it can utilize dieldrin as an energy source. Focht
and Alexander (1971) found a Hydrogenomonas species
which can grow on diphenylmethane, a DDT-like compound, to yield phenol and benzoic acid. This culture was later found to degrade DDT to p-chloro-
phenylacetic acid, when the culture was subjected
to first an anaerobic condition and then to an
aerobic condition. This particular experiment
will be commented on later.

The basic question about such metabolic
activities of microorganisms on pesticidal chemicals
is why they metabolize such non-nutritional chemicals
at all. It is generally acknowledged that pestici-

131

dal chemicals are very poor sources of carbon and
that these artificially produced chemicals are not
present in large enough quantities for long enough
time periods to warrant evolution of specific
organisms to utilize them (with the exception of
certain microorganisms growing in pesticide factory
discharges, or special laboratory selected strains
as above). To elaborate this point further, it
is hard to believe that microorganisms develop
specific metabolic processes for chemicals which
are present in their surroundings at only ppt to
ppm (part per trillion and million, respectively)
levels.

The answer appears to lie in unique characteristics of pesticidal chemicals which make
them show high biological affinity. In other words,
these chemicals come in contact with biological
systems, including microbial ones, whether they are
ready to metabolize and utilize or not. This process of biological binding can be favorably compared to solvent-water partitioning behavior of
these chemicals in many instances; the solvent
representing the biological system in this case.
Thus the reaction is concentraion-independent, and,
particularly in aqueous media, the most lipophilic
pesticidal residues are eventually expected to be
partitioned into biological systems at all concentrations.

It is understandable that those microorganisms
which receive small quantities of foreign compounds
do not particularly develop biochemical or physiological defense mechanisms, particularly when these
chemicals are not toxic to them. Thus cases for
general microbial populations which receive only
small amounts of pesticidal chemicals infrequently
are quite different from these previously discussed
for microorganisms receiving high amounts of
pesticidal chemicals.

The microorganisms receiving low levels of
pesticidal exposure are likely to utilize either
already existing enzymatic systems to degrade these
chemicals or else transport them to non-vital extra-
or intracellular sites by changing their nature

or, if possible, as they are. Thus such reactions are never meant to derive energy from the chemicals. Martin Alexander of Cornell University uses the term "cometabolism" (e.g. Alexander, 1972) to describe such cases. "Co-metabolism" is defined as the microbial metabolic activities on chemicals from which microorganisms do not primarily receive energy. Such metabolic activities require the utilization of existing enzymatic and other physiological defense systems.

In the past such microbial "defense" mechanisms against non-toxic foreign compounds (e.g., "xenobiotics") have not been thoroughly considered. With some knowledge accumulating in this field, it is hoped that some clear concept of microbial "defense" mechanisms will soon emerge.

METABOLIC ACTIVITIES CAUSING DEGRADATION OF PESTICIDES

Hydrolytic processes

It has been noted that microorganisms generally exhibit strong esterase activities. This is particularly applicable to insecticidal organophosphate and carbamate esters. For instance, the molecule of carbaryl, naphthyl N-methyl carbamate is hydrolyzed by Pseudomonas melophtora to naphthol (Matsumura and Boush, 1968).

The oxidative processes which are important in higher animals in degrading these compounds are less frequently observed. This is probably because of the lack of defined mixed-function oxidase systems in microorganisms. It is sometimes difficult to distinguish the enzymatic hydrolysis process from physical ones, such as pH, catalytic, etc. for liable chemicals, however.

Another interesting possibility is that soil enzymes, in the absence of micorbial action, can also degrade pesticides. Soil enzymes are extracellular enzymes found outside of living soil organisms. They could come from an exoenzymic source produced by living microbes and from enzymes released by the death of soil organisms (Skujins, 1966). Getzin and Rosefield (1968), for instance, found that sterilization of soil samples by auto-claving destroyed 90% of the degradation activity of the soil, while a gamma radiation treatment (4 mrad, at 250,000 rads/hr) hardly reduced its metabolic activity. The authors were able to ex-tract a fraction with 0.2 N NaOH that could actively degrade malathion.

As for the true enzymatic hydrolysis system, Matsumura and Boush (1966) demonstrated that mala-thion can be hydrolyzed by an enzyme preparation from Trichoderma viride. The enzyme system is prepared through an acetone power extraction pro-cedure and is sensitive to DFP at 10^{-6}M, indicating the enzymatic origin of the preparation. Boush and Matsumura (1967) also observed degradation of dichlorvos, diazinon, parathion, DFP and carbaryl by cultures of Pseudomonas melophthora. All organophasphate insecticides were converted into water-soluble products, and carbaryl was mainly metabolized to 1-naphthol in the absence of added cofactors. The latter observation also agrees with the findings by Bollag and Liu (1971) who found 1-naphthol to be the major conversion product of carbaryl by soil microorganisms. Although phorate (Thimet) has two vulnerable sites for oxidative attacks (i.e. P=S and the sulfide bond), it is de-graded only through hydrolytic processes in Pseudo-monas fluorescens and Thiobacillus thiooxidans (Ahmed and Casida, 1958). This is surprising since the latter organisms are known to utilize sulfur as an energy source. In any event 60 to 75% of phorate was hydrolyzed in 8 days by these organisms.

The evidence for hydrolytic degradation of diazinon is circumstantial. Bro-Rasmussen et al. (1968) studied various soil environmental factors for the rate of diazinon degradation and concluded that microorganisms play by far the most important role in determining the rate of overall disappear-ance of diazinon. Konrad et al. (1967), on the other hand, showed that hydrolysis is the major mechanism of diazinon degradation in soil. Laanio

et al. (1972) also found that a hydrolysis product,
2-isopropyl-4-methyl-6-hydroxypyrimidine was the
most abundant product in rice paddy water and soil
that had been treated with ^{14}C-diazinon, particularly during several weeks after the application.

Zayed et al. (1965) found that trichlorfon is
also degraded through hydrolytic processes in
Aspergillus niger, Penicillium notatum, and a
Fusarium species. The metabolic products found
were 0-methyl-2,2,2-trichloro-1-hydroxyethyl phosphonic acid and probably 2,2,2-trichloro-1-hydroxy-
phosphonic acid.

Fenitrothion (Sumithion) is also degraded
through hydrolytic processes by Bacillus subtilis,
though in this particular bacterium species a reductive metabolism of this compound is much more pronounced (Miyamoto et al., 1966). The hydrolytic
metabolic products identified by these workers are
desmethylfenitrothion, didesmethylfenitrothion,
dimethylphosphorothioate, and to a lesser extent,
desmethylaminofenitrothion. Interestingly enough,
no fenitroxon (Sumioxon) was observed, indicating
that oxidative desulfuration does not take place
under the culture condition in this species, or that
fenitroxon is quickly degraded by esterases, though
the absence of fenitroxon metabolites makes the
latter probability unlikely. Zectran[R], mexacarbate,
is mostly degraded by microorganisms via hydrolytic
processes to 4-dimethylamino-3,5-xylenol (Benezet
and Matsumura, 1973b). Among 12 microbial isolates
tested, 9 of them produced this hydrolysis product,
while in 5 isolates 4-N-desmethylation was the
major metabolic system.

Oxidative Activities

Oxidative metabolism is also known to take place
on these insecticidal chemicals, but the extent of
such metabolic activities appears, when judged by
the number of examples so far found, to be limited
as compared to those found in herbicidal degradation
(see e.g. Kearney et al., 1967; Bollag, 1972).

This is rather surprising, since these insecticidal
carbamic and phosphorus esters, particularly the
former compounds, are known to undergo extensive
oxidative reactions in higher animals and plants.
This general lack of oxidative reactions in the
microbial world against these insecticides becomes
more noticable when one realizes that there is no
confirmed report on conversion of P=S to P=O (i.e.
desulfuration) among phosphorothioates so far
examined; this reaction is omnipresent among other
biological systems. Although it might mean that
"oxons" are once formed, and further degraded by
hydrolytic enzymes, this conspicuous absence of
"oxons" among microbial metabolites of thiophosphates suggests the basic difference between microbial metabolism and others. Since epoxidation of
cyclodiene insecticides is well known among microbial species, the above phenomenon should not be
regraded as the general lack of any oxidative
system.

While there are only a few examples of metabolic
studies in this regard, two oxidative reactions seem
to commonly take place in microbial systems: these
are oxidation of thioethers to sulfoxides and sulfones, and the other is N-dealkylation of alkylamines (see the following section).

Other oxidative reactions known to occur are
β-oxidation, oxidation of alcohols and aldehydes,
expoxidation, etc. In contrast to the animal and
plant systems, ring hydroxylation processes are
observed less frequently. Thus it is not too
uncommon that scientists find two different pathways for animals and microorganisms for the same
pesticidal chemical; the former showing ring-
hydroxylating and the latter exhibiting hydrolytic
activities.

For instance, the only hydroxylation reactions
so far observed on insecticidal chemicals are the
ones observed by Liu and Bollag (1971a, b) on
carbaryl. Since there are a number of reports on
microbial hydroxylation reactions on herbicidal
chemicals, it is likely, however, that a greater
incidence of such oxidative reactions will be
reported in the near future.

Reductive System Including
Dechlorination Reactions

Reductive reactions are, on the other hand, known to frequently occur in microbial species. Thus denitrothion and EPN are converted to amino-fenitrothion and amino EPN by Bacillus subtilis (Miyamoto et al., 1966), and the major microbial metabolic product of parathion is aminoparathion (Cook, 1957; Ahmed et al., 1958). In addition to these hydrogenation reactions .other major types of reduction activities are particularly important in the microbial world for chlorinated hydrocarbon insecticides. Examples can be found in the dechlorination reaction on DDT to produce TDE (DDD, e.g. Finley and Pillmore, 1963), then to DDMS and DDNS (Matsumura et al., 1971a).

The enzymatic basis of the microbial dechlorination reaction has been studied by French and Hoopingarner (1970). These workers incubated DDT in vitro with various subcellular fractions of Escherichia coli and found that TDE production was highest in the system where both the membrane and the cytoplasm were present. The enzyme system is located in the cell membrane and requires reduced FAD. It is operated under anaerobic conditions inasmuch as that even the addition of any tricarboxylic acid cycle intermediates to the system inhibits the process. These reductive dechlorination systems are apparently present in many microbial systems. Thus even a strain of Hydrogenomonas species which has specially been selected to degrade only DDM analogs (but not DDT) in an aerobic condition (Focht and Alexander, 1971) exhibits the ability to dechlorinate DDT (probably to DDM) when it is subjected to anaerobic conditions. The net result being total degradation of DDT by this strain by this successive change in culturing conditions.

DDT analogs are not the only group of compounds that go through extensive dechlorination reactions. Gamma-BHC is known to be converted into gamma-BTC (gamma-tetrachlorocylohexene) (Tsukano and Kobayashi, 1972).

137

Metabolic Processes Causing
Toxic Terminal Residues

In the foregoing section I have deliberately
summarized the reactions that are mainly involved
in detoxication of pesticidal chemicals. Doubt-
lessly this is the most important area of microbial
action. Nevertheless another aspect of microbial
action requires serious attention. That is, microorganisms, in the process of metabolic conversion
of pesticidal chemicals, can produce compounds of
higher toxicities and stability. Such chemicals
are collectively called "terminal residues" (see
Matsumura, 1972).

Isomerization Reactions

A characteristic reaction associated with
microbial metabolism is the rearrangement process,
such as the intramolecular bridge formation (e.g.,
photodieldrin and photoaldrin formation, Figure 1.
Rosen et al., 1966; Robinson et al., 1966), the
rearrangement process of epoxyrings to form ketones,
aldehydes and alcohols (Matsumura et al., 1968,
1971b).

In endrin and to a lesser extent dieldrin,
the major reaction products are ketones which are
formed as a result of isomerization of the epoxy
ring. In addition, certain microorganisms are
capable of forming photodieldrin from dieldrin
(Matsumura et al., 1970). Such an isomerization
reaction appears to be a very common one in the
case of endrin Figure 2. For instance, Patil et al.
(1970) examined 20 common soil isolates of microorganisms for their metabolic abilities against
endrin, aldrin, DDT, gamma-BHC and propoxur. They
found that all of them could degrade DDT and endrin,
while only 13 degraded aldrin and none degraded
either gamma-BHC or propoxur. All of these isolates
were capable of forming ketoendrin from endrin
(Matsumura et al., 1971b).

The significance of such rearrangement reactions is not known. It is, however, not likely
that the microorganisms are able to derive any
energy from the processes. The rearrangements

138

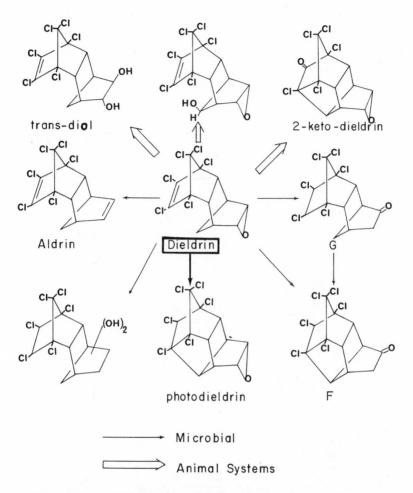

trans-diol

2-keto-dieldrin

Aldrin

Dieldrin

G

photodieldrin

F

———————▶ Microbial

⇨ Animal Systems

Figure 1. Metabolic fate of dieldrin in microorganisms in comparison to mammalian systems.

could, at least, give the microorganisms the chance to degrade the compounds further. In most cases such reactions yield more polar compounds than the parent molecules. Indeed Korte and his associates (Korte, 1970) have shown that photodieldrin can be degraded relatively rapidly by Aspergillus flavus and Penicillium notatum to 2 hydrophilic products. It is important to stress here that so far none of these stable metabolic products have been proven

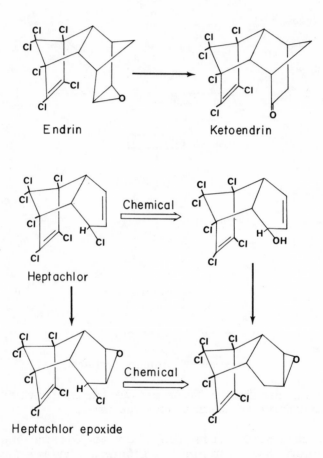

Figure 2. Major microbial metabolic processes for
endrin and heptachlor. The term "chemical" indicates that such processes take place by chemical,
and not by microbial, reactions.

to be less toxic than the parent molecules against
non-mammalian systems. For instance Batterton
et al. (1971) showed that photodieldrin, metabolites

TABLE 1. Toxicities of conversion products of cydo-
dine insecticides on a fresh water blue-green algae
species.

Insecticide	LC-50[1]:ppb
Endrin	310
Ketoendrin	220
Dieldrin	540
Photodieldrin	450
Metab. F	560
Metab. G.	580
Aldrin	>1000
Photoaldrin	>1000

[1]The data expressed in the initial concentration of
each compound in the medium that gave a 50% reduction in the population (Batterton et al., 1971).

F and G, and ketoendrin are about as toxic as
dieldrin and endrin, respectively (Table 1) against
a fresh water blue-green algae species. Wang et al.
(1971) found that photoaldrin and photodieldrin are
more neurotoxic than aldrin or dieldrin in the
American cockroach (Table 2). Another intriguing
example of intra-molecular isomerization is that of
gamma-BHC to alpha-BHC (Benezet and Matsumura, 1973a).
This isomerization reaction is catalyzed by NAD and
to a lesser extent by FAD. The production of gamma-
BTC (Figure 3) has been observed along with that of
alpha-BHC. This process requires the change in the
direction of one chlorine atom from the axial to
the equatorial position. These authors postulated
that such a transformation is possible, with initial
dehydrogenation of the same bond, since the latter
process would favor the formation of the alpha-isomer.
The importance of such microbial action may not be
apparent at first. However, recently two groups

141

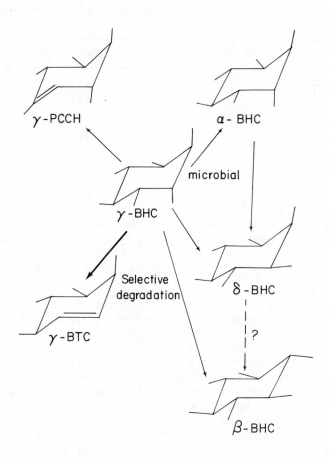

Figure 3. Microbial metabolism of BHC. The term "selective degradation" means that impurities (e.g. S and B-isomers) if present in the original formulation, may remain as a result of extensive degradation of gamma-BHC.

of scientists (Goto et al., 1972; Nagasaki et al., 1972) have independently demonstrated that alpha-BHC is the most tumorigenic member of the BHC family against mice as judged by its ability to cause hepatoma at about 200 to 500 ppm levels in the diet for 24 weeks.

Oxidative Reactions

One of the most thoroughly studied microbial oxidation systems is the epoxidation process on cyclodiene insecticides: e.g. heptachlor to heptachlor epoxide, aldrin to dieldrin, etc. So far as known, such reactions invariably produce more stable and more toxic teminal residues. The system is omnipresent among microbial, plant and animal systems. Strangely, another well-established activation system of desulfuration (i.e. P=S to P=O) on insecticidal thiophosphates has hardly been documented in the microbial systems as mentioned before. There are two other oxidative systems which are acting as 'activating' reactions on organophosphate and carbamate insecticides. One is the oxidation of thioethers to sulfoxides and sulfones, and the other is N-dealkylation of alkylamines. Coppedge et al. (1967) compared degradation of Temik in cotton plants and soil. In soils, they found Temik sulfoxide, sulfone, nitrile sulfoxide, and oxime sulfoxide, indicating that oxidation of the thioether bond had taken place along with hydrolysis and further conversion of the oxime to the nitrile.

Ahmed and Casida (1958) found that a yeast species, Torulopsis utilis and a green alga, Chlorella pyrenoidosa could oxidize phorate (Thimet) to the corresponding sulfoxide.

Williams et al. (1972) determined the residues of fensulfothion, 0,0-diethyl 0-(p-(methylsulfinyl) phenyl) phosphorothioate and its sulfone analog in muck soil in which carrots were grown. Such reactions of sulfur oxidation among microbial species are not surprising when one considers the presence of numerous microorganisms which are specialized in deriving energy from these particular reaction processes.

143

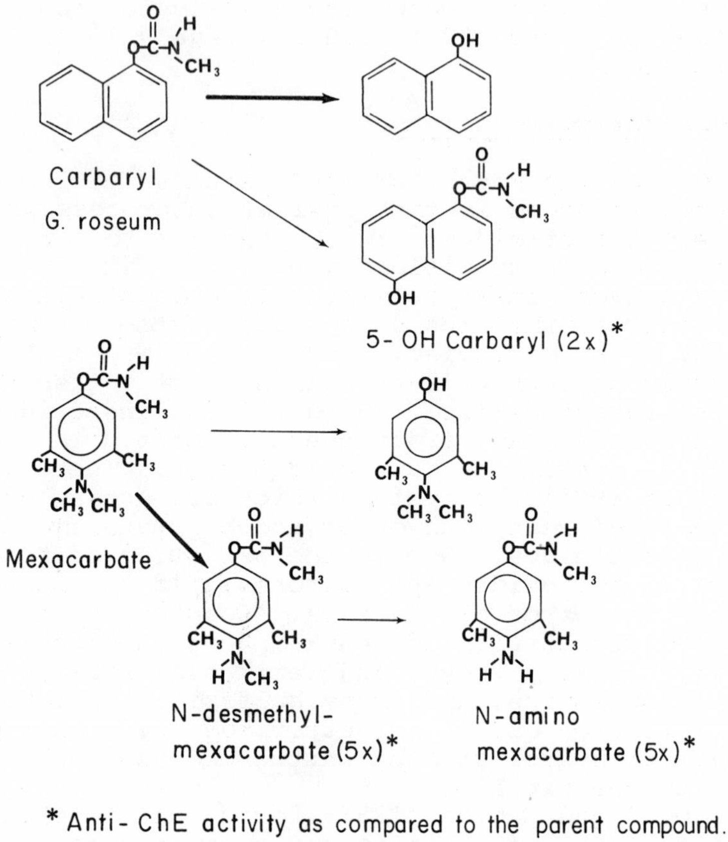

Carbaryl

G. roseum

5- OH Carbaryl (2x)*

Mexacarbate

N-desmethyl-
mexacarbate (5x)*

N-amino
mexacarbate (5x)*

*Anti- ChE activity as compared to the parent compound.

Figure 4. Microbial metabolic processes on carbamate insecticides causing 'activation' of molecules.

An N-dealkylation reaction has also been reported to take place. Liu and Bollag (1971a) isolated a soil fungus Gliocladium roseum from soil which had been treated with carbaryl for 4 weeks. This fungus was found to metabolize carbaryl to 3 major metabolites. They were N-hydroxymethyl carbaryl, 4- and 5-hydroxy-carbaryl. After 7 days of incubation they found

7,500 cpm of radioactive carbaryl remaining out of
12,000 cpm, in contrast to 410, 360 and 696 cpm of
the corresponding metabolites, respectively, in the
growth medium. They noted that the fungus further
metabolized these intermediates. The same workers
(1971b) demonstrated that N-desmethylcarbaryl forms
along with N-hydroxymethylcarbaryl in Aspergillus
terreus and to a lesser extent with A. flavus.
Benezet and Matsumura (1973b) found that Zectran[R],
mexacarbate, is largely degraded by hydrolytic and
4-N-alkylation (Figure 4) processes by several microorganisms. A few microorganism species exclusively
utilized the latter process. One of the bacterium
species, HF-3, in particular produces no hydrolytic
metabolite, in contrast to Trichoderma viride which
exclusively produces the hydrolysis product, 4-
dimethylamino 3,5-xylenol. There is a good probability that the N-desmethylation process is related
to energy production by microorganisms, since both
of these cultures produced N-desmethylation products
in larger quantities in the absence of an added
carbon source as compared to the corresponding
levels of these N-dealkylation products under the
standard growing conditions with mannitol.

It is noteworthy that many of these oxidation
products have already been shown to be more potent
chloinesterase inhibitors (Oonnithan and Casida,
1968).

Other oxidative reactions which create toxic
metabolic products are the formation of dicofol and
FW-152 from DDT (Figure 5 - the former two compounds
are marketed as acaricidal compounds), and β-oxidation of the fatty acid of phenoxyalkanoate herbicides. The latter processes are known to produce
the toxic phenoxyacetic acids such as 2,4-D and
2,4,5-T.

Hydrolysis

Hydrolytic processes are generally regarded as
degradative reactions, though a few examples of
terminal residue formation are known.

One of the most conspicuous examples is that of
epoxy-ring opening of cyclodiene insecticides. The
process has been shown to occur in microorganisms

(Wedemyer, 1968; Matsumura and Boush, 1967). Subsequently Wang and Matsumura (1970) and Wang et al.
(1971) showed that such "diols" are neurotoxic by
using cockroaches (Table 2). Hydrolysis of organophosphates and carbamates could also produce environmentally unwelcome residues. For example, formation

TABLE 2. Comparative neurotoxicities of dieldrin
analogs.

	Latent Periods	Neuro-Symptoms
Dieldrin	50 min.	2
Photodieldrin	30 min.	4
Aldrin	30 min.	3
Photoaldrin	30 min.	4
trans-diol	5 min.	4

From Wang et al. (1971) against the nervous system
of the American cockroach.

of 1-naphthol from carbaryl does not create environmental problems while 1-naphthol is not an anti-
cholinesterase agent. Miyazaki et al. (1969, 1970)
showed that two acaricidal compounds, chlorobenzilate
and chloropropylate, are hydrolyzed by a yeast species,
Rhodotorula gracilis, to yield 4,4'-dichlorobenzilic
acid (DBA) which is further metabolized to form 4,4'-
dichlorobenzophenone (DBP), a stable terminal residue.

Selective Degradation

Whenever the initial technical pesticidal products contain many isomers or impurities, the problem of differential degradation becomes important.
Probably the most celebrated case of such impurities
becoming the center of attention is that of chlorinated dibenzo-p-dioxins. Tetrachlorodibenzo-p-dioxin
(TCDD) was initially discovered in commercial preparations of 2,4,5-T at levels ranging from 1 to 10
ppm. Its toxicity against the guinea pig is cited
as around 0.6 μg/kg, and is one of the most toxic
synthetic compounds known.

A recent study by Miller et al. (1973) indicated that the growth of coho salmon fingerlings was
markedly reduced even after exposure to less than 1
ppt levels of TCDD in water. Studies in our laboratory (Matsumura and Benezet, 1973) showed that TCDD
is extremely resistant against microbial attack.
Considering that degradation of 2,4,5-T by various
microorganisms (see Kearney et al., 1967) appears to
take place with relative ease, it is possible that
TCDD could accumulate as a result of differential
degradation of 2,4,5-T. At the time of this writing it is not, however, certain whether such accumulation of TCDD in wildlife does take place in nature
or not. The analytical problem of detecting TCDD
must be solved before one can reach a firm conclusion
on this matter. In an analogous situation, other
types of chlorinated dibenzo-p-dioxins have been
found in commercial preparations of pentachlorophenol
(PCP). The average dioxin concentrations found in

TABLE 3. Dioxin contents of commercial PCP

Abbreviation	Contents
PCP	85-90%
OCDD	1980 ppm
HCDD	19 ppm
TCDD	<0.05 ppm

From Johnson et al. (1973).

147

commercial PCP preparation in the U.S. is shown
in Table 3 (from Johnson et al., 1973). Also present are another toxic group of impurities, chlorinated dibenzofurans (Plimmer, 1973). None of these
compounds have been examined for their suscepti-
bilities toward microbial attack, but the fact that
they persisted long enough in commercial preparations
of fats, tallows and greases to cause chick edema
disease incidents indicate that they too are stable
chemicals. Another example of selective, or differential degradation is BHC. It has been shown
that α-, β- and δ-BHCs accumulate in nature as a
result of heavy use of technical BHC in the rice
field in Japan (Tatsukawa et al., 1972; Tanabe,
1972) beyond their proportion expected from their
original composition. Although the proportion of
microbial contribution through isomerization
(Benezet and Matsumura, 1973a) is not clear, certainly significant amounts of these isomers must
have accumulated in the environment as a result of
selective degradation of gamma-BHC.

Other Reactions

One of the most interesting reactions is the
formation of DDCN (Figure 5). This reaction was
reported simultaneously by two groups of workers
through isolation of the product from sewage sludges
(Albone et al., 1972, Jensen et al., 1972). The
former workers incubated in a vessel radiolabelled
and non-radioactive DDT with anaerobic sewage sludge
from a water treatment plant in Bristol, Britain for
88 days at 37°C. Minced beef was added to the system
to promote microbial activities. The latter workers
incubated DDT with the sludge at 20°C for up to 8
days under nitrogen atmosphere, and found that by 24
hours, approximately 60% of DDT was consumed and
apparently no further degradation took place. At
24 hours of incubation the percentages of metabolic
products formed were approximately 28 for DDD, 8 for
DDCN, 5 for DDMU, and 2 for DBP. They reasoned that
DDCN formed directly from DDT in a similar chemical
reaction as the formation of benzonitrile from α-
trichlorotoluene and ammonium chloride at high
temperature. The significant point is that these

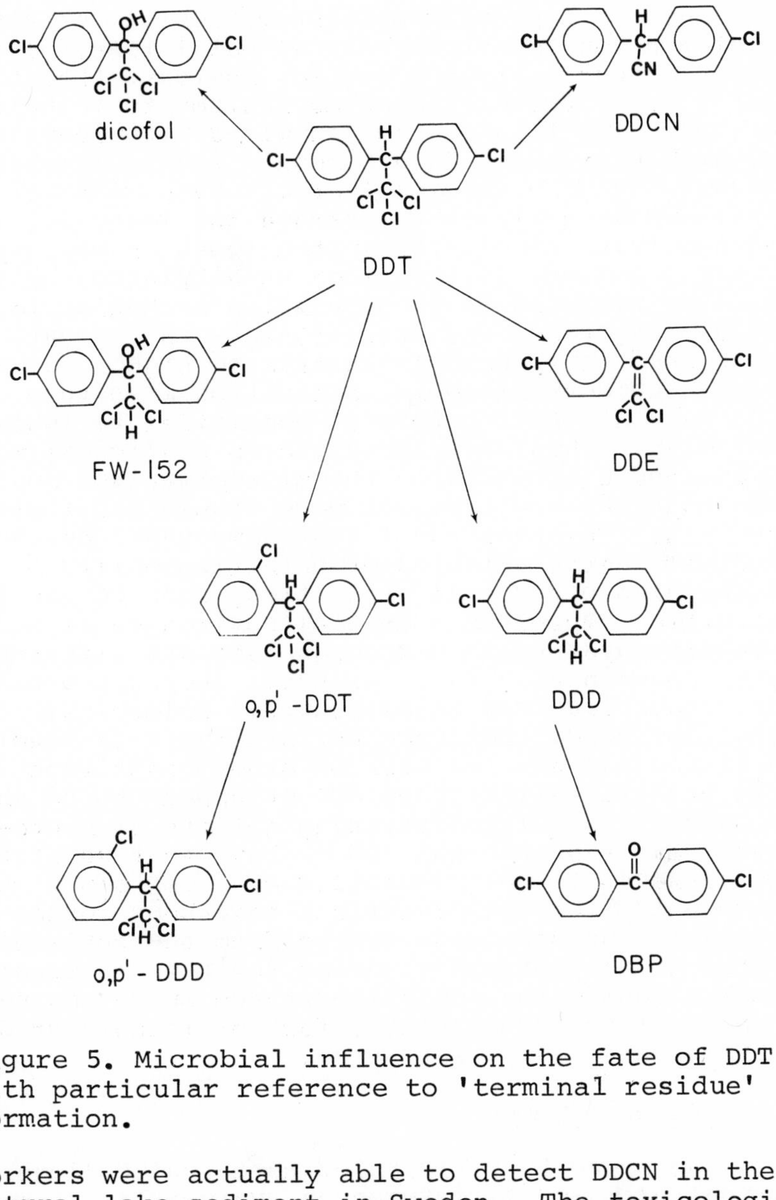

Figure 5. Microbial influence on the fate of DDT with particular reference to 'terminal residue' formation.

workers were actually able to detect DDCN in the natural lake sediment in Sweden. The toxicological significance of DDCN formation in the environment is not apparent. Jensen et al. (1972), point out that it is known as a biocide for soil pests.

149

Another type of important microbial activity is alkylation reaction on heavy metal ions, particularly mercury. Recent studies indicate that there are at least two different mechanisms to methylate mercury. The first scheme involves methylcobalamin (Vitamin B_{12}) which is a commonly found microbial product that can chemically react even with mercuric ions, (Wood et al., 1968; Yamada and Tonomura, 1971) and homocystein-mediated system found in Neurospora crassa (Landner, 1971). Such an alkylation system could be regarded as a conjugation mechanism for those microorganisms, but certainly they create unexpected environmental hazards to higher animals.

In summary microbial activities in nature certainly affect the fate of pesticidal residues in many ways. Physically they tie up pesticidal molecules, and biochemically the microorganisms modify them to either harmless or more stable and toxic residues. Whenever the latter compounds possess chemical characteristics of being lipophilic or having high biological affinities, such conversion activities represent potential environmental hazards. Metabolic systems in microorganisms are different from those in animals or plants. They can metabolize many otherwise near indestructable molecules. On the other hand, there are certain types of chemicals (e.g. lignin, and the bulk of other constituents of soil organic matter) they do not appear to be able to handle. Nevertheless, adaptability of microorganisms is phenomenal and we have just scratched the surface of their capabilities. Certainly many unexpected microbial reactions have been found; some favorable and some undesirable from the environmental standpoint. Because of their omnipresence, massive action and their importance in the maintenance of the total biota, further intense studies on this subject are warranted.

Acknowledgement

Supported by Division of Research, College of Agricultural and Life Sciences, University of Wisconsin, Madison and in part by research grants, R-801060 and EP-00812 from the Environmental Protection Agency, Washington, D.C.

References

Ahmed, M. K., J. E. Casida, and R. E. Nichols. 1958. J. Ag. Food Chem. 6: 740.

Ahmed, M. K., and J. E. Casida. 1958. J. Econ. Entomol. 51: 59.

Albone, E. S., G. Eglinton, N. C. Evans, and M. M. Rehead. 1972. Nature 240: 420.

Alexander, M. 1972. In "Environmental Toxicology of Pesticides," p. 365, (Matsumura, F., G. M. Boush, and T. Misato, Eds.), Academic Press, N.Y.

Batterton, J. C., G. M. Boush, and F. Matsumura. 1971. Bull. Environ. Contam. Toxicol. 6: 589.

Benezet, H. J., and F. Matsumura. 1973a. Nature 243: 480.

Benezet, H. J., and F. Matsumura. 1973b. Manuscript in preparation.

Bixby, M., G. M., Boush, and F. Matsumura. 1971. Bull. Environ. Contam. Toxicol. 6: 491.

Bollag, J. M. 1972. Critical Rev. Microbiol. 2 issue 1:35, Laskin, A. I., and H. Lechevalier. CRC Press, Cleveland.

Bollag, J. M., and S. Y. Liu. 1971. Soil. Biol. Biochem. 3: 337.

Boush, G. M., and F. Matsumura. 1967. J. Econ. Entomol. 60: 918.

Bro-Rasmussen, F., E. Noddegaard, and K. Voldum-Claussen. 1968. J. Sci. Food Ag. 19: 278.

Cook, J. W. 1957. J. Ag. Food Chem. 5: 859.

Coppedge, J. R., D. A. Lindquist, D. L. Bull, and H. W. Dorough. 1967. J. Ag. Food Chem. 15: 902.

Cserjesi, A. J., and E. L. Johnson, 1972. Cand. J. Microbiol. 18: 45.

Finley, R. B., and R. E. Pillmore. 1963. Am. Inst. Biol. Sci. Bull. 13: 41.

Focht, D. D., and M. Alexander. 1971. J. Ag. Food Chem. 19: 20.

French, A. L., and R. A. Hoppingarner. 1970. J. Econ. Entomol. 63: 756.

Getzin, L. W., and I. Rosefield. 1968. J. Ag. Food Chem. 16: 598.

Goto, M., M. Hattori, and T. Miyagawa. 1972. Chemosphere 1: 153.

Jensen, S., R. Goethe, and M. O. Kindstedt. 1972. Nature 240: 421.

Johnson, R. L., P. J. Gehring, and R. J. Kociba. 1973. Chlorinated dibenzodioxins and penta-chlorophenol. Environ. Health Perspectives. National Inst. Environ. Health, Research Triangle, N.C. (in press).

Kearney, P. C., D. D. Kaufman, and M. Alexander. 1967. In: "Soil Biochemistry", Vol. 1, (McLaren and G. H. Peterson, Eds.), p. 318, Marcel Dekker, N.Y.

Konrad, J. G., D. E. Armstrong, and G. Chesters. 1967. Agronomy J. 59: 591.

Korte, F. 1970. J. Assoc. Offic. Analyt. Chem. 35: 988.

Laanio, T. L., G. Dupuis, and H. O. Esser. 1972. J. Ag. Food Chem. 20: 1213.

Landner, L. 1971. Nature 230: 452.

Liu, S. Y., and J. M. Bollag. 1971a. J. Ag. Food Chem. 19: 487.

Liu, S. Y., and J. M. Bollag. 1971b. Pesticide Biochem. Physiol. 1: 366.

Matsumura, F., and G. M. Boush. 1966. Science 153: 1278.

Matsumura, F., and G. M. Boush. 1967. Science 156: 959.

Matsumura, F., and G. M. Boush. 1968. J. Econ. Entomol. 61: 610.

Matsumura, F., G. M. Boush, and A. Tai. 1968. Nature 219: 965.

Matsumura, F., K. C. Patil, and G. M. Boush. 1970. Science 170: 1206.

Matsumura, F., K. C. Patil, and G. M. Boush. 1971a. Nature 230: 325.

Matsumura, F., V. G. Khanvilkar, K. C. Patil, and G. M. Boush. 1971b. J. Ag. Food Chem. 19: 27.

Matsumura, F. 1972. In: "Environmental Toxicology of Pesticides", p. 525, (Matsumura, F., G. M. Boush, and T. Misato, Eds.), Academic Press N.Y.

Matsumura, F., and H. J. Benezet. 1973. Studies on the bioaccumulation and microbial degradation 2,3,7,8-tetrachlorobenzo-p-dioxin. Environ. Health Sci. Research Triangle, N.C. (in press).

Miller, R. A., L. A. Norris, and C. L. Hawkes. 1973. Acute and chronic toxicity of w,3,7,8-tetrachlorodibenzo-p-dioxin (dioxin) in aquatic organisms. Environ. Health Perspectives. National Inst. Environ. Health Sci. Research Triangle, N.C. (in press).

Miyamoto, J., K. Kitagawa, and Y. Sato. 1966. Jap. J. Expt. Med. 36: 211.

Miyazaki, S., G. M. Boush, and F. Matsumura. 1969. Appl. Microbiol. 18: 972.

Miyazaki, S., G. M. Boush, and F. Matsumura. 1970. J. Ag. Food Chem. 18: 87.

Nagasaki, H., S. Tomii, T. Mega, M. Murakami, and N. Ito. 1972. Gann (Cancer) 63: 393.

Oonnithan, E. S., and J. E. Casida. 1968. J. Ag. Food Chem. 16: 28.

Patil, K. C., F. Matsumura, and G. M. Boush. 1970. Appl. Microbiol. 19: 879.

Plimmer, J. R. 1973. Technical pentachloropenol: The origin and analysis of base-insoluble contaminants. Environ. Health Perspectives, National Inst. Environ. Health. Research Triangle, N.C. (in press).

Raghu, K., and I. C. MacRae. 1966. Science 154: 264.

Robinson, J., A. Richardson, B. Bush, and K. E. Elgar. 1966. Bull. Environ. Contam. Toxicol. 1: 127.

Rosen, J. D., D. J. Sutherland, and G. R. Lipton. 1966. Bull. Environ. Contam. Toxicol. 1: 133.

Skujins, J. J. 1966. "Soil Biochemistry", (ed. A. D. McLaren and G. H. Peterson), Marcel Dekker Inc., New York. p. 371-414.

Tanabe, H. 1972. In: "Environmental Toxicology of Pesticides" p. 239, Matsumura, F., G. M. Boush, and T. Misato, Eds. Academic Press.

Tatsukawa, R., T. Wakimoto, and T. Ogawa. 1972. In: "Environmental Toxicology of Pesticides" p. 229, (Matsumura, F., G. M. Boush, and T. Misato, Eds.) Academic Press, N.Y.

Tsukano, U., and A. Kobayashi. 1972. Ag. Biol. Chem. 36: 116.

Tweedy, B. G., C. Loeppky, and J. A. Ross. 1970. Science 168: 482.

Wang, C. M., and F. Matsumura. 1970. J. Econ. Entomol. 63: 1731.

Wang, C. M., T. Narahashi, and M. Yamada. 1971. Pesticide Biochem. Physiol. 1: 84.

Wedemyer, G. 1968. Appl. Microbiol. 16: 661.

Williams, I. H., M. J. Brown, and G. Finlayson. 1972. J. Ag. Food Chem. 20: 1219.

Wood, J. M., F. S. Kennedy, and C. G. Rosen. 1968. Nature 220: 173.

Yamada, M. and K. Tonomura. 1971. J. Ferment. Technol. 50: 159.

Zayed, S.M.A.D., I. Y. Mostafa, and A. Hassan. 1965. Archiv. Für Mikrobiologie (Berlin) 51: 118.

DETOXICATION OF ACARICIDES BY ANIMALS

Charles O. Knowles

Department of Entomology, University of Missouri
Columbia, Missouri 65201

Abstract

Acaricide chemicals undergo metabolic transformations in animals similar to those of other
xenobiotics. These transformations include
hydrolysis, oxidative desulfuration, aromatic
hydroxylation, aliphatic hydroxylation, thioether
oxidation, N- and O-dealkylation, reduction, glycoside and sulfate syntheses, and possibly others,
depending upon the molecular configuration of the
acaricide and the animal. Although hydrolysis or
oxidation often result in formation of metabolites
that are more toxic than the parent compound, most
acaricide biotransformations in animals yield products of markedly reduced toxicity. Thus, they are
detoxication mechanisms and could play an important
role in survival of animals exposed to acaricides.

Introduction

Acaricides are used to control mites that infest
plants and mites and ticks that are ectoparasites of
certain animals. Thus, non-target animals can be
exposed to acaricides either directly by treating
animals parasitized by acarines or indirectly in a
manner similar to that of other chemical pest control agents used for plant protection. There are
numerous factors that facilitate survival of animals
exposed to acaricides, and it seems probable that
detoxication is important.

Marked structural diversity exists among the
acaricides, and presently we possibly are using more
different classes of chemicals as acaricides than
as any other group of pest control agent (Knowles
1973; Knowles et al., 1972). The purpose of this

paper is to discuss the metabolism by animals of
some members of the different chemical classes of
acaricides and to emphasize, where available data
permit, those transformations that constitute detoxication. The term "detoxication" as used in
this paper denotes those reactions that result in
the formation of products less toxic than the
parent acaricide.

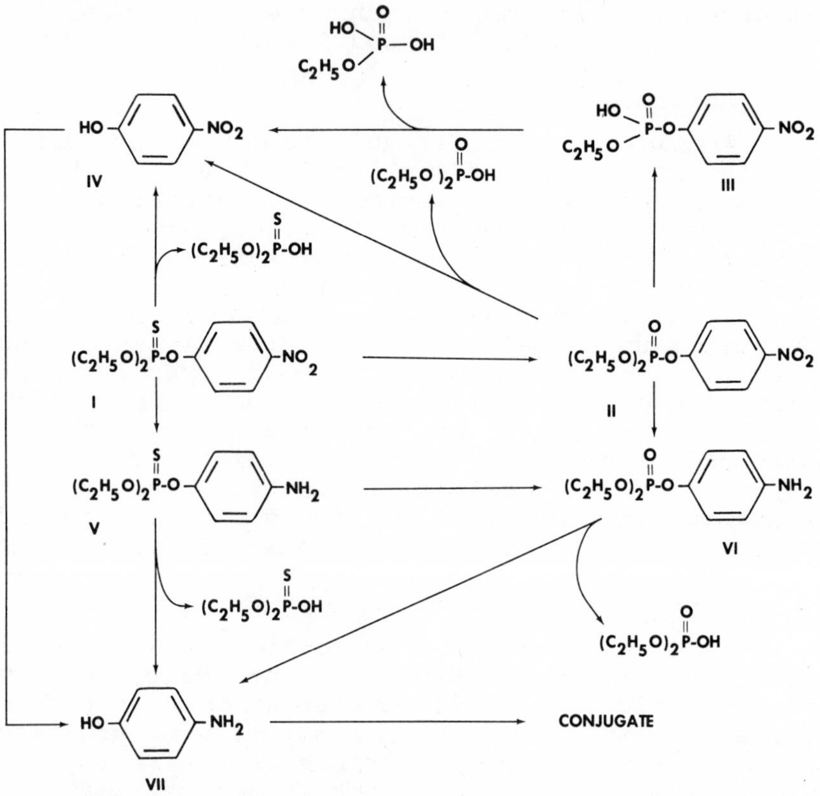

Figure 1. Metabolic paths for parathion.

ORGANOPHOSPHATES
Parathion

Many organophosphorus esters, although primarily insecticidal, possess significant acaricidal

activity. Parathion is a good example (Fig. 1).
Its metabolic fate in animals has been studied
extensively (Dahm, 1970; O'Brien, 1960) and is summarized below. Parathion (I) is converted to paraoxon (II) by oxidative desulfuration; this reaction
is not a detoxication, as paraoxon is the actual
toxicant (O'Brien, 1960). However, the other reactions given in Fig. 1 can be regarded as detoxication mechanisms. They include oxidative cleavage
of parathion (I) to p-nitrophenol (IV) and diethyl
phosphorothioic acid, cleavage of paraoxon (II)
to p-nitrophenol (IV) and diethyl phosphoric
acid, de-ethylation of paraoxon (II) to de-ethyl
paraoxon (III), and reduction of parathion (I)
and paraoxon (II) nitro groups to give aminoparathion (V) and aminoparaoxon (VI), respectively. Addtional reactions, such as conversion

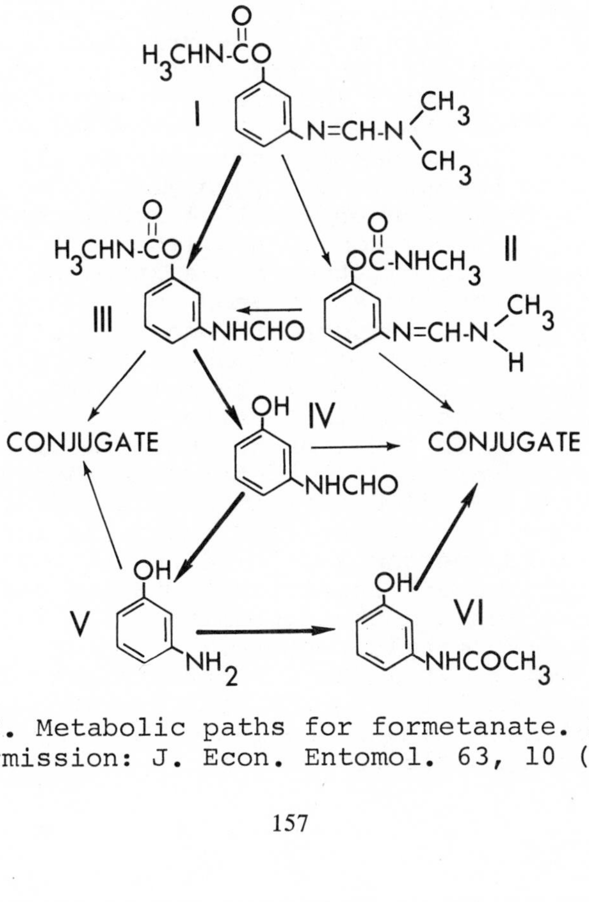

Figure 2. Metabolic paths for formetanate. Reprinted
with permission: J. Econ. Entomol. 63, 10 (1970).

of de-ethyl parathion (III) to p-nitrophenol (IV)
and monoethyl phosphoric acid, aminoparathion (V)
to p-aminophenol (VII) and diethyl phosphorothioic
acid, aminoparaoxon (VI) to p-aminophenol (VII) and
diethyl phosphoric acid, p-nitrophenol (IV) to
p-aminophenol (VII), and conjugation of p-aminophenol (VII) with glucuronic acid, also occur.

Thus, oxidation, hydrolysis, and conjugation
are involved in parathion detoxication by animals.

CARBAMATES
Formetanate

The metabolism of formetanate, an N-methylcarbamate insecticide and acaricide, has been
studied in vitro and in vivo in rats (Ahmad and
Knowles, 1970; Knowles, 1970; Sen Gupta and Knowles,
1970a) and in houseflies, Musca domestica L.
(Arurkar and Knowles, 1971). Rats metabolize
formetanate (I) directly to 3-formamidophenyl
methylcarbamate (III) or indirectly to Compound
III via an N-demethyl intermediate (II) (Fig. 2).
It is not known whether the N-dealkylation of
formetanate (I) to demethylformetanate (II) proceeds via an oxidative or hydrolytic mode (Knowles,
1970). 3-Formamidophenyl methylcarbamate (III) is
hydrolyzed to 3'-hydroxyformanilide (IV) which is
subsequently deformylated to m-aminophenol (V).
m-Aminophenol (V) is acetylated to yield 3-hydroxy-
acetanilide (VI). Glucuronic and sulfuric acid
conjugates of several of the above metabolites also
are present in rat urine. The metabolic path for
formetanate in house flies differs slightly from
that in rats. In addition to the formation of
demethylformetanate (II), 3-formamidophenyl methylcarbamate (III), 3'-hydroxyformanilide (IV), and
m-aminophenol (V), houseflies hydrolyze formetanate
at the N-methylcarbamyl-ester linkage to yield
3-dimethylaminomethyleneiminophenol and deformylate
3-formamidophenyl methylcarbamate (III) to yield
3-aminophenyl methylcarbamate.

The metabolites demethylformetanate, 3-form-
amidophenyl methylcarbamate, and 3-aminophenyl
methylcarbamate retain the intact carbamyl-ester
grouping and should be regarded as potential toxi-

cants. However, they are much weaker inhibitors of human plasma and housefly head cholinesterase than is formetanate (Knowles and Ahmad, 1971b; Sen Gupta and Knowles, 1970a); so their formation during metabolism probably can be regarded as detoxication. Formetanate detoxication reactions consist of hydrolysis, N-demethylation, acetylation, and glu-curonide and ethereal sulfate syntheses.

Aldicarb

The metabolism of aldicarb, a carbamoyl oxime insecticide and acaricide, has been reviewed by Fukuto (1970). When aldicarb (I) is administered to rats (Andrawes et al., 1967; Knaak et al., 1966), cows (Dorough and Ivie, 1968; Dorough et al., 1970) or insects (Bull et al., 1967; Metcalf et al., 1966) the following metabolites are detected: aldicarb sulfoxide (II), aldicarb sulfone (III), aldicarb oxime (IV), oxime sulfoxide (V), oxime sulfone (VI), nitrile sulfoxide (VII), and nitrile sulfone (VIII, mammals only) (Fig. 3).

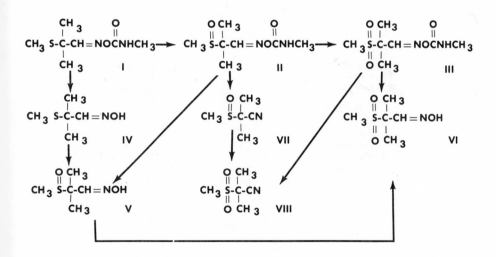

Figure 3. Metabolic paths for aldicarb.

159

Aldicarb sulfoxide (II) and aldicarb sulfone (III) formed by sequential thioether oxidation are toxic; the other metabolites generally are nontoxic. Therefore, hydrolysis is the major detoxication mechanism for aldicarb in animals.

CHLORINATED HYDROCARBONS
Endosulfan

Endosulfan is an insecticide with good acaricidal properties. Its metabolic fate has been investigated in rats and mice (Deema et al., 1966; Lindquist and Dahm, 1957; Schupahn et al., 1968), sheep (Gorbach et al., 1968), houseflies (Barnes and Ware, 1965), and a locust (Ballschmiter and Tölg, 1966). Generally endosulfan (I) is converted to endosulfan diol (II), endosulfan ether (III), and endosulfan hydroxyether (IV) (Fig. 4). By an alternate pathway endosulfan (I) is converted to endosulfan sulfate (V) and endosulfan lactone (VI) (Fig. 4). Unidentified compounds, probably conjugates, are present.

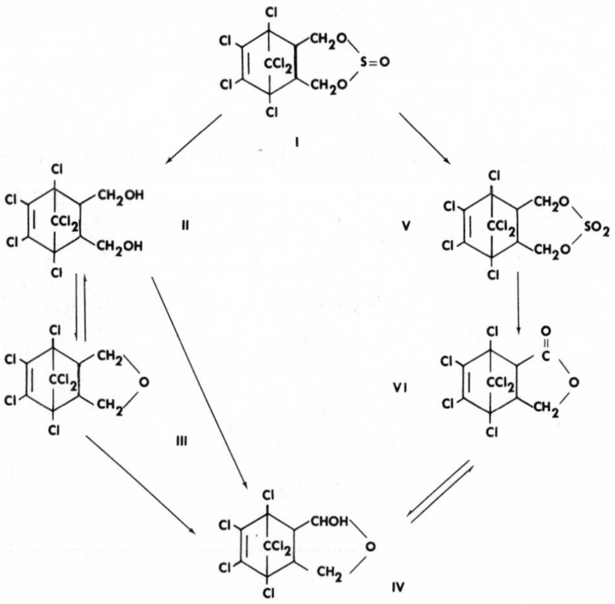

Figure 4. Metabolic paths for endosulfan.

160

Endosulfan sulfate (V), which is formed by oxidation of endosulfan (I), is toxic; so its formation does not constitute a detoxication. The other metabolites apparently are nontoxic.

DIPHENYL ALIPHATICS
Chlorobenzilate, Chloropropylate, Acarol and Dicofol

The metabolic fate of chlorobenzilate, chloropropylate, and Acarol in vitro by rat hepatic subcellular fractions has been elucidated by Knowles and Ahmad (1971a). Fig. 5 shows the degradation of chlorobenzilate or ethyl 4,4'-dichlorobenzilate by the microsomal fracton. After a 4-hr incubation period appreciable metabolism of chlorobenzilate (CB) has occurred. Metabolites are 4,4'-dichlorobenzilic acid (DBA), 4,4'-dichlorobenzhydrol (DBH), 4,4'-dichlorobenzophenone (DBP), and p-chlorobenzoic acid (CBA). Also, DBA (II) is a chlorobenzilate metabolite in the dog, sheep, and cow (Bartsch et al., 1971; St. John and Lisk, 1973). The path for chloropropylate or isopropyl 4,4'-dichlorobenzilate degradation by rat liver is similar to that of CB, except that cleavage of the isopropyl ester link proceeds more slowly than does cleavage of the ethyl ester bond (Knowles and Ahmad, 1971a). Acarol or isopropyl 4,4'-dibromobenzilate is even more resistant to degradation than is chloropropylate (Knowles and Ahmad, 1971a).

Al-Rubae and Knowles (1972) studied the metabolism of chloropropylate and Acarol by two-spotted spider mites, Tetranychus urticae (Koch), and houseflies. Chloropropylate (I) is converted sequentially to DBA (II), DBH (III), DBP (IV), and CBA (V) (Fig. 6). Acarol metabolism is slightly slower than that for chloropropylate. However, the metabolic path is identical to chloropropylate, except that metabolites contain bromine in position 4 of the benzene rings instead of chlorine.

Dicofol or 1,1-bis(4-chlorophenyl)-2,2,2-trichloroethanol, also known as Kelthane, is metabolized by rats to DBP, DBH, and 1,1-bis(4-chlorophenyl)-2, 2-dichloroethylene (DDE) (Brown et al., 1969).

161

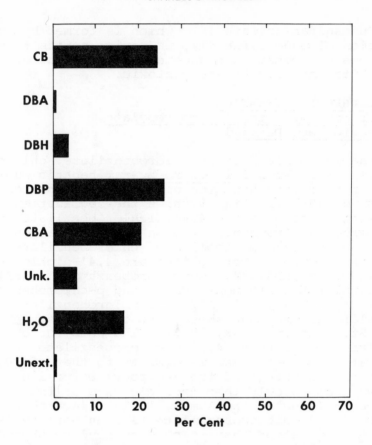

Figure 5. Metabolism of chlorobenzilate by rat liver,
microsomal fraction. Chlorobenzilate (CB) was incubated with enzyme preparation for 4 h, and analysis
of metabolism was conducted. DBA = 4,4'-dichloro-
benzilic acid; DBH = 4,4'-dichlorobenzhydrol; DBP =
4,4'-dichlorobenzophenone; CBA = p-chlorobenzoic
acid; unk. = unknown metabolite(s); H_2O = water
soluble compounds; and unext. = unextractable radioactive material.

     It is difficult to make conclusions relative to
detoxication mechanisms of diphenyl aliphatic acaricides. Although it is tempting to suggest that
toxicity is dependent upon the intact parent molecule
(Knowles, 1973), it should be mentioned that benzo-

162

phenone is toxic to certain mites (Eaton and Davies, 1950) and that chlorobenzilate, chloropropylate, Acarol, and dicofol each produce a halogenated benzophenone metabolite (Brown et al., 1969; Knowles and Ahmad, 1971a).

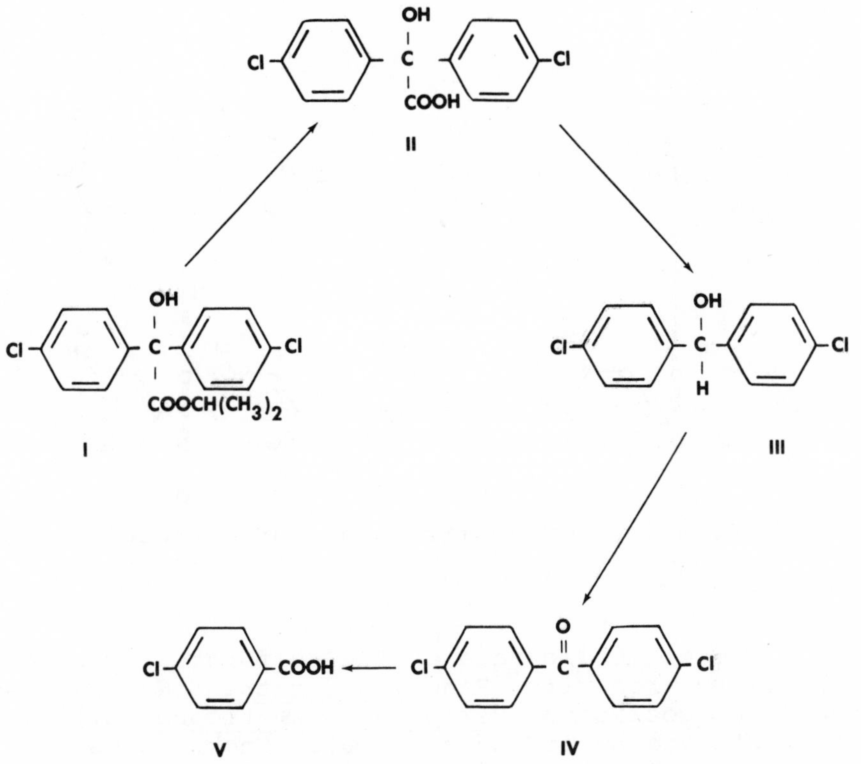

Figure 6. Metabolic paths for chloropropylate.

SULFIDES
Tetrasul

Verschuuren (1969) investigated the metabolism of the sulfide tetrasul in rats. The major pathways are oxidation of the sulfide (I) to the sulfoxide (II) and sulfone (III) and hydroxylation at the 3 position of the monochlorinated ring (IV) (Fig. 7).

Also, there is evidence for breakdown of the molecule on either side of the sulfur atom.

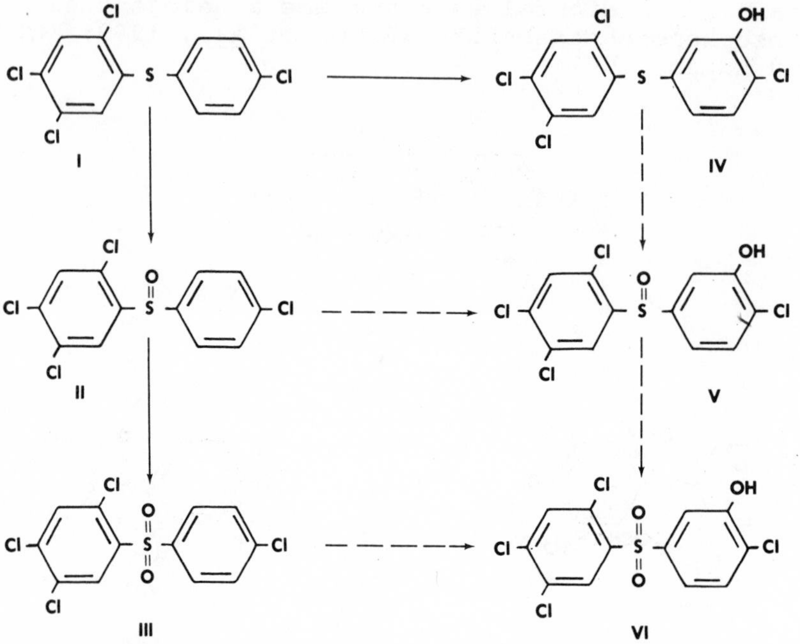

Figure 7. Metabolic paths for tetrasul.

SULFONATES

Ovex

The metabolic fate of the sulfonate, ovex, in the citrus red mite, Panonychus citri McGregor, and American cockroach, Periplaneta americana (L.), has been studied by Tomizawa (1960). Cockroaches convert ovex (I) to p-chlorobenzenesulfonic acid (II), but mites do not appreciably alter the acaricide (Fig. 8).

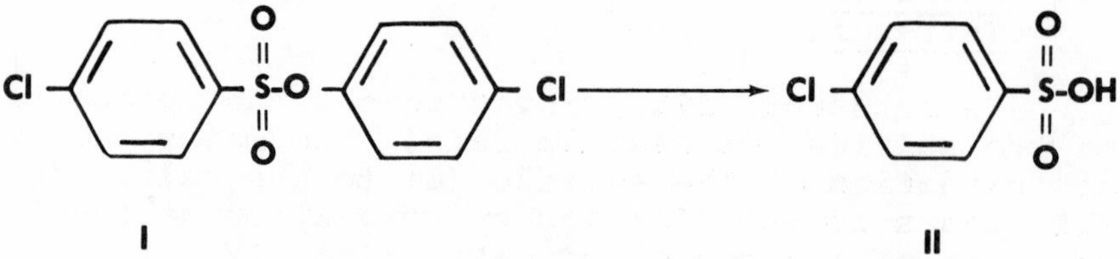

Figure 8. Metabolic path for ovex.

164

ORGANOFLUORINES
Fluenethyl

Fluenethyl, an organofluorine acaricide used
in Europe, contains two potential toxaphores, the
monofluoroethyl (Pianka and Polton, 1965) and
biphenyl moieties (Eaton and Davies, 1950). Johannsen and Knowles (1974a, b) studied fluenethyl action
and metabolism in the mouse, housefly, and two-
spotted spider mite. Fluenethyl (I) is hydrolyzed
in vivo and in vitro to biphenylacetic acid (BAA,
II) and monofluoroethanol (III) in all systems
examined (Fig. 9). In addition to the parent compound (I), BAA (II), biphenyl (IV), 2-hydroxybiphenyl
(V), 4-hydroxybiphenyl (VI), 4,4'-dihydroxybiphenyl
(VII), and 3,4-dihydroxybiphenyl (VIII) are present
in urine of fluenethyl-treated mice (Fig. 9). BAA
(II) and the hydroxylated biphenyls are found in
mouse urine in the free form and as conjugates with
glucuronic and sulfuric acids. Fluenethyl was labeled
with tritium in the aromatic portion of the molecule;
thus the fate of the fluorine-containing moiety (III)
could not be ascertained following initial cleavage
of the acaricide. However, the metabolism of monofluoroethanol (III) in vitro by rat liver slices has
been reported (Treble, 1962).

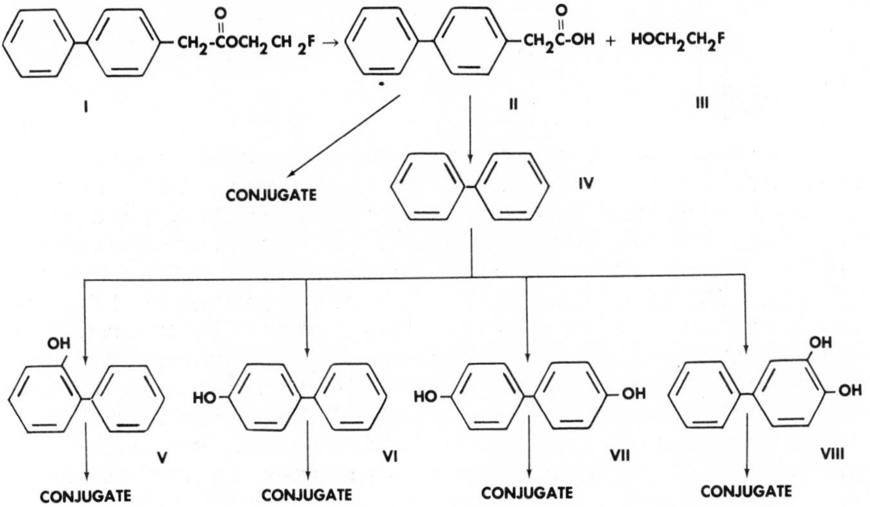

Figure 9. Metabolic paths for fluenethyl.

Metabolism of fluenethyl also is effected by houseflies and two-spotted spider mites. Although quantitative differences are apparent, qualitatively the metabolites are identical to the free compounds isolated from mouse urine, with the exception that the 2-hydroxybiphenyl (V) is not present in spider mites. Thus, aromatic hydroxylation and glucuronide and ethereal sulfate syntheses are important detoxication mechanisms for fluenethyl acaricide.

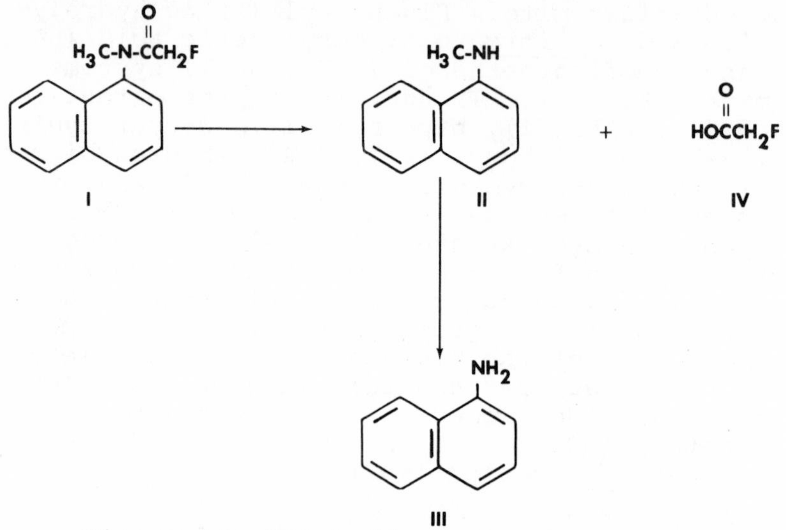

Figure 10. Metabolic paths for Nissol.

Nissol

Nissol or MNFA is an organofluorine acaricide used primarily in Japan. It hydrolyzes to N-methyl-1-naphthylamine (II) and monofluoroacetic acid (IV) in rats, guinae pigs, houseflies, and two-spotted spider mites (Knowles and Shrivastava, 1971; Noguchi et al., 1968) (Fig. 10). 1-Naphthylamine (III) and unidentified polar metabolites, possibly hydroxylated derivatives, also are present. The metabolic fate of monofluoroacetic acid (IV) in the rat was investigated by Gal et al. (1961). In addition to the parent compound (IV) fluorocitrate and several unidentified metabolites are present in rat urine.

Fenazaflor

Fenazaflor metabolism and excretion by mice, rats, and houseflies has been investigated by Bowker and Casida (1969). Fenazaflor (I) is readily hydrolyzed to 5,6-dichloro-2-trifluoromethylbenzimidazole (II) and subsequently hydroxylated at various positions in the benzene moiety (III, IV, V) (Fig. 11). The benzimidazole (II) is conjugated as an N-glucuronide in mice and rats and as an N-glucoside in houseflies. Conjugates of the hydroxylated benzimidazoles (III, IV, V) also are present in mouse and rat urine.

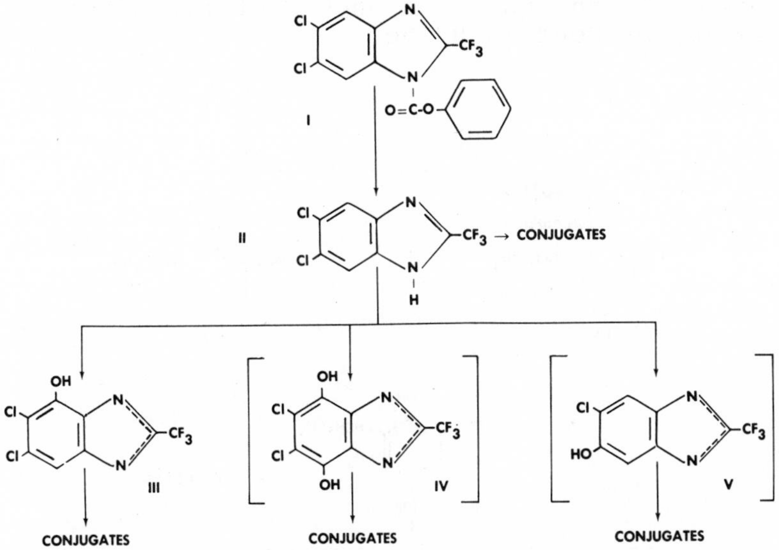

Figure 11. Metabolic paths for fenazaflor.

Since 5,6-dichloro-2-trifluoromethylbenzimidazole (II) uncouples oxidative phosphorylation in mammals (Ilivicky and Casida, 1969) and spider mites (Corbett and Wright, 1970), the initial hydrolysis of fenazaflor (I) to the benzimidazole (II) is not a detoxication mechanism. Detoxication of the benzimidazole (II) occurs primarily by aromatic hydroxylation and conjugation.

NITROPHENOL DERIVATIVES
Dinobuton

Bandal and Casida (1972) studied the metabolism of dinobuton, one of several nitrophenol derivatives active as acaricides, in mice and rats. The acaricide (I) is rapidly hydrolyzed to 2-sec-butyl-4,6-dinitrophenol (DNBP, III) either directly or via an intermediate (II) in both animal species (Fig. 12). Rats reduce DNBP (III) nitro groups to yield Compounds (IV and V; they also N-acetylate Compound V. Rats and mice oxidize either of the methyl groups in the sec-butyl side chain of DNBP (III) to yield Compounds VI and VII. Conjugates of Compounds III through VII and numerous uncharacterized metabolites also are present in urine.

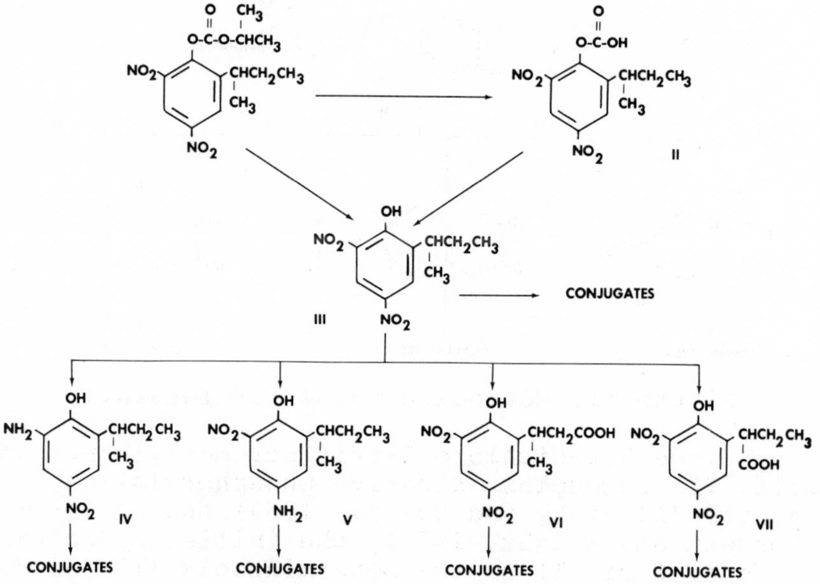

Figure 12. Metabolic paths for dinobuton.

Hydrolysis of dinobuton (I) to DNBP (III) is not a detoxication, since this latter compound is a potent uncoupler of oxidative phosphorylation in mammals (Ilivicky and Casida, 1969). Thus, dinobuton detoxication consists of reduction of nitro groups, oxidation of side chain methyl groups, acetylation, and conjugation.

QUINOXALINE DERIVATIVES
Oxythioquinox

Aziz and Knowles (1973b) reported that oxythio-quinox (I) is converted to 6-methyl-2,3-quinoxaline-dithiol (QDSH, II) by two-spotted spider mites (Fig. 13). Since QDSH (II) is toxic to mice, rats, and spider mites (Aziz and Knowles, 1973b; Carlson and DuBois, 1970), this reaction is not a detoxication.

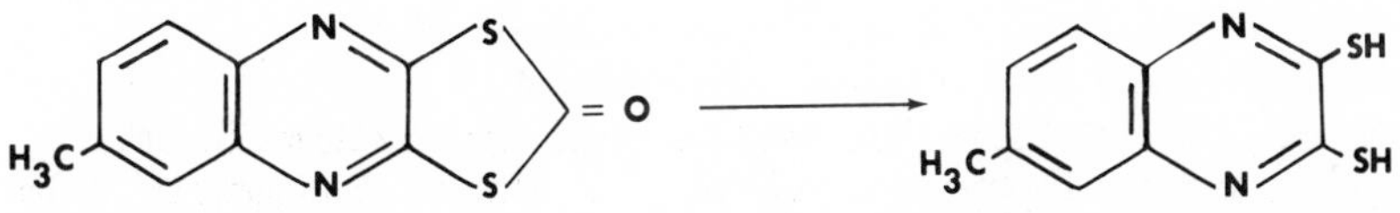

Figure 13. Metabolic path for oxythioquinox.

FORMAMIDINES
Chlordimeform

Chlordimeform metabolism has been investigated in the rat, dog, and goat (Ahmad and Knowles, 1971a; Knowles 1970; Knowles and Sen Gupta 1970; Sen Gupta and Knowles, 1970b), in the two-spotted spider mite (Knowles et al., 1972), in the cattle tick, Boophilus microplus (Canestrine) (Knowles and Schuntner, 1974; Schuntner, 1971), and in the housefly (Knowles and Shrivastava, 1973) (Fig. 14). Chlordimeform (I) undergoes oxidative N-demethylation to form demethyl-chlordimeform (II) in all animals studied; this reac-tion is not a detoxication, since demethylchlordime-

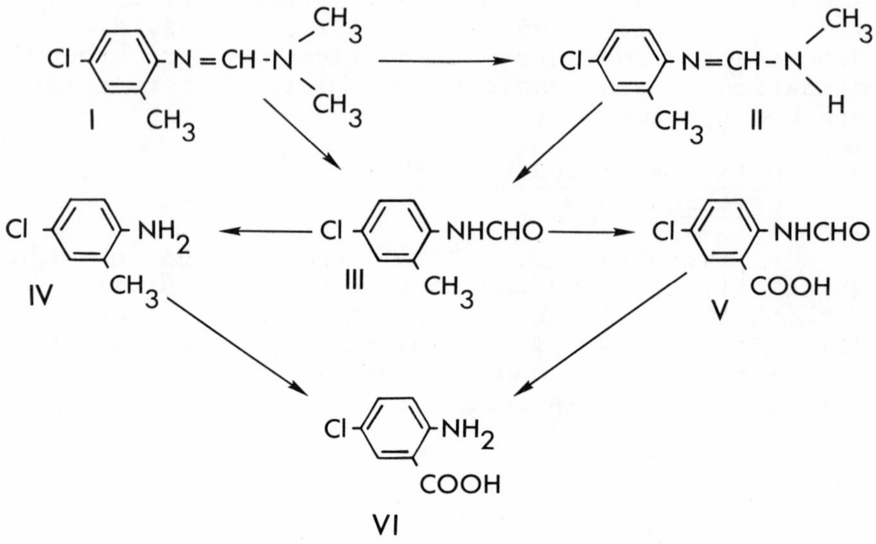

Figure 14. Metabolic paths for chlordimeform.
Reprinted with permission: J. Econ. Entomol. 63:
856 (1970).

form also is a potent acaricide (Aziz and Knowles,
1973a; Knowles and Roulston, 1972, 1973; Knowles
et al., 1972; Sen Gupta and Knowles, 1969). 4'-
Chloro-o-formotoluidide (III) is the next metabolite
in the sequential degradation of chlordimeform.
Although in most cases it is difficult to discern to
what extent the 4'-chloro-o-formotoluidide is derived
directly from chlordimeform (I) or from demethyl-
chlordimeform (II), there is evidence that most is
formed in the cattle tick via the demethyl derivative
(II) (Knowles and Schuntner, 1974). The 4'-chloro-
o-formotoluidide is subsequently deformylated to
4-chloro-o-toluidine (IV) or oxidized at the ring
methyl moiety to yield N-formyl-5-choloroanthranilic
acid (V). 5-Chloroanthranilic acid (VI) could form
by oxidation of .4-chloro-o-toluidine (IV) or by
deformylation of N-formyl-5-chloroanthranilic acid

(V). Rat liver formamidase (EC no. 3.5.1.9) will
catalyze deformylation of Compound III to IV and
Compound V to VI (Ahmad and Knowles, 1971b). The
anthranilic acid derivatives (V and VI) have been
identified in mammalian urine but not in houseflies,
ticks, and mites. 4'-Chloro-2'-methyl-acetanilide
also is present in rat urine. Conjugates of certain
of these chlordimeform metabolites are present in
most animals.

Therefore, chlordimeform detoxication proceeds
by hydrolysis, oxidation, acetylation, and conjugation.

PHENYLHYDRAZONES
Banamite

Banamite or benzoyl chloride (2,4,6-trichloro-
phenyl) hydrazone is a relatively new synthetic
organic acaricide (Kaugars et al., 1973), and its
metabolic fate in two-spotted spider mites has been
investigated by Knowles and Aziz (1972). The
initial transformation of Banamite (I) in mites
involves replacement of the benzoyl chlorine by
hydroxyl to yield an unstable enol derivative (II)
(Fig. 15). This enol compound (II) is subsequently
converted to benzaldehyde 2-(2,4,6-trichlorophenyl)
hydrazone (BATH, III) or to benzoic acid 2-(2,4,6-
trichlorophenyl) hydrazide (BOTH, VI). BATH (III)
is hydrolyzed to benzaldoxime (IV) and 2,4,6-tri-
chloroaniline (TCA, V); BOTH (VI) is hydrolyzed to
benzoic acid (VII) and 2,4,6-trichlorophenylhydra-
zine (TCH, VIII). Several unidentified materials
also are present; at least two are probably con-
densation products. Of the compounds isolated and
identified during metabolism studies, the parent
compound (I) and TCH (VIII) are toxic to two-
spotted spider mites. Thus, conversion of Banamite
(I) to benzaldoxime (IV) and TCA (V) via enol (II)
and BATH (III) intermediates constitutes a sequence
of detoxication reactions. Conversion of Banamite
(I) via the alternate pathway yields a toxic
metabolite (TCH, VIII) (Fig. 15).

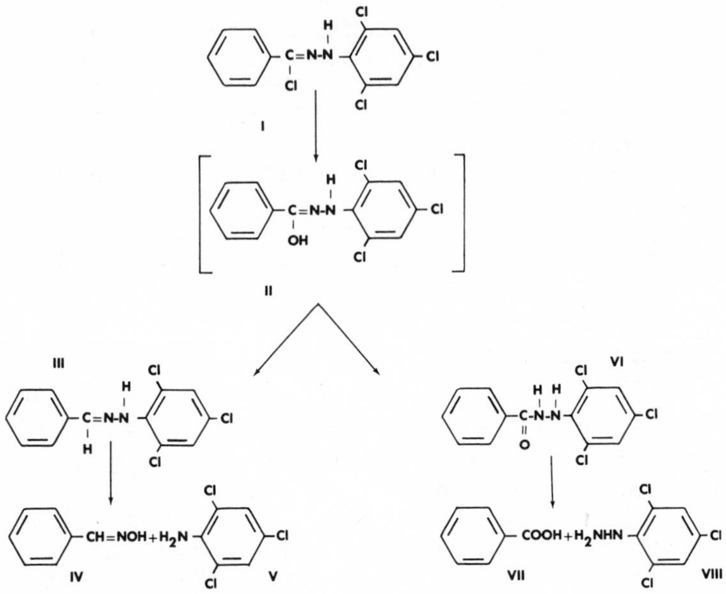

Figure 15. Metabolic paths for Banamite.

CONCLUSIONS

Acaricides are metabolized both by target and nontarget animals. Differences in acaricide metabolism among species are apparent but are usually quantitative rather than qualitative. Moreover, the metabolic paths for acaricides in animals are similar to those of other xenobiotics. In some cases metabolic attack on the acaricide molecule results in the formation of toxic products. However, the majority of acaricide biotransformations result in the formation of innocuous polar compounds. The transformations can be regarded as detoxication mechanisms and probably are important in the survival of animals exposed to acaricides. Table 1 lists examples of some of the detoxication mechanisms that have been ascribed to these chemicals. They include hydrolysis, aromatic hydroxylation, aliphatic hydroxylation, dealkylation, reduction, acetylation, and glycoside and ethereal sulfate syntheses. Because of the diversity that exists with regard to the molecular configuration of acaricides, it seems evident that other detoxication mechanisms may be present.

TABLE 1. Probable Detoxication Mechanisms by Animals for Acaricide Chemicals

| | | Reaction Reference[b] | |
Mechanism	Acaricide[a]	Figure	Conversion of Compound
Hydrolysis	Chlordimeform	14	I to III
	Chloropropylate	6	I to II
Aromatic hydroxylation	Fluenethyl	9	IV to V, VI, VII, VIII
	Fenazaflor	11	II to III
Aliphatic hydroxylation	Chlordimeform	14	III to V; IV to VI
	Dinobuton	12	III to VI & VII
Dealkylation	Formetanate	2	I to II
Reduction	Parathion	1	I to V; II to VI
	Dinobuton	12	III to IV & V
Acetylation	Formetanate	2	V to VI
Glycoside synthesis	Formetanate	2	VI to c
	Parathion	1	VII to c
	Fenazaflor	11	II to c II to d
Ethereal sulfate synthesis	Formetanate	2	VI to e
	Fluenethyl	9	V, VI, VII VIII to e

[a]Representative examples. [b]Refers to figures in text. c = glucuronide. d = glucoside. e = sulfate.

Acknowledgements

This paper is a contribution from the Missouri Agricultural Experiment Station, Columbia. Journal series number 6868.

References

Ahmad, S. and C. O. Knowles. 1970. J. Econ. Entomol. 63: 1690-1692.

Ahmad, S. and C. O. Knowles. 1971a. Comp. Gen. Pharmacol. 2: 189-197.

Ahmad, S. and C. O. Knowles. 1971b. J. Econ. Entomol. 64: 792-795.

Al-Rubae, A. Y. and C. O. Knowles. 1972. J. Econ. Entomol. 65: 1600-1603.

Andrawes, N. R., H. W. Dorough and D. A. Lindquist. 1967. J. Econ. Entomol. 60: 979-987.

Arurkar, S. K. and C. O. Knowles. 1971. Trans. Mo. Acad. Sci. 5: 43-47.

Aziz, S. A. and C. O. Knowles. 1973a. Nature (Lond.) 242: 417-418.

Aziz, S. A. and C. O. Knowles. 1973b. J. Econ. Entomol. 66: 1041-1045.

Ballschmiter, K. H. and G. Tolg. 1966. Angew. Chem. 78: 775-776.

Bandal, S. K. and J. E. Casida. 1972. J. Agr. Food Chem. 20: 1235-1245.

Barnes, W. W. and G. W. Ware. 1965. J. Econ. Entomol. 58: 286-291.

Bartsch, E., D. Eberle, K. Ramsteiner, A. Tomann and M. Spindler. 1971. Residue Revs. 39: 1-93.

Bowker, D. M. and J. E. Casida. 1969. J. Agr. Food Chem. 17: 956-966.

Brown, J. R., H. Hughes and S. Viriyanondh. 1969. Toxicol. Appl. Pharmacol. 15: 30-37.

Bull, D. L., D. A. Lindquist and J. R. Coppedge. 1967. J. Agr. Food Chem. 15: 610-616.

Carlson, G. P. and K. P. DuBois. 1970. J. Pharmacol. Exptl. Therap. 173: 60-70.

Corbett, J. R. and B. J. Wright. 1970. Pestic. Sci. 1: 120-123.

Dahm, P. A. in "Biochemical Toxicology of Insecticides" (R. D. O'Brien and I. Yamamoto, eds.). Academic Press, New York, 1970. p. 51.

Deema, P., E. Thompson and G. W. Ware. 1966. J. Econ. Entomol. 59: 546-550.

Dorough, H. W. and G. W. Ivie. 1968. J. Agr. Food Chem. 16: 460-464.

Dorough, H. W., R. B. Davis and G. W. Ivie. 1970. J. Agr. Food Chem. 18: 135-142.

Eaton, J. K. and R. G. Davies. 1950. Ann. Appl. Biol. 37: 471-489.

Fukuto, T. R. 1970. Drug Metab. Revs. 1: 117-151.

Gal, E. M., P. A. Drewes and N. F. Taylor. 1961. Arch. Biochem. Biophys. 93: 1-14.

Gorbach, S. G., D. E. Christ, H. M. Kellner, G. Kloss and E. Borner. 1968. J. Agr. Food Chem. 16: 950-953.

Ilivicky, J. and J. E. Casida. 1969. Biochem. Pharmacol. 18: 1389-1401.

Johannsen, F. R. and C. O. Knowles. 1974a. J. Econ. Entomol., in press.

Johannsen, F. R. and C. O. Knowles. 1974b. Comp. Gen. Pharmacol., in press.

Kaugars, G., E. C. Gemrich and V. L. Rizzo. 1973. J. Agr. Food Chem. 21: 647-650.

Knaak, J. R., M. Tallant and L. J. Sullivan. 1966. J. Agr. Food Chem. 14: 573-578.

Knowles, C. O. 1970. J. Agr. Food Chem. 18: 1038-1047.

Knowles, C. O. "Abstracts of Papers,: 166th Meeting, ACS, August 1973.

Knowles, C. O. and S. Ahmad. 1971a. Can. J. Physiol. Pharmacol. 49: 590-597.

Knowles, C. O. and S. Ahmad. 1971b. Pest. Biochem. Physiol. 1: 445-452.

Knowles, C. O. and S. A. Aziz. 1972. Unpublished data.

Knowles, C. O. and W. J. Roulston. 1972. J. Aust. Entomol. Soc. 11: 349-350.

Knowles, C. O. and W. J. Roulston. 1973. J. Econ. Entomol. 66: 1245-1252.

Knowles, C. O. and C. A. Schuntner. 1974. J. Aust. Entomol. Soc., in press.

Knowles, C. O. and A. K. Sen Gupta. 1970. J. Econ. Entomol. 63: 856-859.

Knowles, C. O. and S. P. Shrivastava. 1971. Unpublished data.

Knowles, C. O. and S. P. Shrivastava. 1973. J. Econ. Entomol. 66: 75-79.

175

Knowles, C. O., S. Ahmad and S. P. Shrivastava in "Pesticide Chemistry", Gordon and Breach, London, 1972. p. 77.

Lindquist, D. A. and P. A. Dahm. 1957. J. Econ. Entomol. 50: 483-486.

Metcalf, R. L., T. R. Fukuto, C. Collins, K. Borck, J. Burk, H. T. Reynolds and M. F. Osman. 1966. J. Agr. Food Chem. 14: 579-584.

Noguchi, T., H. Miyata, T. Mori, Y. Hashimoto and S. Kosaka. 1968. Pharmacometrics. 2: 376-382.

O'Brien, R. D. "Toxic Phosphorus Esters", Academic Press, New York and London, 1960. p. 175.

Pianka, N. and D. Polton. 1965. J. Sci. Food Agr. 16: 330-341.

Schuntner, C. A. 1971. Aust. J. Biol. Sci. 24: 1301-1308.

Schupahn, I., K. Ballschmiter and G. Tolg. 1968. Z. Naturforsch., B. 23: 701-706.

Sen Gupta, A. K. and C. O. Knowles. 1969. J. Agr. Food Chem. 17: 595-600.

Sen Gupta, A. K. and C. O. Knowles. 1970a. J. Econ. Entomol. 63: 10-14.

Sen Gupta, A. K. and C. O. Knowles. 1970b. J. Econ. Entomol. 63: 951-956.

St. John, L. E., Jr. and D. J. Lisk. 1973. J. Agr. Food Chem. 21: 655-646.

Tomizawa, C. 1960. Botya-Kagaka. 25: 47-51.

Treble, D. H. 1962. Biochem. J. 82: 129-134.

Verschuuren, H. G. 1969. Arch. Int. Pharmacodyn 182: 438.

DETOXICATION OF FOREIGN CHEMICALS BY INVERTEBRATES

M. A. Q. Khan, R. H. Stanton and G. Reddy
Department of Biological Sciences
University of Illinois at Chicago Circle
Chicago

Detoxication systems have been well studied in vertebrates in connection with drug biotrans-formation (Williams, 1959; Brodie and Maickel, 1962) and in insects in connection with insecticide metabolism (see Smith, 1968). Most of these xenobiotics are non-polar and lipophilic in nature and are converted to ionized (polar) or water-soluble compounds which can then be excreted as they are or after their conjugation. This article will review the present status of knowledge of main detoxication and conjugation systems of insects and other invertebrates.

DETOXICATION SYSTEMS

The primary metabolism of a foreign chemical takes place in the cytoplasm of the cell. The detoxification systems can be located in the cytoplasmic fluid (soluble enzymes) or may be bound to the endoplasmic reticulum (microsomal enzymes). The soluble enzymes include: DDT-dehydrochlorinase, esterases and reductases. The microsomal enzymes may include some of the esterases and connugation systems, but they mainly consist of the multi-function oxidases. Both enzyme systems are capable of catalyzing various types of conjugations of a xenobiotic with endogenous molecules).

I. Esterases: These soluble enzymes attack ester bonds of various insecticides. The bonds attacked are 1) in the case of organophosphates

(OP): phosphoryl, carboxyester, carboxyamide; 2) in
the case of methylcarbamates: carbamic ester; 3) in
pyrethroids: pyrethrate carbomethoxy group,
chrysenthemate cyclopropanecarboxylic ester, etc.
These esterases (especially OP-hydrolases) have
been reported to be present in houseflies, mites,
ticks and mosquitoes (O'Brien, 1967). Such
enzymes can be quite specific towards optical and
geometric isomers of OPs and the isomers of primary
alcohols with chrysenthemates (Casida, 1969). Some
of these can be non-specific--for example, those
attacking the methylcarbamate, carbaryl (Wilkinson,
1968).

(i) <u>Phosphatases</u>. Esterases atacking
phosphorous ester or anhydride bonds have been
widely studied in connection with OPs. These
phosphatases can be: a) Less common ones which
catalyze dealkylations, e.g.

$$\begin{matrix} CH_3O \\ CH_3O \end{matrix} \diagup P(S)O-X \longrightarrow$$

$$\begin{matrix} CH_3O \\ HO \end{matrix} \diagup P(S)O-X.$$

Some other examples of this kind
of esteric cleavage are Ronel, methyparathion and
sumithion. Although located mostly in the soluble
subcell fraction of rat liver, in insects the
activity may be equally distributed in mitochondrial, microsomal and soluble subcell fractions,
as seen in the rice stem borer (Shishido and Fukami,
1963). <u>In vitro</u> activity has been demonstrated for
DFP, TEPP and dichlorovos by insect enzymes sensitive to SH-inhibitors (Kreuger and Casida, 1961).
They are commonly present to some extent in all
organisms but they play only a minor role in
detoxication (O'Brien, 1967). b) Commonest phosphatases which split off the leaving group (X) and
form corresponding dialkyl phosphates along with
various thioanalogs from phosphorothionates,
phosphorothiolates and phosphorodithioates. The
two sites of attack of these phosphatases are as
follows:

$$-P-S-C$$
$$\downarrow$$
$$-P:OH + HSC \longrightarrow -PSH + HO-C$$

Due to highly active phosphatases, most OPs have a half-life of but a few hours in insects.

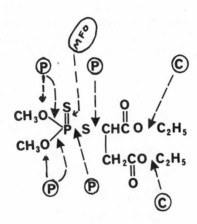

Figure 1. Sites of attacks of phosphatase (P), carboxylesterase (C) enzymes on Malathion (O'Brien, 1967).

(ii) <u>Carboxyesterases.</u> The carboxyl ester bonds of OPs are hydrolyzed by carboxylesterases. Malathion is converted to mono- and di-acids along with dimethylphosphorothioate which results from phosphatase attack (Fig. 1). There are both qualitative and quantitative differences among insects. White peach scale enzyme is very active while that of lady beetles is inactive. Also different isozymes may be involved in the same insect since malathion, malaoxon, acethion and acetoxon appear to be metabolized by different enzymes (O'Brien, 1967). Among insects, the malation-resistant mosquito larvae (<u>Culex</u> and <u>Aedes</u>) have been shown to degrade malathion mainly by carboxyesterases (Matsumura and Brown, 1963).

(iii) <u>Amidases.</u> Another group of esterases attacks acid-amide bonds (CONR$_2$ group) as in

179

dimethoate: $(CH_3O)_2 \cdot P(S)CHC(O)NHCH_3 \longrightarrow$ $(CH_3O)_2P(S)SCHCOOH$ (Fig. 2). Furthermore, an OP compound can be attacked by other esterase enzymes resulting in more than one product in addition to the degradation by a particular esterase.

(iv) Esterases also attack other insecticides. Methylcarbamate insecticide, carbaryl, is decarbamylated by esterases which have not yet been characterized <u>in vitro</u> in invertebrates. The esteratic hydrolysis of pyrethroids is shown in (Fig. 3).

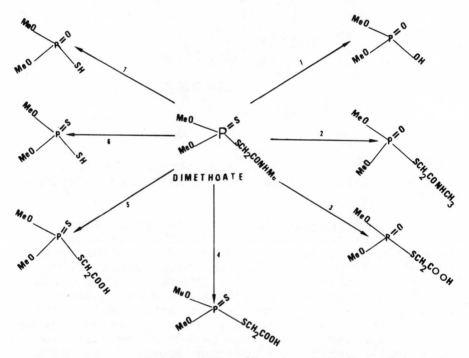

Figure 2. Pathways of metabolism of dimethoate (Bull and Adkinson, 1963; Ichida et al., 1964, 1965) showing O-desulfuration (1,2,3,7) with attacks on various sites of the leaving groups ($-SCH_2CONHCH_3$) which involve bonds P-S (1); PS-C (6,7); PSCH$_2$CON-C (2); PSCH$_2$CO-N (3,4,5).

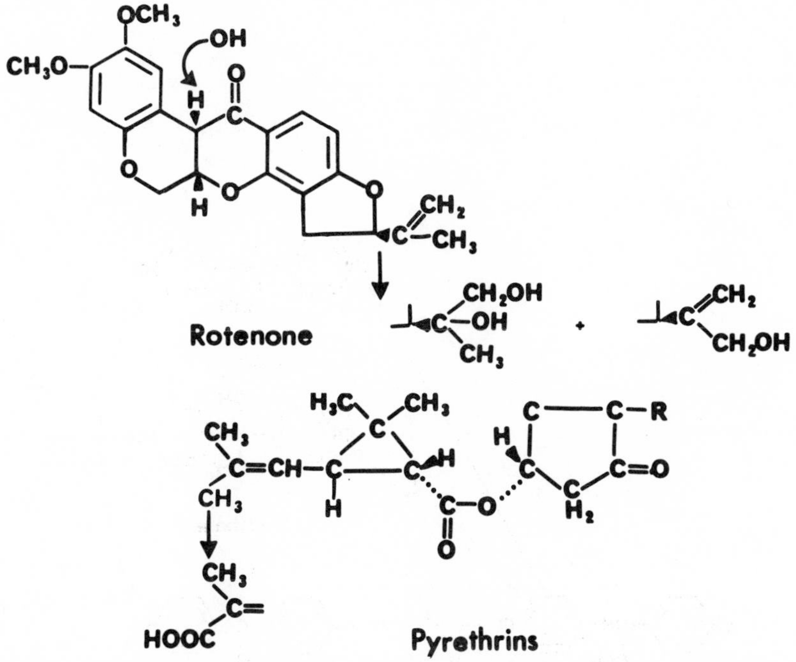

Figure 3. Metabolism of rotenone and pyrethrins in insects (See Casida, 1969)

Reports on the distribution of esterases in aquatic invertebrates include mosquitoes (Trebatosky and Haynes, 1969; Mills and Lang, 1972) and lobster (Homarus americanus) (Mellet et al., 1969; Barlow and Ridgeway, 1971).

II. DDT-Dehydrochlorinase: This soluble enzyme is one of the most important mechanisms by which insects detoxify the insecticide DDT to DDE (Fig. 4). In the presence of reduced glutathione and nitrogen it attacks only p,p'-DDT and its analog, p,p'-DDD. In houseflies it is four times more active towards tribromo analog (CBr$_3$) and fifteen times more active towards dibromo (CHBr$_2$) and monochlorobromo (CHClBr) analogs, while it is least active against DDD (Lipke and Kearns, 1959; Berger and Young, 1962). α and γ-BHC and penta-chlorocyclohexane are reported to be attacked by this or a similar enzyme at high GSH concentrations (Ishida and Dahm, 1965). The enzyme has been

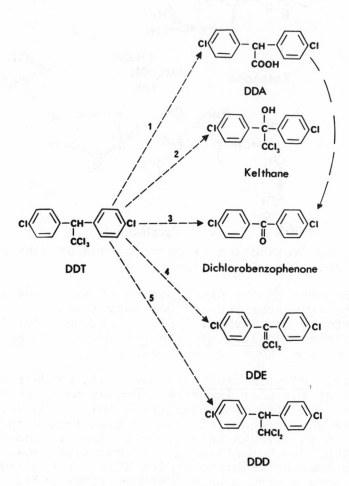

Figure 4. Pathways of metabolism of DDT in body lice (1), <u>Drosophila</u> (2,3); <u>Musca</u> (4) and micro-organisms (5) (O'Brien, 1967)

reported from various insects, e.g. houseflies (Lipke and Kearns, 1959); pink bollworm (Bull and Adkinson, 1963), Aedes (Abedi et al., 1963) Culex mosquitoes (Kimura et al., 1965) and the Mexican bean beetle (Chattoraj and Kearns, 1958). It has also been characterized in vitro in the leach, Hirudinia sp. (Kimura and Keegan, 1967) and appears to be present in Daphnia (Neudorf and Khan, unpublished data). In vivo data on the residues of DDT and its metabolite, DDE, in invertebrates indicate that DDT-Dehydrochlorinase may be present in food chain organisms. DDT and Methoxychlor can both be dehydrochlorinated (in vivo) by the salt marsh caterpillar, Estigmene acrea (Kapoor et al., 1970). Johnson et al. (1971) recovered DDE along with DDT after a three-day exposure of aquatic invertebrates to ^{14}C-labelled DDT. Amounts of DDE recovered (% of total radioactivity) were: about 20 in Chironomus sp. larvae (Diptera), Palaemonetes kadiakenis (Decapoda), Gammarus fasciatus (Amphipoda) and Daphnia magna (Cladocera); 28 in niads of Libellula sp. (Odonata); and 85 in nymphs of Hexagenia bilineata (Ephemeroptera). In cases of low DDE recovery, other products such as DDD, DTMC and DBP were formed. Residues of DDE and DDT in earthworms (see Pimental and Goodman, 1974) may indicate the presence of in vivo dehydrochlorination mechanisms in this invertebrate.

III. Glutathione S-Transferases: These enzymes cleave organic thiocyanates and OPs with O-methyl, O-aryl and O-pyrimidinyl groups. The latter form, as in the case of O-methyl OP, a demethylated product and S-methyl-GSH. These substrate specific enzymes are common among vertebrates. Among invertebrates, glutathione S-aryltransferases are of common occurrence (Cohen et al., 1964).

In the housefly, soluble fractions fortified with glutathione degrade parathion (Oppenoorth et al., 1972), and diazinon (Lewis, 1969). The enzyme catalyzes the reaction between glutathione and such halogen compounds as benzylbromide or dichloronitrobenzene. Insect enzyme has low affinity for bromosulphalein and aappears to have two groups

183

in its active site (Cohen et al., 1964). In insects, the metabolism of BHC to dichlorophenylglutathione may result from the interaction between penta-chlorocyclohexene with GSH (Clark et al., 1966).

IV. <u>Microsomal Enzymes</u>: Commonly called "mixed-function oxidases" (MFO), these membrane bound enzymes catalyze a variety of chemical reactions. Some of these are shown in Table I.

Table 1. Some of the substrates and their reactions which are catalyzed by MFO of invertebrates, <u>in</u> <u>vivo</u> and <u>in</u> <u>vitro</u>. The housefly MFO can perform almost all of these reactions.

Reaction	Substrates
Epoxidation	aldrin, photoaldrin, isodrin, etc. (Khan et al., 1970,1972a)
Epoxide hydration	cyclodienes (Brooks and Harrison, 1969)
Sulfoxidation	Mesurol, Temik, Phorate (Casida, 1969)
Cyclic ether cleavage	Benzodioxoles: piperonyl butoxide, sesamex (Casida, 1969)
Oxidative hydrolysis	OPs: EPN, Paraoxon, Diazinon (Dahm, 1970; Yang et al., 1972; Casida, 1969; Carlson, 1972)
N-dealkylations	hempa (Akov and Borkovec, 1968); N-methyl- and N,N-di-methylcarbamates (Casida, 1969); p-chloro-N-methylani-line and dimethylaminopyrene (see Wilkinson and Brattsten, 1972)
O-dealkylations	Methoxychlor (Khan et al., 1970); Baygon (Casida, 1969)
O-desulfurations	phosphorothionates: Guthion, Parathion, Schradan (Casida, 1969; Wilkinson and Brattsten, 1972)

TABLE 1 (CONTD)

Hydroxylations	Naphthalene (Schonbrod et al., 1968); aniline, Biphenyl, Baygon (Hook et al., 1968; Wilkinson and Brattsten, 1972); Dihydrocyclodienes (Brooks and Harrison, 1969); DDT. alkyl-benzenes, pyrethroids (Casida, 1969; Wilkinson and Brattsten, 1972)
Reductions	parathion (Lichtenstein and Fuhremann, 1972; nitrobenzene (Wilkinson and Brattsten, 1972)

As early as 1961, the involvement of these enzymes in the detoxication of xenobiotics was demonstrated in invertebrates (Agosin et al., 1961; Brodie and Maickel, 1962). Since then almost all investigations of this system in invertebrates have been confined to terrestrial insects. Excellent reviews on insect MFO have recently been published by Casida (1969), Hodgson and Plapp (1970) and Wilkinson and Brattsten (1972). Insects studied for the MFO characterization belong to a few orders which are of economic and health importance such as; diptera (houseflies, mosquitoes, blowflies), orthoptera (locusts, cockroaches) and lepidoptera (caterpillars). Most of the synthetic organic insecticides are metabolized by the MFO of insects (Casida, 1969). The reactions catalyzed (Table 1) can be generalized as follows:

1) Aliphatic oxidations. Methyl groups of toluene and p-nitrotoluene are oxidized in intact insects (Chakrabarty and Smith, 1964; Reddy and Krishnakumaran, 1974). Farnesol is oxidized to farnesic acid in Tenebrio larvae (Emmerich et al., 1965). During the hydroxylation of methyl groups of O-cresyl phosphates cyclization can take place whereby cyclic saligenin phosphate is formed (Fig. 5) (Eto et al., 1963).

185

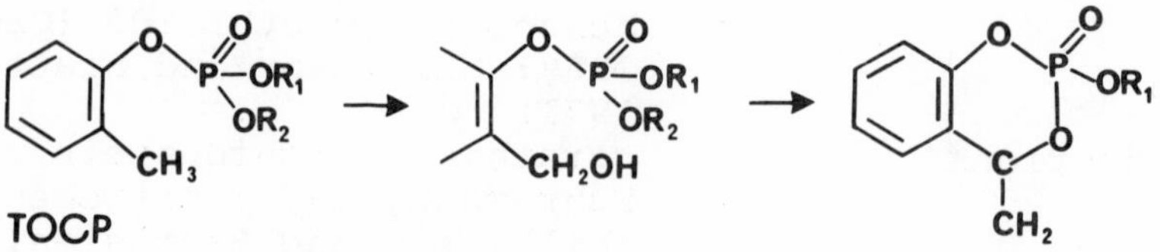

Figure 5. Metabolism of a tri-o-cresylphosphate leading to the formation of cyclic saligenin phosphate (Eto et al., 1964).

Higher alkylbenzenes are also hydroxylated in flies, locusts and caterpillars (Chakrabarty and Smith, 1967). These hydroxylations occur only at the terminal carbon atom (the penultimate and the α-methylenic position) adjacent to the aromatic ring. The oxidation of DDT to kelthane (Fig. 4) is an example of an α-methylenic oxidation (Tsukamoto, 1961).

2) <u>Aryl hydroxylations</u>. Chlorobenze, carbaryl and naphthelene are hydroxylated by locusts and flies (Smith, 1964a; Dorough and Casida, 1964). Oxidation of nicotine to cotinine occurs in several insects including tobacco wireworms, cigarette beetles, houseflies and grasshoppers (Self et al., 1964).

3) <u>N-demethylations</u>. Hydroxylation of N-methyl groups may involve the formation of an N-oxide or N-methylol. In the demethylation of methylamides and N-methylcarbamates the stable N-methylol is formed. Examples are the demethylation of carbaryl and dimetilan (Dorough and Casida, 1964; Zubairi and Casida, 1965). The OP, bidrin, and its

demethyl derivative azodrin are demethylated in
flies, cockroaches, bollworms, boll weevils and
tobacco budworms (Fig. 6). Some insects can
metabolize alkylamines by demethylamination to
methylamine and a hydroxy compound seen in the
case of Zectran (Fig. 7) (Williams et al., 1964).

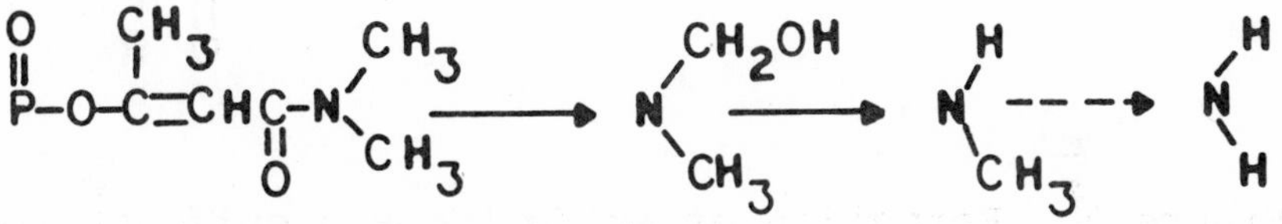

Figure 6. In vivo N-demethylation of a phosphora-
midate (Bidrin) by insects (Hall and Sun,
1965; Menzer and Casida, 1965)

187

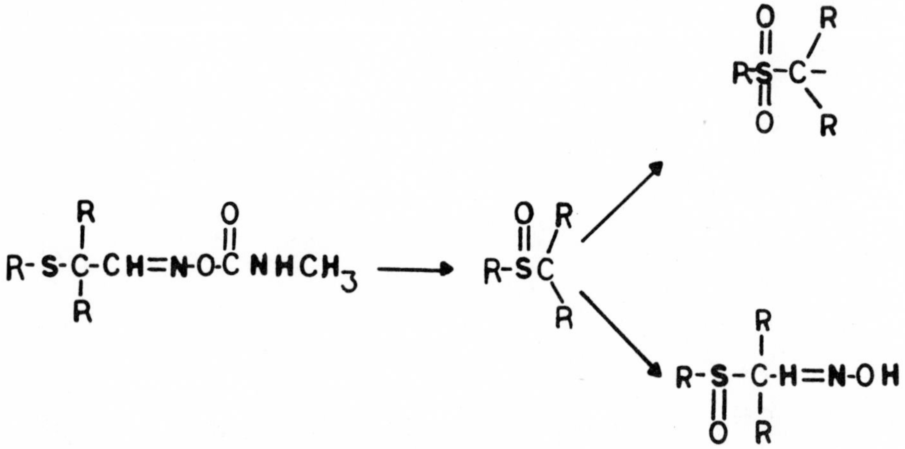

Figure 7. Formation of sulfoxide and sulfone from
"Temik" by insects (Metcalf et al., 1966)

4) <u>Epoxide hydration</u>. Dieldrin has been reported to be converted to mono- and dihydroxy analogs
in the mosquitoes <u>Culex</u> (Oonithan and Miskus, 1964)
and <u>Aedes</u> and also in houseflies (Korte et al.,
1962; Gerolt, 1965). <u>In vitro</u> hydration has been
demonstrated by housefly MFO (Brooks and Harrison,
1969).

5) <u>Oxidation of sulfur compounds</u>. These rapid
reactions involving oxidative desulfuration of
thionophosphates and oxidation of thioethers to

188

sulfoxides and sulfones have been reported in insects (O'Brien, 1962) and mites (Matsumura and Voss, 1964). Disyston or Temik are metabolized to sulfoxide and sulfone in boll weevils and bollworms (Fig. 7) (Bull, 1965; Metcalf et al., 1958).

6) <u>Oxidation of pyrethroids and rotenone.</u> These insecticides are oxidatively detoxified by insect MFO. The sites attacked by MFO are shown in Fig. 8 (Casida, 1969).

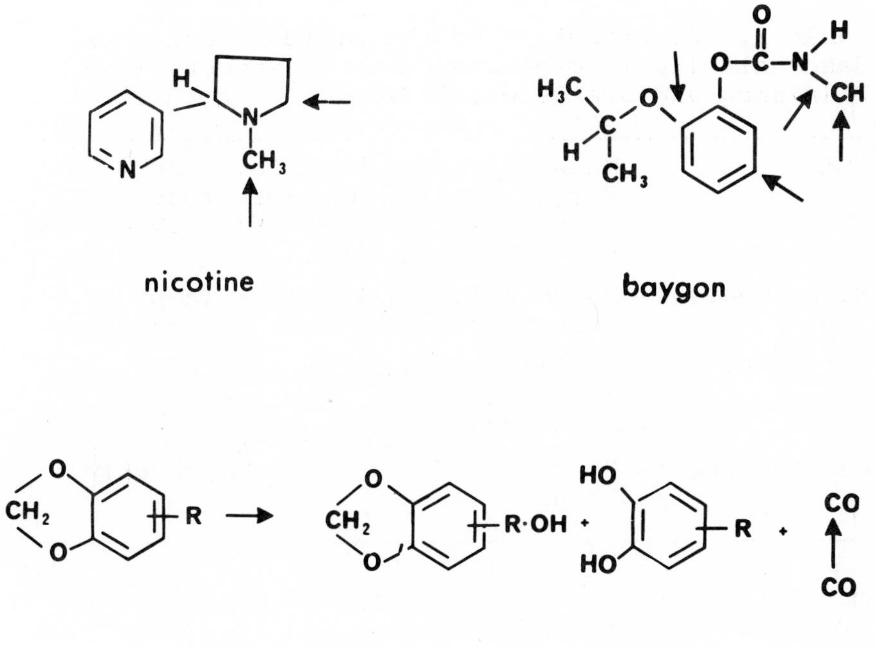

nicotine   baygon

Figure 8. Sites (arrows) of attack by insect MFO on nicotine, Baygon and methylene dioxy synergists (see Casida, 1969).

189

Housefly MFO can metabolize a number of insecticides (DDT, aldrin, parathion, carbaryl, Baygon, Metacil, rotenone, pyrethroids, etc.). It is not clear whether these reactions are catalyzed by the same enzyme with non-specific binding sites or by several enzymes with relatively specific binding sites; but in either case the reactions are coupled with NADPH oxidations. Recent reviews on in vitro characterization of these enzymes in insects have been written (Terriere, 1968; Hodgson and Plapp, 1970; Wilkinson and Brattsten, 1972). Their distribution in insects is not confined only to one tissue or organ as in vertebrates. The most active organs are fat body and excretory organs (Table 2);but fat body, because of its large mass, may be most important in insects so far as the total detoxication per insect is concerned (see Wilkinson and Brattsten, 1972).

Table 2. Distribution of the mixed-function oxidase activity in organs/systems of insects (see Wilkinson and Brattsten, 1972).

Gut	Housefly; Honeybee; Colorado Potato beetle; American roach; locust; larvae of sawfly, caddisfly; moths; cattle grub.
Malp. Tubules	House cricket; roaches: Tampa Madagascar, American; locust.
Fat Body	Blowfly; cabbage looper; caddisfly larva; roaches: American Madagascar; cattle grub.
Gastric Caeca	Roaches: Madagascar, American; locust.

Brodie and Maickel (1962) reported the in vivo metabolism of drugs injected into a fresh water crayfish (Astacidae) and the marine lobster, Homarus americanus. Based on the percent recovery of the drug after 24 hours, aminopyrine, chloropromazine, hexobarbitol and thiopentol were metabolized to 25, 20, 65 and 39 percent, respective-

ly. The enzymes were located in the microsomal
fraction of the hepatopancreas and showed much
lower levels of activity than the MFO of other
animals.

Since microsomal mixed-function oxidase catalyzes the epoxidation of aldrin to dieldrin, this
in vivo reaction which is common in aquatic invertebrates has been used an an indicator of MFO
activity. Khan et al. (1972b) found almost all of
the fresh water invertebrates they tested epoxidize
aldrin in vivo, although the rates of epoxidation
varied (Table 3). They demonstrated the in vitro
epoxidation by using tissue homogenates of the
crayfish (Cambarus), the snail (Lymnaea) and the
mussel (Anodonta). The activity, undetected in
gills, muscles, mantle and gonads, was present in
hepatopancreas, alimentary canal and kidneys. Most
hepatopancreas activity was in the microsomal
fraction (Table 4). The microsomal MFO activity in
these invertebrates is very sensitive to pH (Fig. 9),
temperature and buffer molarity. Crayfish MFO can
catalyze epoxidation of aldrin, hydroxylation of
photoisodrin and benzopyrene, and O-demethylation
of methoxychlor (Khan et al. 1972b). The levels of
MFO activity in these animals are extremely low
when compared with terrestrial insects. In the
Fiddler Crab, Uca pugnax, using aldrin epoxidation,
they are 2-times higher in the green gland than in
gills, claw muscles or gut. The lowest activity
was found in the hepatopancreas (Burns, personal
communication). The in vivo metabolism of naphthalene by the marine crab, Maia squinado has also
been reported (Corner et al., 1973).

There are only two reports regarding in vitro
MFO activity in fresh water insect larvae. The MFO
in a propoxur-selected strain of Culex pipiens
fatigans can metabolize the N-methylcarbamate
insecticides, propoxur, carbaryl, carbofuran and
aldicarb (Shrivastava et al., 1971). The oxidations
involve ring hydroxylation (of benzene, naphthalene,
furan), N-methyl hydroxylation, O- and N-dealkyla-
tions as well as thioether oxidation to sulfoxide
and sulfone. Very low levels of in vitro activity
were also observed using larvae of susceptible

Table 3. Pick-up of Aldrin and its Subsequent Epoxidation by Freshwater Invertebrates (Khan et al., 1972a).

Animal	Insecticide absorbed: ng/animal			Epoxidation of aldrin
	aldrin	dieldrin	Total	% dieldrin/animal
1. Hydra littoralis (Coelentrate)	45.02	1.20	46.25	2.59
2. Dugesia (plannarian)	23.01	0.24	23.25	1.03
3. Leech (Annelid)	34.14	0.54	35.65	1.51
4. Asellus (Crustacea, isopod)	25.02	0.59	25.61	2.30
5. Gammarus (Crustacea, amphipod)	19.98	1.52	21.50	7.07
6. Daphnia pulex (Crustacea, Cladocera)	27.16	1.64	28.80	5.69
7. Cyclops (Crustacea, copepoda)	26.23	1.13	27.36	4.13
8. Cambarus (Crustacea, Decapoda)	86.43	8.01	94.44	8.48
9. Aeschna (Insecta, Odonata)	48.59	16.11	64.70	24.90
10. Aedes aegypti (Insecta, Diptera)	95.06	69.82	164.88	42.35
11. Anodonta (Mollusk, pele-cypoda)	553.89	130.81	684.70	19.10
12. Lymnaea palustis (Mollusk, Gastropoda)	69.15	13.95	83.10	16.79

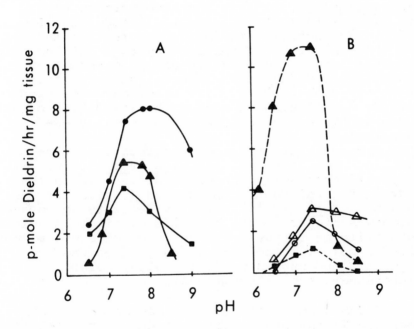

Figure 9. Effect of pH on microsomal aldrin epoxidase from various organs. A, crayfish: ●-● green gland,▲ -▲ liver,■ -■ gut; B. clam:▲- ▲ liver, o-o gut; snail▲---▲ liver, ■ --■ gut (Khan et al., 1972a).

strains of C. pipiens fatigans and of other
mosquitoes, C. tarsalis, C. peus, Anopheles albimanus,
Aedes aegypti and A. triseriatus. The enzymes in
the resistant C. p. fatigans differ from the MFO
of other animals in their optima of buffer molarity
(1 M), pH (neutral) and temperature (25°C). They
are very unstable and the activity, unlike that in
other insects, can not be restored by BSA
(Shrivastava et al., 1971).

The levels of MFO activity in aquatic invertebrates and C. p. fatigans larvae are very low.
However, the MFO of fresh water caddisfly larvae,
Limnephilus sp., exhibit the same pattern of
activity as terrestrial insects (Krieger and Lee,
1973). The activity is located in the gut and
fat body and can be stabilized by BSA. It has
somewhat broader temperature and pH optima than
those reported for other insects, however it is
inactivated above 30°C. The reactions catalyzed
include epoxidation of aldrin, hydroxylation of di-
hydroisodrin and demethylation of p-chloro-N-
methylamine.

MFO activity has also been reported in an
annelid, the earthworm, Lumbricus terrestris. The
enzyme is more active in expoxidizing aldrin than
hydrolyzing radioactive parathion (the latter was
metabolized in vivo). Activity detoxifying parathion was higher in the brain (3.14 picomole acidic
metabolite/mg tissue/hr) than in calciferous glands
(1.88 p-mole), integument (0.84 p-mole) and crop,
nephridia and esophagus (about 0.4 p-mole)
(Nakatsugawa and Nelson, 1972).

Metabolism of naphthalene has recently been
reported in the crab, Maia squinado (Corner et al.,
1973) and studies of the mixed-function oxidase in
marine invertebrates recently have been conducted
by Pohl et al. (1974).

V. Reductions. Some reductive reactions have
been reported to be catalyzed by insect MFO (Rose,
cited by Wilkinson and Brattsten, 1972). However,
such reduction of parathion to aminophenol is
anaerobically catalyzed by the soluble enzyme of the
housefly (Lichtenstein and Fuhremann, 1972). Re-

ductive dechlorination of BHC and DDT in insects may
be due to microbial activity (Khan et al., 1974).
The hepatopancreas of the quahaug, Mercenaria
mercenaria, shows no oxidative metabolism of the
insecticide, EPN, or such other xenobiotics as
p-nitroanisole, aminopyrine and hexobarbital.
However, the in vitro reduction of p-nitrobenzoic
acid to p-aminobenzoic acid takes place at 34-35°C
(pH 6.0). This activity was present in mantle,
gill, foot and gonads as well as the hepatancreas
(Carlson, 1972).

VI. Detoxication of Cyanide. Formation of
thiocyanates occurs in molluscs, parasitic
helminthes and larvae of the insect, Gasterophilus
equi (Smith, 1964b). Rhodanase is present in
blowflies (Calliphora vomitoria) (Parson and
Rothchild, 1962) and the CN group can be incorporated into the protein of Sitophilus granarius
(Bond, 1961).

CONJUGATION OF METABOLITES

After a foreign chemical is initially metabolized by one or more of the above detoxication
systems, the metabolite(s) can be conjugated with a
carbohydrate or peptide, etc. before it is excreted.
The conjugation reactions are more rapid than the
detoxication reactions (Perry, 1964; Smith, 1968)
(Table 5).

Table 5. Some examples of the conjugation reactions of xenobiotics in invertebrates.

Glucose:	B-glucoside: flies (naphthalene); locusts (DNOC).
H_2SO_4:	ethereal sulfate: flies (Naphthol), locusts (DNOC), spiders (p-amino-benzoic acid), grass grubs (biphenyls).
Acetic acid:	acetylation of amino groups; locusts (DNOC, chlorophenyl cysteine), Drosophila (hydroxytyramine).
Glycine:	acid conjugates: nicotine to nico-tinuric acid.
Cysteine or GSH	aromatic and aliphatic halogen and

TABLE 5 (CONTD.)	nitro groups: locusts (benzylbromide, dichloronitrobenzene), flies (BHC, PCH).
Amine	acids form amide bond.

Glucose conjugation. In invertebrates foreign compounds with a functional group generally form β-glucosides with sugars. These have been reported for many insects (Gassner and Acara, 1966; Smith, 1968; Mehendale and Dorough, 1972) although some insects can also form β-glucuronides (Ishiguro and Linzen, 1966; Zayed et al., 1965; Terriere et al., 1961). In vitro conjugation of o-aminophenol has been found in Helix, Arion and Limax (Dutton, 1962). The system is located in the 20,000 g/15 min pellet. Some carbamate insecticides can be directly attacked by the microsomal conjugating system in the tobacco hornworm (Manduca sexta); the enzyme being almost equally effective in fat body and gut (Mehendale and Dorough, 1972).

Ethereal sulfate formation. Conjugation of phenols with sulfates and formation of N-sulfates or phenylsulfamates are common among insects and many Arachnids (Hithcock and Smith, 1964; Hithcock, 1965), mussels, sea urchins, holothurians, crabs (Alsop, 1965; Hithcock, 1965) and the marine gastropods, Murex and Purpura (Bouchilloux and Roche, 1965). Soluble fractions from the gut of the Southern Army worm (Prodenia eridania) conjugate p-nitrophenol and various steroid hormones (Yang and Wilkinson, 1972).

Acetylations. Both aliphatic and aromatic amines can be acetylated in insects such as locusts, silkworms, wax moths and blowflies (Calliphora) (Karlson and Ammon, 1963; Smith, 1964b).

Formation of Peptides. Arginine conjugation of aromatic acids (p-nitro-and p-amino-benzoic acids) is common in millipeds (Hitchcock and Smith, 1964). Terrestreial woodlice (Oniscus and Armadillio spp), houseflies and rice moths use glycine for conjugation (Smith, 1962; Allsop, 1965).

Phosphate formation Formation of phosphate esters of phenols is very common in houseflies, blowflies (Lucilia) and larvae of the beetle, Costelytra zealandria (Smith, 1962).

Acknowledgements

Support from a grant (ES-00808) from the National Institute of Environmental Health Sciences is acknowledged. Thanks are due to Miss Janice Rajecki and Mr. R. I. Morimoto for their assistance in drawing figures.

REFERENCES

Abedi, Z. H, J. R. Duffy and A. W. A. Brown. 1963. J. Econ. Entomol. 56: 511

Agosin, M., D. Michaeli, R. Miskus, S. Nagasawa and W. H. Hoskins. 1961. J. Econ. Entomol. 54: 340.

Akov, S. and A. B. Borkovec. 1968. Life Sci. 7: 1215.

Alsop, T. 1965. Detoxication in invertebrates. M. S. Thesis, Victoria University, Wellington, New Zealand.

Barlow, J. and G. J. Ridgway. 1971. J. Fish. Res. Bd. Can. 28: 15.

Berger, R. S. and R. G. Young. 1962. J. Econ. Entomol. 53: 533.

Bond, E. J. 1961. Can. J. Zool. 39: 1793.

Bouchilloux, S. and J. Rocke. 1965. Bull. Soc. Chim. Biol. 37: 37.

Brooks, G. T. 1969. In: Residue Rev. 27: 81.

Brooks, G. T. and A. Harrison. 1969. Biochem. Pharmacol. 18: 557.

Brodie, B. B. and R. P. Maickel. 1962. In: Metabolic Factors Controlling Duration of Drug Action. (B. B. Brodie and E. G. Erdos, Eds.) Pergamon Press. 324 pp.

Bull. D. L. 1965. J. Econ. Entomol. 58: 249.

Bull. D. L. and P. L. Adkinson. 1963. J. Econ. Entomol. 56: 641.

Burns, K. Personal communication. Woodshole Oceanographic Inst., Woodshole, Mass.

Carlson , G. P. 1972. Comp. Biochem. Physiol.
43: 295.
Casida, J. E. 1969. In: Microsomes and drug oxida-
tions. (J. R. Gillette et al., Eds.) Academic
Press. 517 pp.
Chakrabarty, J. and J. N. Smith. 1964. Biochem. J.
93: 389.
Chakrabarty, J. and J. N. Smith. 1967. Biochem. J.
102: 498.
Chattoraj, J. and C. W. Kearns. 1958. Bull. Entomol.
Soc. America, 4: 95.
Clark, A. G., M. Hithcock and J. N. Smith. 1966.
Nature, 209: 103.
Cohen, A. J., J. N. Smith and H. Turbert. 1964.
Biochem. J. 90: 457.
Corner, E. D. S., C. C. Kilvington and S. C. M.
O'Hara. 1973. J. Marine Biol. Assoc. of United
Kingdom. 53: 819.
Dahm, P. A. 1970. In: Biochemical toxicology of
insecticides. (R. D. O'Brien and I. Yamamoto,
Eds.) Academic Press. 318 pp.
Dorough, H. W. and J. E. Casida. 1964. J. Agri.
Food. Chem. 12: 249.
Dutton, G. J. 1962. Compar. Biochem. Physiol. 7: 39.
Emmerich, H., G. Drews, K. Trautmann, and P.
Schmialek.1965. Z. Naturforsch. 20B: 211.
Eto, M., S. Mutsuo and Y. Oshina. 1963. Agri.
Biol. Chem. (Toyko) 27: 870.
Gassner, T. and M. Acara. 1966. Feder. Proceed.
25: 658.
Gerolt, P. H. 1965. J. Econ. Entomol. 58: 849.
Hall, W. E. and Y. P. Sun. 1965. J. Econ. Entomol.
58: 845.
Hithcock, M. and J. N. Smith 1964. Biochem. J. 93:
392.
Hitchcock,M. 1965. cited by J. N. Smith. 1968.
Adv. Compar. Physiol. Biochem. 3: 173.
Hodgson, E. and F. W. Plapp, Jr. 1970. J. Agri.
Food. Chemist. 18: 1048.
Hook, G. E. R., J. W. Jordan and J. N. Smith. 1968.
In: Enzymatic oxidations of toxicants (E.
Hodgson, ed). North Carolina State University
220 pp.
Ishida, M. and P. A. Dahn. 1965. J. Econ. Entomol.
58: 602.

Ishiguro, I. and B. Lingen. 1966. J. Insect. Physiol.
    12: 267.
Johnson, B. T., C. R. Saunders, H. O. Saunders and
    R. S. Campbell. 1971. J. Fish. Res. Bd. Canada.
    28: 705.
Kapoor, I. P., R. L. Metcalf, A. S. Hirwe, P. Lu,
    J. R. Coats and R. Y. Nystrom. 1970. J. Agri.
    Food Chem. 20: 1.
Karlson, P. and H. Ammon. 1963. Z. Physiol. Chem.
    33: 161.
Khan, M. A. Q., M.L. Gassman, and S.H. Ashrafi.1974. In:
    Environmental Dynamics of Pesticides (V. H.
    Freed and R. Hague, eds.) Plenum Publishing Co.
    (in press)
Khan, M. A. Q., W. Coello, A. A. Khan and H. Pinto.
    1972a. Life Sci. 11: 405.
Khan, M. A. Q., A. Kamal, R. J. Wolin and J.
    Runnels. 1972b. Bull. Environ. Contam. Toxicol.
    8: 219.
Khan, M. A. Q., J. L. Chang, D. J. Sutherland, J.
    D. Rosen and A. Kamal. 1970. J. Econ. Entomol.
    63: 1807.
Kimura, T., J. R. Duffy and A. W. A. Brown. 1965.
    Bull. World Health Org. 32: 557.
Kimura, T. and H. L. Keegan. 1967. Amer. J. Trop.
    Med. 16: 688.
Korte, F., G. Ludwig and J. Vogel. 1962. Ann. Chem.
    656: 135.
Kreuger, H. R. and J. E. Casida. 1961. J. Econ.
    Entomol. 54: 239.
Krieger, R. I. and P. W. Lee. 1973. J. Econ. Entomol.
    66: 1.
Lewis, J. B. 1969. Nature. 224, 917.
Lichtenstein, E. P. and T. W. Fuhremann. 1972.
    Science. 172: 589.
Lipke, H. and C. W. Kearns. 1959. J. Biol. Chem.
    234: 2129.
Matsumura, F. and A. W. A. Brown. 1963. Mosq. News.
    23: 26.
Matsumura, F. and G. Voss. 1964. J. Econ. Entomol.
    57: 911.
Mehendale, H. M. and H. W. Dorough. 1972. J. Insect
    Physiol. 18: 981.
Mellett, L. B., S. M. El Dareer, D. P. Rall and
    R. H. Adamson. 1969. Archs. Inst. Pharmacology
    177: 60.

Menzer, R. E. and J. E. Casida. 1965. J. Agr. Food Chem. 13: 102.

Metcalf, R. L., T. R. Fukuto, and R. B. March. 1958. J. Econ. Entomol. 50: 338.

Mills, B. J. and C. A. Lang. 1972. J. Geront. 27: 333.

Nakatsugawa, T. and P. A. Nelson. 1972. In: Environmental toxicology of pesticides. (F. Matsumura, G. M. Boush and T. Misato, Eds.) Acad. Press. 637 pp.

Neudrof, S. and M. A. Q. Khan. 1974. submitted to Bull. Environ. Contam. Toxicol.

O'Brien, R. D. 1962. In: Metabolic factors controlling duration of drug action. (B. B. Brodie and E. G. Erdos, Eds.) Macmillan, N. Y., 324 pp.

O'Brien, R. D. 1967. Insecticide: action and metabolism, Academic Press. 332 pp.

Oonithan,E. S. and R. Miskus. 1964. J. Econ. Entomol. 57: 425.

Oppenoorth, F. J., S. El Bashir, N. W. H. Houx and S. Voerman. 1972. Pest. Biochem. Physiol. 2: 262.

Parsons, J. and M. Rotschild. 1962. J. Ins. Physiol. 8: 285.

Perry, A. S. 1964. In: The physiology of insecta. (M. Rockstein, ed.) vol. III: 286, Academic Press.

Pimental, D. and N. Goodman. 1974. See this Book.

Pohl, R. J., J. R. Bend, A. M. Guarino and J. R. Disp. Fouts. 1974. Drug (in press)

Reddy, G. and A. Krishnakumaran. 1974. Insect. Biochem. In press.

Schonbrod, R. D., M. A. Q. Khan, L. C. Terriere and F. W. Plapp, Jr. 1968. Life Sciences 7: 681.

Self, L. S., F. E. Guthrie and E. Hodgson. 1964. Nature 204: 200.

Shisido, T. and J. Fukami. 1963. Botyu-Kagaku 28: 69.

Shrivastava, S. P., M. Tsukamoto and J. E. Casida. 1969. J. Econ. Entomol. 62: 483.

Shrivastava, S. P., G. P. Georgiou and T. R. Fukuto. 1971. Entomologia Experiment et. Appli. 14: 333.

Smith, J. N. 1962. Ann. Rev. Entomol. 7: 465.

Smith, J. N. 1964a. In: comparative Biochemistry (M. F. Lorkin and H. S. Mason, Editors) Vol. VIm 403. Academic Press.

Smith, J. H. 1964(b). J. New Zealand Inst. Chem. pp. 153.

Smith, J. N. 1968. Adv. Comp. Physiol. and Biochem.
    3:173.
Terriere, L. C., R. B. Boose and W. T. Roubal.
    1961. Biochem. J. 79: 620.
Terriere, L. C. 1968. Ann. Rev. Entomol. 13: 75.
Trebatoski, A. M. and J. F. Haynes. 1969. Annal.
    Entomol. Soc. Amer. 62: 327.
Tsukamoto, M. 1961. Botyu-Kagaku 26: 74.
Wilkinson, C. F. 1968. In: Enzymatic oxidations
    of toxicants. (E. Hodgson, Ed.). North Carolina
    State University. 228 pp.
Wilkinson, C. F. and L. B. Brattsten. 1972. Drug
    and metabolism Rev. 1: 153.
Williams, R. T. 1959. Detoxication Mechanisms.
    Chapman & Hall.,London.900 pp.
Williams, E.,R. W. Maickle and C. T. Redman. 1964.
    J. Agri. Food Chem. 12: 453.
Yang, R. S. H., G. Pelliccia and C. F. Wilkinson.
    1973. Biochem. J. 136: 817.
Yang, R. S. H. and C. F. Wilkinson. 1972. Biochem.
    J. 130: 487
Zayed, S. M. A., A. Hassan and T. M. Hussein. 1965.
    Z. Naturforsch 20B: 587.
Zubairi, M. Y. and J. E. Casida. 1965. J. Econ.
    Entomol. 58: 403.

THE DISPOSITION OF XENOBIOTICS BY FISHES

Richard H. Adamson and Susan M. Sieber

Laboratory of Chemical Pharmacology, National
Cancer Institute, National Institutes of Health,
Bethesda, Maryland 20014

Abstract

The mechanisms for termination of xenobiotic
activity in fishes include biliary excretion, renal
excretion, gill excretion, and metabolism. Xenobiotic metabolism occurs by both microsomal and
nonmicrosomal enzymes. Among the pathways fish
utilize in metabolizing xenobiotics are: glucuronic
acid conjugation, glycine conjugation, thiocyanate
synthesis, hydrolysis, reduction of azo- and nitro-
groups, N-oxidation, hydroxylation, demethylation,
and o-dealkylation.

Introduction

The fate of xenobiotics[1] (foreign compounds)
in fish has received increased attention during the
past eight years. This increased attention has
resulted from an increased awareness of environmental pollution by mercury, pesticides, polychlorinated biphenyls and other synthetic compounds; from the increased emphasis on oceanography
and the marine environment; because the world fish
catch is leveling off and even declining; and
because comparative physiology and comparative
pharmacology are now both acceptable as well as
necessary scientific endeavours.

---

[1]This term was introduced by Professor R. Tecwyn
Williams over two decades ago. See Vol. 1, No. 1
of Xenobiotica.

Xenobiotic disposition by fish has been studied because of the above reasons as well as the fact that fish alone comprise more than half the vertebrate animal species on earth, and because studies of xenobiotic disposition and metabolism by fish may shed further light on the evolution of these mechanisms and reasons for their development. These reasons have been previously summarized (Adamson et al., 1965; Adamson, 1967) and reiterated by Dewaide (1971). The reader is referred to previous summaries on xenobiotic metabolism by fish (Adamson et al., 1965; Dixon et al., 1967; Adamson, 1967; Buhler and Rasmusson, 1968a; Buhler and Rasmusson, 1968b; Dewaide, 1971; Adamson, 1972; Adamson and Guarino, 1972; Adamson and Davies, 1973).

Pattern of Xenobiotic Metabolism

The general pattern of xenobiotic metabolism for all animals including fish can be written in the following form:

phase I   phase II
Xenobiotic → Oxidation, red. Synthetic → Conjugated
            or hydrolysis   reaction   metabolite

The reaction of both phases is catalyzed by enzymes either microsomal or non-microsomal and qualitative and quantitative differences in these enzymes explain many of the species variations found with regard to metabolism of xenobiotics. Many xenobiotics (foreign compounds) are metabolized by only phase I reactions or by phase II reactions, many undergo both reactions and some compounds are metabolized only to a minor extent or not at all.

Phase I Pathways of Metabolism in Fish

The first phase of xenobiotic metabolism by fish consists of reactions in which the xenobiotic undergoes reduction, oxidation or hydrolysis or a combination of these reactions.

The enzymes responsible for reduction of an azo linkage or reduction of a nitro group exist in several species of fish (Adamson et al., 1965; Adamson, 1967; Buhler and Rasmusson, 1968a). Table I summarizes the azo reductase activity found in the liver of several fish and the temperature at which the in vitro assay was performed. All fish liver assayed contained azo reductase activity and this activity generally was highest at the environmental temperature of the species studied. Also, the addition of flavinadenine dinucleotide, riboflavin-5-phosphate at concentrations of 10^{-3} to 10^{-4}M stimulated the basal level of reduction threefold.

TABLE 1. Azo-reductase activity

Fish	Temp °C	Activity*
Lemon Shark	26	0.61
Dogfish	37	0.33
Stingray	26	0.76
Skate	37	0.16
Hagfish	37	0.13
Lungfish	37	1.2
Barracuda	26	0.76
Yellow-tail Snapper	26	0.78
Rat	37	5.88

*μmoles product formed/g liver/hr.
Data from Adamson et al. (1965); Adamson (1967).

TABLE 2. Nitro-reductase activity

Fish	Temp °C	Activity
Lemon Shark	26	0
Dogfish	37	0
Skate	37	0.49
Barracuda	26	0.50
Yellow-tail Snapper	26	0.66
Pacific Lamprey	25	0.02
Northern Pike	25	0.14
Steelhead Trout	25	0.18
Carp	25	0.33
Coarsescale Sucker	25	0.63
Rat	37	2.08

*μmoles product formed/g liver/hr.
Data from Adamson et al. (1965); Buhler and Rasmusson (1968a).

In addition to azo reductase activity, nitro reductase activity has been found in the liver of several fish. Nitro reductase activity was found (Table 2) in elasmobranchs and salt and fresh water teleosts. The nitro reductase system was localized primarily in the soluble fraction of the cell, it required NADPH and was inhibited by oxygen. Evidence was obtained which indicated that the fish liver nitro reductase system contained essential sulfhydryl groups and a carbon monoxide-sensitive component (Adamson et al., 1965; Buhler and Rasmusson, 1968a). Reduction of the 4-nitro group of parathion to a metabolite with antichlolinesterase activity has been reported to take place by a liver enzyme system in sunfish and bullheads (Hitchcock and Murphy, 1966).

Oxidation of xenobiotics can occur by various pathways including aromatic hydroxylation, aliphatic hydroxylation, deamination, o-dealkylation, N-dealkylation, N-oxidation and sulfoxidation. Several of these pathways have been found in several fish both from in vivo and from in vitro studies (Adamson, 1967). Thus, the hydroxylation of biphenyl and of aniline has been reported (Creaven et al., 1965; Buhler and Rasmusson, 1968b), the o-dealkylation of alkoxybiphenyls by trout liver preparations occurs and is more efficient at 37°C that at 20°C (Creaven et al., 1967). O-dealkylation of phenacetin and N-dealkylation of aminopyrine occurs by the hepatic microsomal system of several species of fish (Buhler and Rasmusson, 1968b; Dewaide, 1971). N-oxidation also occurs by fish and a reaction of importance is the oxidation of trimethylamine to trimethylamine-N-oxide. The oxidation of trimethylamine to trimethylamine-N-oxide is accomplished by hepatic microsomes and requires NADPH and molecular oxygen. This enzyme system occurs in several species and among fish is present in both fresh and salt water fish including some elasmobranchs The N-oxidation of trimethylamine to trimethylamine-N-oxide is a true detoxication mechanism (Baker et al., 1963; Adamson, 1972). Data on aniline hydroxylase activity and aminopyrine demethylase activity in several species of fish is presented in Table 3. Other oxidations of various xenobiotics have been reported from both in vivo and in vitro studies (Adamson, 1967), and most recently hydroxylation of aniline and demethylation of (d)-benzphetamine has been shown to take place by the hepatic enzymes of skate, flounder and dog-fish (Bend et al., 1972).

TABLE 3. Aniline hydroxylase and aminopyrine de-methylase activity in liver of various fish species

	Aniline hydroxylase activity*	Aminopyrine demethylase activity*
Blue gill	0.027	0.006
Carp	0.08	0.031
Yellow Perch	0.087	0.034
American Shad	0.069	0.082
Largescale Sucker	0.165	0.051
Steelhead Trout	0.030	0.012
Rat	0.30	0.40

*μmoles product formed/g liver/hr.

Xenobiotic metabolism by hydrolysis is confined to esters and amides and is an important reaction in the inactivation and quite often the activation of drugs. This pathway is of particular importance in the metabolism and detoxication of insecticides, especially the organophosphate insecticides. Although this reaction has not been fully studied in fish, the hydrolysis of some of the insecticides and of succinylcholine by various fish is known (Murphy, 1966; Adamson and Guarino, 1972).

TABLE 4. Compounds used in conjugation reactions

Source of conjugating agent	Conjugating agent
Carbohydrate	Glucuronic acid (sometimes replaced by glucose, ribose or N-acetyl-glucosamine)
Amino Acid	Glycine (sometimes replaced by orni-thine, arginine, agmatine, glycyl-taurine, glycylglycine, or serine) Glutathione (mercapturic acid synthesis) Methionine (methylation)
Miscellaneous	Acetyl (acetylation) Sulfate (ethereal sulfate synthesis)

Phase II Pathways of Metabolism in Fish

The phase II reactions in which a conjugated metabolite of the xenobiotic is formed is not only concerned with the xenobiotic or its phase I products, but also with the conjugating agent which is provided by the body, usually derived from carbohydrate, protein, or fat metabolism. A list of 15 types of conjugating agents is given in Table 4, but many of these are rarely used by any species and generally the six important reactions are thought to be glucuronide formation, glycine conjugation, mercapturic acid synthesis, methylation, acetylation, and ethereal sulfate synthesis. Five of these reactions have been demonstrated to occur in various fish in vivo or by in vitro studies, the exception being mercapturic acid synthesis (Adamson, 1967; Adamson and Davies, 1973). The synthesis of glucuronides is an extremely important pathway in the conjugation of foreign compounds and the types of compounds which can be conjugated with glucuronic acid include carboxylic acids, alcohols (primary, secondary and tertiary), phenols, primary amines, hydroxylamines and some thio-compounds. A list of some of the xenobiotics which are conjugated as glucuronides by various fish is found in Table 5.

TABLE 5. Glucuronic acid conjugation of various xenobiotics by fish*

Xenobiotic	Species conjugating with glucuronic acid
o,m,p-Aminobenzoic Acid	Dogfish, goosefish, flounder
Phenol Red	Dogfish
o-Aminophenol	Trout
p-Nitrophenol	Seventeen species of fish including carp, trout, salmon, eel, perch

*Data from Adamson (1967); Dewaide (1971).

Factors Influencing Xenobiotic Metabolism by Fish

Factors which one must take into account in studying the detoxication and metabolism of xenobiotics by fish, either in vivo or in vitro, include environmental temperature, optimal conditions for enzyme assay, seasonal variation, exposure to prior xenobiotics and holding in captivity (Adamson, 1967; Dewaide, 1971).

Excretion of Xenobiotics by Elasmobranchs

Although foreign compounds are only excreted to a limited degree across the dogfish gill (Table 6), various xenobiotics are excreted by the kidney and into the bile of various elasmobranchs and teleosts (Adamson, 1967; Adamson and Guarino, 1972; Guarino et al., 1972). Table 7 summarizes the distribution of various xenobiotics in the plasma, hepatic and renal compartment of the dogfish. Further studies on the gill, urinary and biliary excretion of different xenobiotics should be undertaken with various fish species.

TABLE 6. Excretion of various xenobiotics across the gill of the spiny dogfish

Xenobiotic	% Dose excreted per hour
Pentobarbital	1
Sulfadiazine	1
DDT	1
p-Aminobenzoic Acid	1
Antipyrine	2

References

Adamson, R. H. 1967. Fed. Proc. 26:1047-1055.
Adamson, R. H. 1972. Foreign nitrogenous compounds their effects and metabolism. In: Nitrogen Metabolism and The Environment, (J. W. Campbell and L. Goldstein, eds.). Academic Press, N.Y. pp. 209-233.

TABLE 7. Distribution of xenobiotics in plasma, hepatic and renal compartments of the spiny dogfish*

Xenobiotic	Plasma 4 hr.	24 hr.	Liver 4 hr.	24 hr.	Bile 4 hr.	24 hr.	Kidney 4 hr.	24 hr.	Urine 4 hr.	24 hr.
Salicylic Acid	9.41	5.06	3.04	1.32	0.05	0.05	0.71	0.58	2.63	22.82
Penicillin	6.40	1.15	15.70	5.55	6.05	23.96	2.96	0.34	10.41	27.46
Decamethonium	16.50	3.52	2.67	6.07	0.01	0.08	11.12	28.42	17.65	35.85
Bromobenzene	0.28	0.14	22.20	20.60	0.03	0.04	0.05	0.02	0.16	0.11
DDT	4.30	1.81	34.55	48.28	0.17	0.15	1.59	0.30	0.17	0.15
Methyl Mercury	6.85	4.05	29.30	28.10	0.02	0.03	5.85	2.90	0.10	0.29

*Distribution in terms of percent of administered dose of ^{14}C-labeled xenobiotic in indicated compartment. Values are mean percent of 2-6 dogfish/time period.

Adamson, R. H. and D. S. Davies. 1973. Comparative aspects of absorption, distribution, metabolism and excretion of drugs. In: Comparative Pharmacology: Volume II Section 85 International Encyclopedia of Pharmacology and Therapeutics, (M. J. Michelson, ed.). Pergamon Press, Oxford and New York. pp. 851-911.

Adamson, R. H., R. L. Dixon, F. L. Francis, and D. P. Rall. 1965. Proc. Nat. Acad. Sci. 54: 1386-1391.

Adamson, R. H., and A. M. Guarino. 1972. Comp. Biochem. Physiol. 42A:171-182.

Baker, J. R., A. Struempler, and S. Chaykin. 1963. Biochim. Biophys. Acta 71:58-64.

Bend, J. R., R. J. Pohl, and J. R. Fouts. 1972. Bull. Mt. Desert Island Biol. Lab. 12:12-15.

Buhler, D. R., and M. E. Rasmusson. 1968a. Arch. Biochim. Biophys. 25:223-239.

Buhler, D. R., and M. E. Rasmusson. 1968b. Comp. Biochem. Physiol. 25:223.

Creaven, P. J., D. V. Parke, and R. T. Williams. 1965. Biochem. J. 96:879-885.

Creaven, P. J., D. V. Parke, and R. T. Williams. 1967. Life Sci. 6:105-111.

Dewaide, J. H. 1971. Metabolism of xenobiotics -- Comparative and kinetic studies as a basis for environmental pharmacology. Ph.D. Thesis, Drukkerij Leijn, Nijmegen, The Netherlands.

Dixon, R. L., R. H. Adamson, and D. P. Rall. 1967. Metabolism of drugs by elasmobranch fishes. In: Sharks, Skates and Rays, (P. W. Gilbert, R. F. Mathewson and D. P. Rall, eds.). Johns Hopkins Press, Baltimore, Md. pp. 547-552.

Guarino, A. M., P. M. Briley, J. B. Anderson, M. A. Kinter, S. Schneiderman, L. D. Klipp, and R. H. Adamson. 1972. Bull. Mt. Desert Island Biol. Lab. 12:41-43.

Hitchcock, M. and S. D. Murphy. 1966. Fed. Proc. 25:687.

Murphy, S. D. 1966. Proc. Soc. Expt. Biol. Med. 123:392-398.

COMPARATIVE STUDIES OF CYTOCHROME P-450 AND ITS INTERACTION WITH PESTICIDES

Ernest Hodgson

Department of Entomology
North Carolina State University
Raleigh, North Carolina

Abstract

Cytochrome P-450 is known to occur in many plants and animals and is frequently associated with xenobiotic metabolism. The significance of this mixed function oxidase as a general system for detoxication is considered and special reference is made to its interactions with pesticides.

Ligand binding can be investigated by optical difference spectroscopy and structure-activity relationships in the production of different spectral interactions are summarized and discussed. Induction of cytochrome P-450 by xenobiotics is well-known and the findings specific to pesticides are discussed. Different forms of the cytochrome have been demonstrated in animals induced by xenobiotics (including pesticides) and in insects different forms of the cytochrome occur in genetically different strains. The biochemical genetics of molecular variants of cytochrome P-450 is reviewed and its possible relationship to resistance to toxicants considered.

Paper number 4213 of the Journal Series of the North Carolina State University Agricultural Experiment Station, Raleigh, North Carolina.

Introduction

Since Garfinkel (1958) and Klingenberg (1958) independently demonstrated the CO-binding pigment, later termed cytochrome P-450, in mammalian liver, it has become abundantly clear that it is the key element in the electron transport chain responsible for mixed function oxidase activity toward a large number of xenobiotic substrates and a smaller number of endogenous ones. That is to say, it is the locus for interaction with both the substrate and with molecular oxygen. There have been numerous reviews of this subject, the most recent being the proceedings of a conference held in Palo Alto, California in 1972 (Estabrook et al., 1973).

This presentation will emphasize two aspects; comparative studies of cytochrome P-450 within the various classes and phyla of animals and, more specifically, the interaction of pesticides with this cytochrome. Detailed studies of reaction mechanisms and the mechanism of induction, are the subject of other presentations in this symposium. Although higher plants and microorganisms are proper subjects for comparative studies, they will be largely neglected. Little is known of cytochrome P-450 in the former, while in the latter, although much studied, the studies are not related in any particular way to pesticides. While emphasis will be placed on investigations carried out at North Carolina State University, this emphasis will not preclude the review of the literature necessary to place the work in proper perspective.

One of the advantages a biologist may have over his more chemically oriented colleagues in biochemistry, is the habit of thinking in terms of the time-frame of organic evolution. The recent assault on all forms of life with synthetic organic chemicals has not lasted much over a century - 4 or 5 milliseconds in the day of organic evolution on earth. It is unlikely that so universal an enzyme as cytochrome P-450 arose

independently, in almost every phylum, in response to this challenge. We need, therefore, to
ask the following questions: what selection
pressure caused the selection and survival of
this system and what survival value might it have
to a species?

The food of animals contains many toxicants
frequently derived from plants, which are lipophilic and of low, but appreciable, toxicity.
The most conspicuous examples seen today are the
so-called secondary plant substances - terpenes,
steroids, methylenedioxyphenyl compounds, etc.
Such compounds would become hazards only if they
accumulated to toxic levels in the tissues.
Because of their lipophilicity this would occur
unless the means were at hand to render them more
hydrophilic and thus, more excretable. Examined
in this light, the mixed function oxidase system
is an adaptation to the everyday consumption of
lipophilic food components of low toxicity; the
development of induction providing a measure of
flexibility to permit adaptation to somewhat
higher levels. Even when induced, however, this
system is unable to counteract the deleterious
effects of the sudden intake of large doses of
highly toxic chemicals - such occurrences being
rare and possibly of less importance to the survival of the species. The more specialized cytochrome P-450's of micro-organisms can be visual-
ized as specialized evolutionary developments
from the same common progenitor that gave rise
to the cytochrome used by animals for detoxication.

This speculation by-passes a problem which
troubles many enzymologists, that of the lack of
specificity of the mixed function oxidase system,
since, given the above premises, a lack of
specificity would be selected for and a highly
specific system would be of little or no use. The
low turnover numbers for all substrates investigated, which has also been of concern, is probably a corollary of this. The wide latitude,

in terms of molecular fit, necessary in an enzyme of low specificity, may preclude the highly organized and precise fit necessary for efficient turnover.

Some support for the above can be found in the studies of Krieger et al. (1971), who showed a higher level of mixed function oxidase activity in polyphagous caterpillars than in oligophagous ones.

Before considering the distribution of cyto-chrome P-450 and its interaction with pesticides, I would like to review the various types of diff-erence spectra which have proven useful in these studies and also certain methodological problems which make comparisons with much of the published work difficult. This subject, particularly as it concerns insects, has recently been reviewed (Hodgson et al., 1974).

Carbon monoxide spectrum. This is the method commonly used to estimate cytochrome P-450 in enzyme preparations. An interaction between CO and the reduced cytochrome yields a difference spectrum with a peak at or about 450 nm. Cyto-chrome P-450 is relatively labile, breaking down to an enzymatically inactive pigment, cytochrome P-420, which under the above conditions, gives rise to a difference spectrum with a peak at 420 nm. This degradation has long been known in mammals (Omura and Sato, 1964a, 1964b, Omura et al, 1965) and insect cytochrome P-450 appears similar (Philpot and Hodgson, 1971a). The method usually used involves the saturation of both sample and reference cuvettes with CO, followed by the addition of dithionite to the sample cuvette (Omura and Sato, 1964a).

Two problems have arisen as a result of this method. One is, that the practice, perhaps inad-vertent, of adding dithionite prior to the addi-tion of CO, (Capdevila et al., 1973a, 1973b, Matthews and Casida, 1970, Morello et al., 1971, Perry and Bucknor, 1970, Perry et al., 1971) results in an underestimate of the amount of cytochrome P-420 present, since Omura and Sato (1964b) demonstrated that cytochrome P-420 is

216

degraded when subjected to dithionite under aerobic conditions. Another problem is the calculation of cytochrome P-420 from the Δ O.D. between 420 nm and 490 nm. Since the 420 nm peak exists as a shoulder on the 450 nm peak, the proper baseline is the hypothetical one - the 450 nm peak alone. Hodgson et al. (1974) illustrated the correct use of this baseline.

Type I and type II spectra. These spectra are obtained with various ligands and oxidized cytochrome P-450 (Schenkman et al., 1967) and have been used a great deal in studies of mammalian cytochrome P-450, while only scattered reports are available of their determination in other animals (Hodgson and Plapp, 1970, Philpot and Hodgson, 1971a, Tate et al., 1973b, 1973c, Capdevila et al., 1973a, 1973b). The type I spectrum has a peak at 385 nm and a trough at 420 nm while the type II has a peak at about 430 nm and a trough at about 393 nm. Unusual spectral perturbations which complicate meaningful interpretation may be caused by: non-linear baseline changes due to turbidity differences between sample and reference cuvettes; mixed interactions, such as the simultaneous formation of type I and type II spectra; denaturation of cytochrome P-450 to cytochrome P-420; native absorbance of added ligands. Recently we have attempted to establish formal guidelines to determine whether or not such problems exist (Mailman et al., 1973). These guidelines are:

1. the isobestic point must remain constant as the concentration of the ligand is changed (e.g. c 404 nm for type I);

2. increasing concentrations of a ligand should show concomitant increases in maxima and decreases in minima;

3. there must be no noticeable absorbance inflection between 500 and 470 nm.

4. the absorbance change at 360 nm should be less than 50 per cent of Δ A at the nearest maximum or minimum and always be positive for type I and negative for type II.

217

The designation of spectral type to spectra determined in the presence of other ligands such as ethyl isocyanide, or with reduced microsomes, particularly when no spectrum is apparent with oxidized microsomes (Capdevila et al., 1973b), is hazardous, since other interpretations are possible.

The n-octylamine spectrum is a special type of type II spectrum which can be demonstrated in two forms, one with a double trough at 410 nm and 394 nm and the other with a single trough at 390 nm.

Ethyl isocyanide spectrum. This represents an interaction between ethyl isocyanide and the reduced form of cytochrome P-450 and characteristically has two peaks in the Soret region, one at 455 nm and the other at 430 nm. The size of these peaks is pH dependent and a pH equilibrium point can be calculated by plotting peak height against pH. Changes in the pH equilibrium point have been used, in studies of induction in mammals, to indicate whether or not a qualitative change has occurred in the induced cytochrome (Sladek and Mannering, 1966). Recent studies (Bell and Hodgson, unpublished observations) have indicated that the formation of these peaks is both time and concentration dependent.

Cytochrome P-420 also exhibits an ethyl isocyanide difference spectrum which has a single peak at 433 nm (Omura and Sato, 1964a), a peak which may obscure the 430 nm peak of cytochrome P-450 and make calculation of equilibrium points difficult. This difficulty serves to underline the importance of making correct estimates of cytochrome P-420 contamination, as discussed above.

Type III spectrum. We have recently related piperonyl butoxide inhibition to the CO-cytochrome P-450 spectrum in mice to a piperonyl butoxide-cytochrome P-450 interaction that prevents CO binding to the cytochrome (Hodgson et al., 1973, Philpot and Hodgson 1971b,c, 1972). This has been confirmed and extended in some respects by Franklin (1971, 1972a, 1972b). Piper-

only butoxide forms a typical type I spectrum
with oxidized microsomes (Matthews et al., 1970,
Philpot and Hodgson, 1971b) and the addition of
dithionite eliminates this. After incubation
with NADPH a spectrum with peaks at 455 and 427
nm appears and dithionite simply serves to increase the size of these peaks. If dithionite is
not added but the preparation allowed to use up
the available NADPH, the spectrum assumes an
oxidized type III form with a single peak at 437
nm. It does not return to the type I form but
can be transformed from oxidized to reduced type
III by the addition of NADPH. This spectrum cannot be displaced by CO or any other ligand
tested.

  Enzyme preparations. The subject of the
proper methodology for the preparation of microsomes is too large to be included here. It is
sufficient to say that a great deal of painstak-
ing and empirical work is involved for those
interested in comparative studies. The commonest
trap into which the comparative biochemist falls
is the wholesale transfer of methods which have
proven successful when working with mammals, to
investigations using other animals. As an example, some of the problems concerned with the preparation of microsomes from houseflies are discussed by Hodgson et al. (1974).

OCCURRENCE OF CYTOCHROME P-450

  Cytochrome P-450 has been identified in
most of the major groups of vertebrates, in
higher plants and in microorganisms (Table 1).
In invertebrates, although mixed function oxidase activity is known in other groups (Khan et
al., 1972a, 1972b), cytochrome P-450 has been
explored only in insects (Table 2). The mixed
function oxidase activity of insects has recently been the subject of an extensive review
(Wilkinson and Brattsten, 1972).

  The cytochrome P-450 of certain mammals,
the rat, mouse and rabbit in particular, have
been explored in considerable detail, refer-

Table 1. Occurrence of cytochrome P-450

Organism	Tissue	References
Mammals*		
Armadillo (Tolypeutes tricinctus	Liver	Machinist et al., 1968
Bat (Myotis velixer)	Liver	Machinist et al., 1968
Bovine (Bos taurus)	Adrenal cortex	Estabrook et al., 1963
Cat (Felix domesticus)	Liver	Machinist et al., 1968
Ground squirrel (Citellus tridecem- lineatus)	Liver	Machinist et al., 1968
Guinea pig	Liver	Flynn et al., 1972
Human (Homo sapiens)	Fetal liver	Yaffe et al.,1970 Ackermann et al., 1972
	Liver	Alvares et al., 1969
	Placenta	Meigs and Ryan, 1968
	Kidney	Jacobsson and Cinti, 1973
Mouse (Mus musculus)	Liver	Abernathy et al., 1971a Flynn et al., 1972
Opossum (Didelphis virginiana)	Liver	Machinist et al., 1968

Table 1 (continued)

Organism	Tissue	References
Pig (Sus scrofa)	Adrenal gland	Machinist et al., 1968
	Kidney	Garfinkel, 1963
		Machinist et al., 1968
	Liver	Garfinkel, 1958
		Machinist et al., 1968
	Lung	Machinist et al., 1968
Rabbit (Oryctolagus cuniculus	Liver	Omura and Sato, 1964a
		Sato et al., 1973
	Lung	Bend et al., 1973
Raccoon (Procyon lator	Liver	Machinist et al., 1968
Rat (Rattus norvegicus)	Adrenal cortex	Harding et al., 1964
	Kidney	Orrenius et al., 1973
	Liver	Klingenberg, 1958
		Lu et al., 1973
	Testes	Machino et al., 1969
Sheep (Ovis musimon)	Liver	Kulkarni and Hodgson, 1973

Birds

Chick (Gallus domesticus	Embryonic Liver	Mitani et al., 1971
	Liver	Machinist et al., 1968

221

Table 1 (continued)

Organism	Tissue	References
Japanese quail (Coturnix coturnix japonica	Liver	Bunyan and Page, 1973
Reptiles		
Alligator snapping turtle (Chelydra serpentina)	Liver Intestine Kidney	Garfinkel, 1963 Garfinkel, 1963 Garfinkel, 1963
Amphibians		
Bullfrog (Rana catesbiana)	Liver Intestine Kidney	Garfinkel, 1963 Machinist et al., 1968 Garfinkel, 1963 Garfinkel, 1963
Fish		
Carp (Carpoides thompson)	Liver	Garfinkel, 1963
Fresh water buffalo fish (Cyprinus carpio)	Liver	Machinist et al., 1968
Largemouth bass (Micropterus salmoides)	Liver	Kulkarni and Hodgson, 1973
Channel catfish (Ictaburus punctatus)	Liver	Machinist et al., 1968

Table 1 (continued)

Organism	Tissue	References
Insects - see Table 2		
Bacteria		
Corynebacterium spp		Cardini and Jurtshuk, 1968
Pseudomas putida		Katagiri et al., 1968
Rhizobium japonicum		Appleby, 1969
Staphlococcus aureus		Joyce and White, 1971 Hammond and White 1970
Fungi		
Candida tropicalis		Lebault et al., 1971
Claviceps purpurea		Ambike and Baxter, 1970
Higher Plants		
Phaseolus vulgaris		Markham et al., 1972
Pisum sativum		Markham et al., 1972
Vinca rosa		Meehan and Coscia, 1973
Zea mays		Markham et al., 1972

Table 1 (continued)

---

*Published work on mammals is so voluminous, particularly in the case of the rat, rabbit and mouse, that the references cited are only illustrative. Access to other investigations can be gained through review articles such as those in Estabrook et al., 1973 and Brodie et al., 1971.

Table 2. Occurrence of cytochrome P-450 in
          insects

Species	Tissue	Reference
Achetus domesticus house cricket	Malphigian tubes	Benke and Wilkinson, 1971
Anthereae pernyi american silkmoth	Midgut	Krieger and Wilkinson, 1970
Blattella germanica german cockroach	Whole body	Ray, 1965
Calliphora erythrocephala blowfly	Fat body	Price and Kuhr, 1971
Drosophila melanogaster (fruitfly)	Whole body	Kulkarni and Hodgson, 1973
Gromphadorhina portentosa madagascar cockroach		Benke et al., 1972
Heliothis zea corn earworm	Abdomen & Thorax	Williamson and Schechter, 1970
Hippelates bishoppi eye gnat	Whole body	Kulkarni and Hodgson, 1973
Hippelates pusio eye gnat	Whole body	Kulkarni and Hodgson, 1973
Macremphytus varianus sawfly	Gut	Krieger et al., 1970
Manduca sexta tobacco hornworm	Midgut	Kulkarni and Hodgson, 1973

Table 2 (continued)

Species	Tissue	Reference
<u>Musca</u> <u>domestica</u> housefly	Whole body, Abdomen	Perry and Bucknor, 1970 Hodgson and Plapp, 1970 Matthews and Casida, 1970
<u>Musca</u> <u>vicina</u> housefly	Whole body	Ray, 1965, 1967
<u>Periplaneta</u> <u>americana</u> american cockroach	Fat body, midgut	Fukami <u>et</u> <u>al</u>., 1969
<u>Prodenia</u> <u>eridania</u> southern armyworm	Midgut	Krieger and Wil- kinson, 1970
<u>Tricoplusia</u> <u>ni</u> cabbage looper	Fat body, gut	Kuhr, 1971

ences in the scientific literature to the cytochrome P-450 of these mammals must number at
least several hundred. The cytochrome P-450 of
certain bacteria has also been explored in detail and recently, a start has been made toward
a detailed examination of the cytochrome P-450
of the housefly, Musca domestica (Capdevila et
al., 1973a, 1973b, Folsom et al., 1970, Folsom
et al., 1971, Hodgson and Plapp, 1970, Hodgson
et al., 1974, Kulkarni et al., 1973a, Perry
and Bucknor, 1970, Perry et al., 1971, Philpot
and Hodgson, 1971, Tate et al., 1973a, 1973b).
In almost all other cases the characterization
of cytochrome P-450 consists only of a determination, via optical difference spectroscopy,
of CO-binding to the reduced cytochrome.

For the last 2 or 3 years we have been
investigating the cytochrome P-450 of the
housefly, Musca domestica, and its role in insecticide resistance. This is discussed in a
later section. We have also looked (Kulkarni
and Hodgson 1973) at cytochrome P-450 from
other animals, determining the type I (benzphetamine), type II (pyridine), type II (n-octylamine) and ethyl isocyanide difference spectra
to obtain an indication of the range of qualitative variations between the cytochromes of
various species.

Table 3 contains several examples of the
type of data obtained. For example, a type I
spectrum cannot be detected with the cytochrome from eye-gnats (Hippelates) using benzphetamine as a ligand. This is similar to the
findings in wild type houseflies but differs
from that in insecticide-resistant houseflies
and in mammals. Unfortunately no information is
available on resistant eye-gnats. Insects appear
to have much larger ethyl isocyanide (455 nm
peak) spectra than mammals although the hornworm
is an exception. N-octylamine spectra also
appear to be larger in insects than in mammals
but a fish, the largemouth bass, differs from
mammals in the same way. This data serves to
illustrate that qualitative differences may be

Table 3. Optical difference spectra of cytochrome P-450 from various mammals, insects and a fish*

Species	Spectra (ΔO.D./unit cytochrome P-450)			
	Pyridine	n-Octylamine	Benzphetamine	Ethyl isocyanide (455nm)
Mouse	0.55	0.59	0.32	0.49
Rabbit	0.78	0.60	0.23	0.50
Rat	0.54	0.43	0.39	0.48
Sheep	0.62	0.56	0.39	0.29
Drosophila melanogaster	0.40	0.75 0.67	0.16	0.96
Hippelates bishoppi	0.39	0.74 0.70	ND	0.92
Hippelates pallipes	0.55	1.02	ND	1.21
Hippelates pusio	0.40	0.71	ND	1.04
Manduca sexta	0.56	**	ND	0.25
Musca domestica (CSMA)	0.43	0.40	ND	1.00
Musca domestica (Fc)	0.75	0.51	0.26	0.58

Table 3. (continued)

Species	Spectra (Δ O.D./unit cytochrome P-450			
	Pyri- dine	n-Octyl- amine	Benzphet- amine	Ethyl iso- cyanide (455nm)
Largemouth Bass	0.49	0.82	0.29	1.12

*Values for insecticide-susceptible (CSMA) and
-resistant (Fc) Musca domestica taken from
Tate et al. (1973), the remaining values from
Kulkarni and Hodgson (1973).
**An unusual spectral interaction described in
a later section.

common between species; a fact which cannot be deduced from an examination of the size of the CO-spectrum.

SUBSTRATE BINDING OF PESTICIDES

Type I binding is known to be caused by many compounds including drugs (Remmer et al., 1966, Schenkman et al., 1967), pesticides (Baker et al., 1972, Kuwatsuka, 1970, Mailman and Hodgson, 1972) and steroid hormones (Cooper et al., 1971). Other reports have concluded that type II binding is caused by aromatic amines (T'sai et al., 1970), aliphatic amines (Jefcoate et al., 1969), isocyanides (Imai and Sato, 1967), certain steroids (Cooper et al., 1971, Jefcoate et al., 1969a) and alcohols (Diehl et al., 1970).

Although Schenkman et al. (1967) suggested that type II binding represented the formation of a ferrihemochrome from the interaction of a basic amine and a ferrihemoprotein, the above references suggest that other compounds may also play a similar role. Several recent reports (Holtzman, 1973, Mailman and Hodgson, 1972, Mailman et al., 1972, Schenkman, et al., 1973) generally support the contention that steric and basic features of nitrogen are of primary importance in determining whether or not a particular ligand will give rise to a type II spectrum.

We have recently carried out a study of the structure-function relationships in the binding of ligands to the oxidized cytochrome P-450 in hepatic microsomes from the mouse (Mailman et al., 1973). Using derivatives of pyridine, pyrrolidine and piperidone as well as benzothiadiazones, imidazoles, amides, amines, alkylnitriles, benzonitriles, phenols, alcohols and other compounds, it was concluded that a type II spectrum was associated with ligands with a nitrogen atom in which sp^2 or sp^3 non-bonded electrons are sterically accessible. The first point is illustrated in Table 4 in which

230

Table 4. Effect of ligand on spectral interaction with cytochrome P-450 in mouse
hepatic microsomes

Ligand	N	Spectral type	Spectral Size (Δ O.D./Unit P-450)
3-methoxypro-pionitrile	sp	I	0.013
3-chlorobenzo-nitrile	sp	I	0.107
pyridine	sp^2	II	0.540
octylamine	sp^3	II	0.910
aniline	sp^3	II	0.452

sp nitrogens are shown to give type I spectra
and sp^2 and sp^3 nitrogen to give type II. Using
methyl derivatives of pyridine it can be seen
(Table 5) that accessibility is important since

Table 5. Effect of substitutions on pyridine-
cytochrome P-450 difference spectra
with mouse hepatic microsomes

Ligand	Spectral type	Spectral size (Δ O.D./ Unit P-450)
---	II	0.540
4-methyl	II	0.620
3-methyl	II	0.654
2-methyl	II	0.380
2,6-dimethyl	II	0.010

231

3 and 4 substitutions have no effect while 2, or particularly 2 or 6 substitution, causes a significant decrease in the size of the spectral shift. Similar findings are seen with carboxyl derivatives except that the sizes of all spectra are reduced, due, presumably, to the decrease in lipophilicity.

A comparison of indole and indoline shows how quite subtle changes may affect spectra formation. Indoline is a strong type II ligand whereas indole is type I. The difference between the two molecules is the unsaturation at carbons 3-4 of indole, causing a 'stiffening' of the molecule. This causes a change in accessibility to the non-bonded nitrogen electrons.

Our results with oxygen compounds bear on the interpretation of the so-called modified type II or inverse type I spectrum. Without going into any detail, the simplest explanation of our data is that oxygen atoms may act much like nitrogen atoms, i.e. as nucleophiles replacing another ligand at the fifth or sixth ligand position of the heme group of P-450 causing a bathacromic shift. It is of lower intensity and shorter wavelength due to the lower nucleophilicity of the groups involved. Although this argues against the 'endogenous substrate displacement' (Diehl et al., 1970, Wilson and Orrenius, 1972) explanation of this spectral type, it is entirely possible that both hypotheses may be true, depending on the ligand and the cytochrome P-450 involved.

In a companion study (Kulkarni et al., 1973a) on the binding spectra of cytochrome P-450 from the abdomens of insecticide susceptible (CSMA strain) and insecticide resistant (Fc strain) houseflies it became apparent that, although the same basic requirements held true for the housefly cytochrome as for the mouse cytochrome, there were interesting differences between insect and mammal and also between one insect strain and another.

Tables 6 and 7 give data for housefly cytochrome P-450 parallel to those shown for the

Table 6. Effect of ligand on spectral interaction with cytochrome P-450 in housefly microsomes

Ligand	N	Spectral type		Spectral size (Δ O.D./Unit P-450)	
		CSMA	Fc	CSMA	Fc
3-methoxypro-pipnitrile	sp	ND*	ND	---	---
3-chlorobenzo-nitrile	sp	ND	I	---	0.053
pyridine	sp^2	II	II	0.520	0.727
octylamine	sp^3	II	II	0.675	0.915
aniline	sp^3	II	II	0.195	0.336

*ND = not detectable

Table 7. Effect of substitutions on pyridine-
cytochrome P-450 difference spectra
with housefly microsomes

Ligand	Spectral type		Spectral size (Δ O.D./Unit P-450)	
	CSMA	Fc	CSMA	Fc
---	II	II	0.520	0.727
4-methyl	II	II	0.478	0.744
3-methyl	II	II	0.491	0.797
2-methyl	II	II	0.118	0.147
2,6-dimethyl	II	I+II	0.109	---

233

mouse in tables 4 and 5.

The lack of type I spectra in susceptible or wild-type flies previously noted (Philpot and Hodgson, 1971a, Tate et al., 1973a, 1973b) was confirmed in the case of 18 more ligands which gave clearly discernable type I spectra with the resistant strain. This difference is probably the most dramatic one which has been recorded between the cytochrome P-450s of different animals.

Many of the differences between housefly and mouse cytochrome P-450 appear to indicate that the heme is more accessible to ligand binding in the former. Such differences include:

1. Some compounds such as 2-ethyl piperidine, propionitrile and n-hexanol give mixed type I and II spectra with mouse microsomes but a type II with housefly microsomes.

2. Some compounds such as 1-cyclohexenyl pyrollidine and sec-butanol are type II with housefly microsomes but type I with mouse microsomes.

3. Compounds such as tetrahydrofuran and tryptophane give type II spectra with housefly microsomes but give no detectable spectra with mouse microsomes.

Jefcoate et al. (1969a, 1969b) noted a double trough in the n-octylamine spectrum with rabbit liver microsomes and related this to high spin and low spin forms of cytochrome P-450. They also speculated that alkylamines were bound to two sites on each form of the cytochrome. The present study confirmed earlier observations on insects (Philpot and Hodgson, 1971a, Tate et al., 1973a, 1973b) that a double trough occurs in the n-octylamine spectrum of CSMA microsomes but a single trough in the case of Fc microsomes.

In houseflies, benzimidazole exhibited a concentration dependent double trough in which a single minimum at 410 nm became a double trough at 410 and 392 nm as the concentration was increased, and finally, a single minimum at 392 nm.

If these findings are interpreted to represent two binding sites for which benzimidazole has either a high affinity (perturbation at 410 nm) or a low affinity (perturbation at 392 nm) then they may help to explain the observation that the range of peak and trough positions in houseflies type II difference is much greater than it is in mouse hepatic microsomes.

The response of both Fc and CSMA microsomes was similar, but certain differences could be noted. Spectral magnitudes relative to the CO-spectrum were always smaller in the CSMA than in the Fc microsomes. Other differences appear to be related to the fact that there is no type I component in the CSMA spectrum (e.g. 1-cyclohexyl-2-pyrrolidinone is type I with Fc microsomes but type II with CSMA microsomes and 2,6-lutidine gives a mixture of types I and II with Fc but type II with CSMA). Whether this is also responsible for the fact that spectral maxima and minima, if they are not identicial, are always at a shorter wavelength in Fc microsomes than in CSMA, is not yet apparent.

Although some of the compounds of the 125 used in the above studies are pesticides, the majority are model compounds chosen for the light they might shed on the structural requirements necessary for the formation of different spectral types. In a separate study (Kulkarni et al., 1973b), the interactions of pesticides with the cytochrome P-450 in the hepatic microsomes of mouse, rabbit, rat and sheep and the abdominal microsomes of CSMA and Fc houseflies were examined.

A selection of the data is shown in Table 8. The information on mice microsomes obtained in this study largely confirms results obtained with this animal in an earlier report (Mailman and Hodgson, 1972). Several points of interest may be noted.

The spectral types obtained are in conformity with the structure-function analysis reported above.

The difference between the susceptible and

235

Table 8.   Optical difference spectra of cyto-
            chrome P-450 from hepatic microsomes
            of mammals and abdominal microsomes of
            the housefly with various pesticides
            as ligands

| Pesticide | Spectral type and size (Δ O.D./Unit P-450) | | | | | |
| | Sheep | | Rabbit | | Rat | |
	Type	Size	Type	Size	Type	Size
p,P'-DDT	I	0.166	I	0.076	I	0.103
TDE	I	0.283	I	0.219	I	0.310
Kelthane	I	0.314	I	0.057	I	0.345
Aldrin	I	0.271	I	0.219	I	0.247
Toxaphene	I	0.250	I	0.257	I	0.354
Carbaryl	I	0.174	I*	0.088	I	0.270
Bux	I	0.449	I	0.196	I	0.326
Guthion	I	0.134	I	0.155	I	0.170
Zinophos	II	0.377	II	0.321	II	0.242
Nicotine	II	0.434	II	0.540	II	0.505
Allethrin	I	0.270	I	0.160	I	0.362
Rotenone	***	0.094	***	0.130	ND	---

Table 8.   (continued)

| Pesticide | Spectral type and size (Δ O.D./Unit P-450) | | | | | |
| | Mouse | | Housefly (Fc) | | Housefly (CSMA) | |
	Type	Size	Type	Size	Type	Size
p,P'-DDT	I	0.112	I	0.120	ND	---
TDE	I	0.330	I	0.100	ND	---
Kelthane	I	0.295	I	0.154	ND	---
Aldrin	I	0.169	I	0.133	ND	---
Toxaphene	I	0.239	I	0.133	ND	---
Carbaryl	I	0.200	I	0.133	ND	---
Bux	I	0.244	I	0.211	ND	---
Guthion	I+II	---	I	0.222	ND	---
Zinophos	II	0.312	II	0.321	II	0.166
Nicotine	II	0.522	II	0.412	II	0.255
Allethrin	I	0.278	**	0.300	**	0.286
Rotenone	ND	---	ND	---	ND	---

*   Spectrum has a second peak at 407 nm in addition to one at 382 nm.
**   Unusual spectrum with a peak at about 418 nm and a trough at 445 nm.
*** Unusual spectrum with a small peak at 417 nm and a large trough at 395 nm.

237

resistant houseflies is again clearly seen, compounds which are type I in other animals or in the resistant strain giving no detectable spectrum in the susceptible strain.

An unusual spectrum is seen with allethrin and some, but not all, other pyrethroids and housefly microsomes. This spectrum has a peak at about 418 nm and a trough at 445 nm. In mammals these compounds give rise to a typical type I spectrum.

Rotenone does not give rise to any detectable spectrum with microsomes from rat, mouse and both types of houseflies. However, with sheep and rabbit microsomes it gives rise to an unusual spectrum with a large trough at 395 nm and a small peak at 417 nm. These results using rotenone confirm those of Kuwatsuka (1970) but are at variance with those of Schenkman et al. (1967).

The data would again tend to support the hypothesis that qualitative differences between different cytochrome P-450s are common since the ratio between spectral size for any given series of ligands is frequently not consistent. For example, a comparison of the spectral size given by the closely related DDT, TDE and Kelthane in the sheep and rat shows Kelthane > TDE > DDT while the same comparison in the rabbit shows TDE > DDT > Kelthane.

Previous studies (Green and Stevens, 1973, Kuwatsuka, 1970, Roth and Neal, 1972, Schenkman et al., 1967, Stevens et al., 1973) involve only a small number of species and compounds and, though interesting, do not provide an adequate basis for comparison.

Several compounds currently under consideration as pesticides, the juvenile hormone analogs, have been shown to form type I spectra with rat liver microsomes and to function as inhibitors of rat liver oxidation of aniline (Mayer et al., 1973).

Most of the pesticides studied are known to be substrates for microsomal mixed function oxidases, both in insects and mammals. The extent to which spectral binding studies can be correlated with metabolism is not clear, although studies in mammals with other substrates would suggest that the relationship is not an obvious one. At present the extreme variations in techniques between different laboratories make comparison difficult and this is an area in which detailed studies are needed.

Mention of qualitative differences between cytochrome P-450s need not, of necessity, imply differences between the cytochromes themselves. The spectra are recorded using microsomes rather than soluble or purified cytochromes and thus the differences could reflect differences in the environment in which the cytochrome is located within the membrane. For example, differences between housefly and mouse microsomes have been referred to above which imply that the heme iron of the former is more accessible to type II ligands than that of the latter while, at the same time, there are scattered pieces of evidence which indicate that the microsomal membrane of the housefly is different from that of the mouse. These include:

1. The phospholipid composition is quite different, the housefly having more phosphatidylethanolamine than phosphatidylcholine (Khan and Hodgson, 1967).

2. The method used by Wilson and Hodgson (1971a, 1971b) to solubilize NADPH-cytochrome c reductase from housefly microsomes was totally ineffective when tested on mammalian microsomes but the enzyme, when purified, was remarkably similar to the corresponding enzyme from mammals.

3. The preparation of subparticles from housefly microsomes using subtilisin yielded a subparticle containing no cytochrome P-450 but in which the cytochrome P-420 was retained. Parallel experiments in mouse microsomes yielded a cytochrome P-450-containing subparticle, with any cytochrome P-420 formed appearing in the soluble fraction (Philpot and Hodgson, unpublished observations).

I would like to report only briefly on what

we have called type III spectra, obtained on the
interaction of piperonyl butoxide and other
methylenedioxyphenyl compounds with the reduced
form of cytochrome P-450 since this has been reviewed recently (Hodgson et al., 197 , Hodgson
et al., 1974, Hodgson and Philpot, 1974).

Following the demonstration that in vivo
administration of piperonyl butoxide to houseflies inhibited the formation of the CO-cytochrome P-450 difference spectrum (Matthews and
Casida, 1970, Perry and Bucknor, 1970, Perry et
al., 1971) Philpot and Hodgson (1971b, 1971c,
1972) related this inhibition to a piperonyl
butoxide-cytochrome P-450 interaction that prevents CO binding to the cytochrome. Franklin
(1971, 1972a, 1972b), in a series of papers,
confirmed this and extended the findings. The
demonstration of this interaction in houseflies
(Philpot and Hodgson, 1971a) suggested that the
effect of this compound is similar in the two
species. It is now clear (Hodgson and Philpot,
1974) that this interaction is important in
insecticide synergism and in the physiological
effects of methylenedioxyphenyl compounds in
mammals.

Piperonyl butoxide forms a typical type I
spectrum with oxidized cytochrome P-450 (Hodgson
and Plapp, 1970, Matthews et al., 1970, Philpot
and Hodgson, 1971b). On incubation with NADPH a
spectrum (type III) appears with peaks at 455
and 427 nm. If the preparation is allowed to
deplete the NADPH, this assumes an oxidized form
with a single peak at 437 nm; it does not reform
the type I spectrum. This spectrum cannot be
displaced by CO or any other ligand tested.

An examination of many different methylenedioxyphenyl compounds revealed (Hodgson et
al., 1973) that in mice most of these compounds
give rise to type I spectra with oxidized
microsomes becoming type III on incubation with
NADPH. Other reduced spectra were observed however, including the formation of the 427 nm peak
alone and the formation of a large peak at 450
nm following reduction with dithionite. A simi-

lar study using housefly microsomes (Kulkarni et al., 1973c) showed that similar spectra were formed in both resistant (Fc) and susceptible (CSMA) strains. The apparent formation of type I spectra in the CSMA strain was interesting, since previous study, summarized above, showed that over fifty different ligands from many chemical classes which gave type I spectra in resistant houseflies and in several mammals, failed to do so in the susceptible or wild-type housefly. Since all but one (sulfoxide) of those formed with methylenedioxyphenyl compounds are very small and difficult to resolve, and considering the unusual spectral interaction of this class of compounds, it is difficult to determine whether or not this represents typical type I binding.

Before leaving the subject of spectral interaction, I would like briefly to comment on one which is being discussed in detail by Dr. Kulkarni* of our group, at this meeting. Although pyridine yields a typical type II spectrum with microsomes from the gut of the tobacco hornworm, n-octylamine and certain other amines cause a very large spectral displacement which appears to be a summation of a cytochrome b_5 spectrum with a normal n-octylamine spectrum. This decreases with time until the normal n-octylamine spectrum remains. Several experiments by a variety of techniques confirm that a reduced cytochrome b_5 spectrum is involved and that the causative agent is to be found not in the microsomes but in the supernatant, well washed microscomes forming only an n-octylamine spectrum. Until now the phenomenon seemed of little general interest, since it occurred in the gut of an insect larva. The observation that a very small quantity of the hornworm supernatant fraction caused the same phenomenon with mouse microsomes raises the possibility that an understanding of this interaction may be of a more general significance.

*Amer. Zool. 13(4): 1309-1310 (1973)

INDUCTION OF CYTOCHROME P-450 BY PESTICIDES

Since the initial observations of Brown et al. (1954) induction of microsomal mixed function oxidase, particularly in mammalian liver, has been much studied. The early observations were the subject of a landmark review by Conney (1967). It was clear by then that all inducers did not induce the same enzyme activities. Some, such as phenobarbital, were more general, while others, such as the polycyclic hydrocarbons, induced a much narrower range of enzyme activities. Differences were also noted in the CO and ethyl isocyanide difference spectra (Alvares et al., 1967, Hildebrandt et al, 1968, Sladek and Mannering, 1966) and, more recently, evidence from solubilized cytochromes strongly indicates that these differences reside in the cytochrome P-450 itself (Lu et al., 1973).

Although early reports implicated pesticides such as chlordane, DDT, hexachlorocyclohexane, dieldrin, aldrin and heptachlor epoxide in the induction of mammalian hepatic mixed function oxidase activity (see Conney, 1967, for references) they have not been studied extensively in this regard and very few studies have dealt with cytochrome P-450 specifically. Pyrethrum, earlier considered non-inducing (Fouts, 1963), is now known to induce high dose levels (Springfield et al., 1973).

DDT and DDT analogs in mammals. Early work by Fouts and co-workers (Cram and Fouts, 1967, Hansen and Fouts, 1968, 1971, Hart and Fouts, 1965) demonstrated that DDT was an inducer of mixed function oxidase activity in the rat, but only marginal or ineffective in the Swiss-Webster mouse. Subsequently, using a different strain of mice (the North Carolina Board of Health strain), Abernathy et al. (1971a) investigated a series of DDT analogs and found that several of these induced aniline hydroxylase activity, cytochrome P-450 and NADPH-oxidase activity. The structural requirements included a halogen on each phenyl ring and three halogens on the α carbon of the ethane bridge. Molecular dimensions for maximum induction were also defined. In a companion study (Abernathy et al., 1971b) neither DDT nor benzpyrene appeared to be a selective inducer, but both appeared to induce an increased level of the same cytochrome P-450 observed in control mice. In a later study, Fouts (1973) found essentially the same thing in Swiss-Webster mice when DDT was administered at a higher level than in the previous work. He suggested that the lack of specificity was due to the necessity of using high dose levels of toxic chemicals and that the induction was, in fact, stress induction mediated through the endocrine system. Abernathy et al. (1971a), however, found no correlation between toxicity and induction when administering DDT analogs to mice of the North Carolina Board of Health strain.

In other mammals (Bunyan and Page, 1973, Davis et al., 1973, Remmer et al., 1968) and in birds (Bunyan and Page, 1973, Bunyan et al., 1972) DDE is equal to or more potent than DDT, while in the Japanese quail DDMU [1,1-di(p-chlorophenyl)-2-chloroethylene] is even more potent than DDE (Bunyan and Page, 1973).

Mirex in mammals. Recently (Baker et al., 1972) we have examined the inductive ability of Mirex, an insecticide used for the control of the fire ant in the southern U. S. A. This compound is the most effective inducer of microsomal mixed function oxidase activity of any pesticide yet tested, being active at the lowest level tested, 1.0 ppm, in diet of mouse, while a somewhat higher level was required in the case of the rat.

A concentration dependent effect, on both the quantity and type of cytochrome P-450, not previously noted for an inducer of cytochrome P-450, was seen. This is illustrated in Table 9. At low doses induction is approximately 2-fold and the ratio of type II to type I binding remains approximately the same as controls, while at high doses induction is much higher, some 6-fold, and there is a distinct change in

Table 9. Effect of dietary Mirex on the level of hepatic cytochrome P-450 and cytochrome P-450 type I and type II optical difference spectra*

Dietary	P-450 (O.D. units/167 mg liver wt.)	Induction (x control)	Type I binding (O.D. units/167 mg. liver wt)	Type II binding O.D. units/167 mg liver wt.)	Ratio Type II/Type I
0.0	0.077	---	0.010	0.046	4.6
1.0	0.138	1.8	0.20	0.078	3.9
25.0	0.156	2.0	0.023	0.095	4.1
100.0	0.458	6.0	0.049	0.395	8.1
250.0	0.451	5.9	0.053	0.327	6.2

* Taken from Baker et al., (1972).

the ratio of type II to type I binding.

Methylenedioxyphenyl compounds in mammals.
These compounds are chiefly known for their ability to function as insecticide synergists, due
to their ability to act as inhibitors of mixed
function oxidases (Hodgson and Philpot, 1974,
Wilkinson, 1971). They are also known to induce
microsomal mixed function oxidase activity and,
although these studies are not extensive, they
do embrace a number of different compounds and
animals. As with other pesticides, few studies
concern themselves specifically with cytochrome
P-450.

After a single injection of piperonyl butoxide, the effect on cytochrome P-450 is biphasic
(Philpot and Hodgson, 1971c). There is first
apparent reduction, due to the formation of the
type III complex, with a return to control values
in about 24 hours, and next an induction which
returns to control values in about 3-4 days.
These investigations also showed that methylenedioxyphenyl compounds may cause qualitative as
well as quantitative changes in the cytochrome
P-450 but that all compounds of this class do
not have the same effect. Piperonyl butoxide
caused a biphasic change in the ethyl isocyanide
equilibrium point and in the ratio of type I to
type II binding, both of which paralleled the
cytochrome P-450 level. Propyl isome, which
also interacts with cytochrome P-450 to form a
type III complex, induced cytochrome P-450 but
caused no changes in either the ethyl isocyanide
equilibrium point or the ratio of type I to type
II binding.

Following induction by safrole, Parke and
Rahman (1971) proposed the induction of a new
hemoprotein to explain a peak at 455 nm in an oxidized minus reduced difference spectrum.
Following the description of the type III interaction, Lake and Parke (1971) indicated that this
explained, in part, the previous findings, but
that a new hemoprotein was still required for a
complete explanation. The use of the oxidized
minus reduced difference spectra imposes a prob-

lem in interpretation since it involves a
simultaneous difference in the spectra of the
unreacted cytochrome, between the oxidized and
reduced type III spectra and between oxidized
and reduced cytochrome b_5. In our hands the oxidized minus reduced spectra described by Parke
and Rahman (1971) can be fully accounted for by
summation of the spectra referred to above,
without the necessity of invoking a new entity.

It is apparent from extensive reviews of
the xenobiotic induction of mixed function oxidase activity (Conney, 1967, Kuntzman, 1969) that
many compounds, other than methylenedioxyphenyl
compounds, have the same effect. It might be
expected that any synergist which functions by
inhibition of mixed function oxidation could also,
on longer exposure, act as an inducer and give
rise to a biphasic curve. This has, in fact,
been demonstrated for NIA 16824[1], and WL 19255
and to a less marked effect with RO5-8019 and MGK
264 (Skrinjaric-Spoljar et al., 1971).

Induction of cytochrome P-450 in insects.
The induction of mixed function oxidase in insects
by DDT, dieldrin and other insecticides, phenobarbital, juvenile hormone analogs, methylbenzenes, etc., has been studied by Terriere and
his co-workers (Terriere, 1973, Terriere et al.,
1971, Terriere and Yu, 1973, Walker and Terriere,
1970, Yu and Terriere, 1971, 1972, 1973) and
others (Brattsten and Wilkinson, 1973, Khan and
Matsumura, 1972, Matthews and Casida, 1970, Plapp
and Casida, 1970). It is apparent that it is
similar, in general, to induction in mammals,
although little is known of the effects on the
cytochrome.

Perry et al. (1971) reported induction of
cytochrome P-450 in the housefly by phenobarbital, butylated hydroxytoluene, and triphenyl
phosphate and Brattsten and Wilkinson (1973)
induction of P-450 in the southern armyworm by
methylbenzenes.

Capdevila et al. (1973a, 1973b) suggested
that a qualitatively different cytochrome P-450
[1]See page 48

is formed in houseflies treated with naphthalene or phenobarbital. This is plausible since induction is known to produce different cytochromes in mammals and, moreover, different cytochrome P-450s have been characterized in genetically different strains of the housefly (Philpot and Hodgson, 1971, Tate et al., 1973a, and Hodgson et al., 1974). However, methodological differences make comparison of these results with others difficult (see Hodgson, 1974, for discussion) and in at least one strain (Orlando), induction with DDT gives rise to an increased level of a cytochrome apparently identical with that from control insects (Tate et al., 1973a).

GENETICS OF CYTOCHROME P-450 AND RESISTANCE TO INSECTICIDES

Work in our laboratory as well as several others had indicated that an increased level of mixed function oxidase activity is associated with the resistance of houseflies to several insecticides (see Wilkinson and Brattsten, 1972 for references). Since this is clearly related to cytochrome P-450 we decided to compare this cytochrome from flies of the susceptible CSMA and from the Rutgers diazinon resistant strain (Philpot and Hodgson, 1971). A comparison of these two strains based on the size and peak position of the CO-, types I, II, III, n-octylamine and the EtNC difference spectra, expressed on a per fly basis, show several points which taken together provide strong evidence for qualitative as well as quantitative differences between the two strains.

It seems appropriate to mention that several of these parameters such as the n-octylamine spectrum and the ethyl isocyanide spectrum were used to support the contention that the cytochrome P-450 from 3-methyl-cholanthrene induced mammals was a different cytochrome from that found in phenobarbital induced mammals (Alvares et al., 1967; Jefcoate et al., 1969a; Shoeman et al., 1969; Sladek and Mannering, 1966).

Another criterion used is that of the peak position, the wavelength of maximum absorption. There were also variations between the two strains in this regard, usually in the direction of 2-3 nm higher in the susceptible strain (e.g. 451 vs. 499 in the CO spectrum, 426 vs 424 in the pyridine type II spectrum).

We do not mean to imply that there is any direct relationship between induced cytochromes in mammals and resistance in insects; only that the differences cannot be explained on the basis of a quantitative change in a single cytochrome.

Perry et al. (1971) also suggested, based on the peak position of the CO spectrum that qualitative differences existed between a susceptible strain and one of several resistant strains examined, Diazinon-R (this strain and Rutgers diazinon resistant are both derived from the same strain). Based primarily on EtNC, Matthews and Casida (1970) suggested qualitative differences might exist between susceptible and resistant strains and, more recently, Capdevila et al. (1973a, 1973b) have suggested, again based on EtNC spectra, that qualitative differences exist between the cytochrome P-450 of normal and phenobarbital or naphthalene induced flies of the Fc resistant strain.

It should also be noted that none of the investigations reported, from this or other laboratories, have demonstrated that changed spectral properties are due to changes in the cytochrome per se. It is possible that the changes noted are due to changes in other constituents of the microsomal membrane.

It occurred to us that since much was known of the genetics of resistance (particularly that due to oxidation metabolism) and we knew that the cytochrome involved could be different in different strains, this was an opportunity at least to approach the molecular biology of insecticide resistance. That is to say, we could try to relate specific genes to specific cytochromes and eventually to understand how the genetic makeup of the insect related to specific cytochromes P-450.

The genetics of the resistant strain we were working with, Rutgers diazinon resistant, was unknown at that time, so we needed to work with strains of known genetics. In the Fc strain, resistance was known to involve a gene on the fifth chromosome, while in the Baygon resistant strain, the gene was known to be on the second chromosome. The use of visible mutant markers (Tsukamoto, 1964) is well known. In our investigations the following recessive markers were used: stubby wings (stw), the gene for which is located on chromsome II; brown body (bwb), chromosome III; ocra eyes (ocra), chromosome V. The cytochrome P-450 of the triply marked susceptible strain (sbo) showed no significant spectral differences from the CSMA susceptible strain.

The initial study (Tate et al., 1973a) was to examine the cytochrome P-450 in flies from as many strains as possible, including some marked strains. The cytochrome P-450 levels were determined for the following strains: CSMA; Fc_{NCSU}; Fc_{Texas}; Dimethoate-R; R-Baygon, bwb, ocra, (R-chromosome II); stw, bwb, R-Fc (R-chromosome V); and stubby winged, bwb, ocra, (sbo) susceptible.

The data showed that cytochrome P-450 levels are highest in the Fc_{NCSU} and Dimethoate-R strains but only slightly higher than susceptible in Fc_{Tex} while no differences from susceptible levels could be seen in the marked Fc or marked Baygon strains. The absorption maximum was shifted to 449 in the two strains with the highest level. A simultaneous increase in microsomal protein occurs with the increase in cytochrome P-450, thus raising the possibility that one effect may be an increase in endoplasmic reticulum.

Analysis of type I (benzphetamine), type II (pyridine), type III (EtNC) and piperonyl butoxide and n-octyalmine spectra revealed that the most obvious difference in these strains is the presence or absence of detectable type I binding. The marked Fc strain, although resembling the susceptible in cytochrome P-450 level and

optimum, does resemble the other Fc strains in
having a type I binding site. The results seem
to indicate that in the Fc strain, the presence
of type I binding is related to resistance associated with chromosome V.

The presence of a double trough in the n-
octylamine spectrum is a susceptible characteristic seen also in Baygon, Fc_{Tex} and marked Fc
but not in Fc_{NCSU}.

Although Baygon has high oxidase activity
(Plapp and Casida, 1969), its P-450 seems to be
essentially the same as that in susceptible
strains, suggesting that the cytochrome is not
rate limiting and that other factors must be
examined.

A small 455 ethyl isocyanide peak seems to
be linked to the presence of a double trough in
the n-octylamine trough.

Recently (Tate et al., 1973) we have used
crossing experiments with marked strains to provide new information on the cytochrome P-450 in
resistant strains. The Rutgers diazinon resistant strain was of unkonwn genetics. We crossed
this with the marked susceptible (sbo) and then
back-crossed the F_1 progeny to the sbo strain.

High P-450, presence of type I binding,
single trough N-octylamine spectrum and low
ethylisocyanide spectrum are all associated with
the presence, in the substrains, of chromosome
II from the resistant strain, i.e. substrains
+++, ++o, +b+ and +bo. In contrast, strains
without resistant chromosomes II (s++, s+o, sb+
and sbo) show susceptible spectral characteristics. LD_{50} determinations confirm that resistance is associated primarily with chromosome
II in this strain.

In a similar examination of the Fc strain,
high P-450 levels are seen in phenotypes containing the second chromosome from the resistant
strain although much of the resistance in this
strain is due to chromosome V (Oppenoorth and
Houx, 1968; Plapp and Casida, 1969). However,
the presence of the Type I spectrum is associated with V, that is substrains +++, +b+, sb+ and

s++. A single-trough n-octylamine spectrum could not be found in the progeny nor did the ethyl isocyanide spectrum show any striking differences between the different phenotypes, suggesting that ancillary factors may be involved in the expression of these last two characters.

It is interesting to speculate on the genetics of cytochrome P-450 in the housefly. Even at this early stage in the investigations it is apparent that at least four genes (3 on chromosome II and one on chromosome V) are required to explain the spectral variants alone. Moreover, the gene on V, required for type I binding, appears to be similar to the gene for the same characteristics on II in another strain, raising the further speculation that a translocation from II to V may have occurred during the development of the Fc strain.

It is apparent that even though resistant flies may be brought about by selection for a small number of genes, the effects are modified in subtle ways by many other genes and by the genetic background of the strain with which experimental crosses are made. Some of these genes may be increasing formation of smooth endoplasmic reticulum and therefore, by force of circumstances, cytochrome P-450, while others may cause specific change in either the cytochrome P-450 molecule or in the way it is bound in the membrane.

It is apparent, however, that the genetics of cytochrome P-450 and the genetics of some types of resistance appear to be inextricably linked and that this type of analysis represents a new tool with which to explore further the mechanism of resistance at the molecular level.

CONCLUSIONS

Cytochrome P-450 and the electron transport enzymes associated with it form a mixed function oxidase system which in many organisms and tissues functions in the detoxication of

toxic compounds. Evolutionary considerations
lead one to the conclusion that the system is
adapted for increasing the polarity of a wide
range of dietary lipophilic toxicants, usually of
relatively low toxicity, but that it can also be
of importance in the detoxication of more toxic
compounds, such as pesticides.

Cytochrome P-450 appears to be fundamentally
similar wherever it occurs but there are also
enough variations that distinct differences can
be seen between species, between tissues and
between genetically different strains of the same
species.

An additional level of flexibility is provided by induction, in which many xenobiotics
can bring about an increase in the enzymes of the
mixed function oxidase system. In many cases,
large dose levels are required, particularly in
insects. In these cases doubts must be raised
concerning the physiological significance of this
phenomenon.

The presence of distinct forms of cytochrome
P-450 in genetically different strains of the
same species, the characteristics of which are
under genetic control, and the presence of analogous forms in induced animals, inclines one to
view that, at some level in the genetic transcription process, these two phenomena are related.

In summary, it may be said that living organisms possess, in the cytochrome P-450 mixed
function oxidase system, a marvellously flexible
process for the oxidation of lipophilic substrates and that the process of evolution adapted
this in many ways, in many organisms, but frequently as an aid to survival in toxic environments.

ACKNOWLEDGEMENTS

These investigations were supported in part
by Grants ES-00044 and ES-00083 from the National Institute of Environmental Health Sciences,
U. S. Public Health Services.
The collaboration, during the last several

years, of many dedicated co-workers is gratefully acknowledged. Their individual contributions are referred to in the text and references.

REFERENCES

Abernathy, C. O., E. Hodgson and F. E. Guthrie. 1971a. Biochem. Pharm. 20:2385-2393.

Abernathy, C. O., R. M. Philpot, F. E. Guthrie and E. Hodgson. 1971b. Biochem. Pharm. 20:2395-2400.

Ackermann, E., A. Rane and J. L. Ericsson. 1972. Clin. Pharm. Therap. 13:652-662.

Alvares, E. P., G. Schilling, W. Levin and R. Kuntzman. 1967. Biochem. Biophys. Res. Commun. 29:521-526.

Alvares, A. P., G. Schilling, W. Levin, R. Kuntzman, L. Brand and L. C. Mark. 1969. Clin. Pharm. Therap. 10:655-659.

Ambike, S. H. and R. M. Baxter. 1970. Phyto-chemistry 9:1959-1962.

Appleby, C. A. 1969. Biochim. Biophys. Acta 172:71-87.

Baker, R. C., L. C. Coons, R. B. Mailman and E. Hodgson. 1972. Environ. Res. 5:418-424.

Bend, J. R., G. E. R. Hook and T. E. Gram. 1973. Drug Metabol. Disposition 1:358-366.

Benke, G. M. and C. F. Wilkinson. 1971. Pestic. Biochem. Physiol. 1:19-31.

Benke, G. M., C. F. Wilkinson and J. N. Telford. 1972. J. Econ. Entomol. 65:1221-1229.

Brattsten, L. B. and C. F. Wilkinson. 1973. Pestic. Biochem. Physiol. 3:393-407.

Brodie, B. B., J. R. Gillette and H. S. Ackerman (editors). 1971. Handbook of experimental pharmacology 28/2. Concepts in biochemical pharmacology. Springer-Verlag, Berlin-New York.

Brown, R. R., J. A. Miller and E. C. Miller. 1954. J. Biol. Chem. 209:211-222.

Bunyan, P. J. and J. M. J. Page. 1973. Chem.-Biol. Inter. 6:249-257.

Bunyan, P. J., M. G. Townsend and A. Taylor. 1972. Chem.-Biol. Inter. 5:13-26.

Capdevila, J., A. Morello, A. S. Perry and M. Agosin. 1973a. Biochem. 12:1445-1451.

Capdevila, J., A. S. Perry, A. Morello and M. Agosin. 1973b. Biochim. Biophys. Acta 314:93-103.

Cardini, G. and P. Jurtshuk. 1968. J. Biol. Chem. 243:6070-6072.

Conney, A. H. 1967. Pharm. Rev. 19:317-362.

Cooper, D. Y., H. Schleyer, S. S. Levin and C. Rosenthal. 1971. Abstracts 162nd Amer. Chem. Soc. Natl. Meeting.

Cram, R. L., and J. R. Fouts. 1967. Biochem. Pharm. 16:1001-1006.

Davis, J. E., M. F. Cranmer and A. J. Peoples. 1973. Anal. Biochem. 53:522-530.

Diehl, H., J. Schadelin and V. Ullrich. 1970. Hoppe-Seylers Z. Physiol. Chem. 351:1359-1371.

Estabrook, R. W., D. Y. Cooper and O. Resenthal. 1963. Biochem. Z. 338:741-755.

Estabrook, R. W., J. R. Gillette and K. C. Leibman. (editors). 1973. 2nd Internatl. Symp. Microsomes and Drug Oxidations. Drug Metabol. Disposition 1:1-486.

Flynn, E. J., M. Lynch and V. G. Zannoni. 1972. Biochem. Pharm. 21:2577-2590.

Folsom, M. D., L. G. Hansen, R. M. Philpot, R. S. H. Yang, W. C. Dauterman and E. Hodgson. 1970. Life Sci. 9:869-875.

Folsom, M. D., R. M. Philpot and E. Hodgson. 1971. Comp. Biochem. Physiol. 39B:589-597.

Fouts, J. R. 1963. Ann. N. Y. Acad. Sci. 104:875-880.

Fouts, J. R. 1973. Drug. Metabol. Disposition 1:380-385.

Franklin, M. R. 1971. Xenobiotica 1:581-591.

Franklin, M. R. 1972a. Xenobiotica 2:517-527.

Franklin, M. R. 1972b. Biochem. Pharm. 21:3287-3300.

Fukami, J., T. Shishido, K. Fukunaga and J. E. Casida. 1969. J. Agr. Food Chem. 17:1217-1226.

Garfinkel, D. 1958. Arch. Biochem. Biophys. 77:
    493-509.
Garfinkel, D. 1963. Comp. Biochem. Physiol. 8:
    367-379.
Green, F. E. and J. T. Stevens. 1973. In:
    Pesticides and the environment: a continuing
    controversy (W. B. Deichmann, editor).
    Intercontinental Medical Book Corp., N. Y.
    and London. pp. 167-178.
Hammond, R. K. and D. C. White. 1970. J.
    Bacteriol. 103:607-610.
Hansen, A. R. and J. R. Fouts. 1968. Toxicol.
    Appl. Pharm. 13:212-219.
Hansen, A. R. and J. R. Fouts. 1971. Biochem.
    Pharm. 20:3125-3143.
Harding, B. W., S. H. Wong and D. Y. Nelson.
    1964. Biochim. Biophys. Acta 92:415-417.
Hart, L. G. and J. R. Fouts. 1965. Arch. Exptl.
    Path. Pharm. 249:486-500.
Hildebrandt, A., H. Remmer and R. W. Estabrook.
    1968. Biochem. Biophys. Res. Commun. 30:
    607-612.
Hodgson, E. and F. W. Plapp. 1970. J. Agr. Food
    Chem. 18:1048-1055.
Hodgson, E. and R. M. Philpot. 1974. Drug
    Metabol. Revs. in press.
Hodgson, E., L. G. Tate, A. P. Kulkarni and F.
    W. Plapp. 1974. J. Agr. Food Chem. in
    press.
Hodgson, E., R. M. Philpot, R. C. Baker and R.
    B. Mailman. 1973. Drug. Metabol. Dispo-
    sition 1:391-398.
Holtzman, J. L. 1973. Fed. Proc. 32:762.
Imai, Y. and R. Sato. 1967. J. Biochem. 62:
    464-473.
Jacobsson, S. V. and D. L. Cinti. 1973. J.
    Pharm. Exptl. Therap. 185:226-234.
Jefcoate, C. R. E., J. L. Gaylor and R. Calabreze.
    1969a. Biochemistry 8:3455-3463.
Jefcoate, C. R. E. and J. L. Gaylor. 1969b.
    Biochem. 8:3464-3472.
Joyce, G. H. and D. C. White. 1971. J.
    Bacteriol. 106:403-411.

Katagiri, M., B. N. Ganguli and I. C. Gunsalus.
    1968. J. Biol. Chem. 243:3543-3546.
Khan, M. A. Q. and E. Hodgson. 1967. J. Insect
    Physiol. 13:653-664.
Khan, M. A. Q. and F. Matsumura. 1972. Pestic.
    Biochem. Physiol. 2:236-243.
Khan, M. A. Q., W. Coello, A. A. Khan and H.
    Pinto. 1972a. Life Sci. 11(2):405-415.
Khan, M. A. Q., A. Kamal, R. J. Wolin and J.
    Runnels. 1972b. Bull. Environ. Contam.
    Toxicol. 8:219-228.
Klingenberg, M. 1958. Arch. Biochem. Biophys.
    75:376-386.
Krieger, R. I. and C. F. Wilkinson. 1970. J.
    Econ. Entomol. 63:1343-1344.
Krieger, R. I., M. D. Gilbert and C. F. Wilkin-
    son. 1970. J. Econ. Entomol. 63:1322-1323.
Krieger, R. I., P. P. Feeny and C. F. Wilkinson.
    1971. Science 172:579-581.
Kuhr, R. J. 1971. J. Econ. Entomol. 64:1373-
    1378.
Kulkarni, A. P. and E. Hodgson. 1973. Cyto-
    chrome P-450 and mixed function oxidase
    activities: comparative aspects. in
    preparation.
Kulkarni, A. P., R. B. Mailman, R. C. Baker
    and E. Hodgson. 1973a. Cytochrome P-450
    difference spectra: type II interactions in
    insecticide resistant and susceptible house-
    flies. Submitted to Drug Metabol. Disposi-
    tion.
Kulkarni, A. P., R. B. Mailman and E. Hodgson.
    1973b. Cytochrome P-450 optical difference
    spectra of insecticides: a comparative
    study. in preparation.
Kulkarni, A. P., R. B. Mailman and E. Hodgson.
    1973c. Interaction of insecticide syner-
    gists with cytochrome P-450 from the house-
    fly, Musca domestica. in preparation.
Kuntzman, R. 1969. Ann. Rev. Pharm. 9:21-36.
Kuwatsuka, S. 1970. Biochemical aspects of
    methylenedioxyphenyl compounds in relation
    to the synergistic action. In Biochemical
    Toxicology of Insecticides (R. D. O'Brien

and I. Yamamoto, editors). Academic Press, N. Y. pp. 131-144.

Lake, B. G. and D. V. Parke. 1971. Biochem. J. 127:23P.

Lebault, J. M., E. T. Lode and M. J. Coon. 1971. Biochem. Biophys. Res. Commun. 42:413-419.

Lu, A. Y. H., S. B. West, D. Ryan and W. Levin. 1973. Drug Metabol. Disposition 1:29-39.

Machinist, J. M., E. W. Dehner and D. M. Ziegler. 1968. Arch. Biochem. Biophys 125:858-864.

Machino, A., H. Inano and B. Tamaoki. 1969. J. Steroid Chem. 1:9-16.

Mailman, R. B. and E. Hodgson. 1972. Bull. Environ. Contam. Toxicol. 8:186-192.

Mailman, R. B., A. P. Kulkarni, R. C. Baker and E. Hodgson. 1973. Cytochrome P-450 difference spectra: effect of chemical structure on type II spectra in mouse hepatic microsomes. Submitted to Drug Metabol. Disposition.

Mailman, R. B., R. C. Baker and E. Hodgson. 1972. Abstracts 162nd Amer. Chem. Soc. Natl. Meeting.

Markham, A., G. C. Hartman and D. V. Parke. 1972. Biochem. J. 130:90P.

Matthews, H. B., and J. E. Casida. 1970. Life Sci. 9(1):989-1001.

Matthews, H. B., M. Skrinjaric-Spoljar, and J. E. Casida. 1970. Life Sci. 9:1039-1048.

Mayer, R. T., A. E. Wade and M. R. I. Soliman. 1973. J. Agr. Food Chem. 21:360-362.

Meehan, T. D. and C. J. Coscia. 1973. Biochem. Biophys. Res. Commun. 53:1043-1048.

Meigs, R. A. and K. J. Ryan. 1968. Biochim. Biophys. Acta 165:476-482.

Mitani, F., A. P. Alvares, S. Sassa and A. Kappas. 1971. Mol. Pharm. 7:280-292.

Morello, A., W. Bleecker and M. Agosin. 1971. Biochem. J. 124:199-205.

Omura, T. and R. Sato. 1964a. J. Biol. Chem. 239:2370-2379.

Omura, T. and R. Sato. 1964b. J. Biol. Chem. 239:2379-2385.

Omura, T., R. Sato, D. Y. Cooper, O. Rosenthal and R. W. Estabrook. 1965. Fed. Proc. 24:1181-1189.

Oppenoorth, F. J., N. W. H. Houx. 1968. Entomol. Exptl. Appl. 11:81-93.

Orrenius, S., A. Ellin, S. V. Jakobsson, H. Thor, D. L. Cinti, J. B. Schenkman and R. W. Estabrook. 1973. Drug. Metabol. Disposition 1:350-356.

Parke, D. V. and H. Rahman. 1971. Biochem. J. 123:9-10P.

Perry, A. S. and A. J. Bucknor. 1970. Life Sci. 9:335-350.

Perry, A. S., W. E. Dale and A. J. Bucknor. 1971. Pestic. Biochem. Physiol. 1:131-142.

Philpot, R. M. and E. Hodgson. 1971a. Chem.-Biol. Inter. 4:399-408.

Philpot, R. M. and E. Hodgson. 1971b. Life Sci. 10:503-512.

Philpot, R. M. and E. Hodgson. 1971c. Chem.-Biol. Inter. 4:185-194.

Philpot, R. M. and E. Hodgson. 1972. Mol. Pharm. 8:204-214.

Plapp, F. W. and J. E. Casida. 1969. J. Econ. Entomol. 62:1174-1179.

Plapp, F. W., Jr., and J. E. Casida. 1970. J. Econ. Entomol. 63:1091-1092.

Price, G. M. and R. J. Kuhr. 1971. Biochem. J. 112:133-138.

Ray, J. W. 1965. Pest infestation research. Her Majesties Stationery Office, London.

Ray, J. W. 1967. Biochem. Pharm. 16:99-108.

Remmer, H., R. W. Estabrook, J. B. Schenkman and H. Greim. 1968. Induction of microsomal liver enzymes. In Enzymatic oxidation of toxicants (E. Hodgson, editor). North Carolina State University.

Remmer, H., J. B. Schenkman, R. W. Estabrook, H. Sasame, J. R. Gillette, S. Narasimhula, D. Cooper and O. Rosenthal. 1966. Mol. Pharm. 2:187-190.

Roth, J. A. and R. A. Neal. 1972. Biochem. 11:955-961.

258

Sato, R., H. Satake and Y. Imai. 1973. Drug Metabol. Disposition 1:6-12.

Schenkman, J. B., H. Remmer and R. W. Estabrook. 1967. Mol. Pharm. 3:113-123.

Schenkman, J. B., D. L. Cinti, P. W. Moldeus and S. Orrenius. 1973. Drug Metabol. Disposition 1:111-119.

Shoeman, D. W., M. D. Chaplin and G. J. Mannering. 1969. Mol. Pharm. 5:412-419.

Skrinjaric-Spoljar, M., H. B. Matthews, J. L. Engel and J. E. Casida. 1971. Biochem. Pharm. 20:1607-1618.

Sladek, N. E. and G. J. Mannering. 1966. Biochem. Biophys. Res. Commun. 24:668-674.

Springfield, A. C., G. P. Carlson and J. J. Defeo. 1973. Toxicol. Appl. Pharm. 24: 298-308.

Stevens, J. T., F. E. Green, R. E. Stitzel and J. T. McPhillips. 1973. Effects of anti-cholinesterase insecticides on mouse and rat liver microsomal mixed function oxidases. In: Pesticides and the environment: a continuing controversy. (W. B. Deichmann, editor) Intercontinental Medical Book Corp., N. Y. and London. pp. 498-501.

Tate, L. G., F. W. Plapp and E. Hodgson. 1973a. Chem. Biol. Inter 6:237-247.

Tate, L. G., F. W. Plapp and E. Hodgson. 1973b. Biochem. Genet. in press.

Terriere, L. C. 1973. The induction of detoxifying enzymes in insects. J. Agr. Food Chem. in press.

Terriere, L. C. and S. J. Yu. 1973. Pestic. Biochem. Physiol. 3:96-107.

Terriere, L. C., S. J. Yu and R. Hoyer. 1971. Science 171:581.

Tsai, R., A. Yu, I. C. Gunsalus, J. Peisach, W. Blumberg, W. M. Orme-Johnson and H. Beinert. 1970. Proc. Natl. Acad. Sci. 66:1157-1167.

Tsukamoto, M. 1964. Botyu-Kagaku 29:51-59.

Walker, C. R. and L. C. Terriere. 1970. Entomol. Exptl. Appl. 13:260-274.

Wilkinson, C. F. 1971. Insecticide synergists
and their mode of action. Proc. 2nd Internatl. I.U.P.A.C. Congr. on Pesticide Chem.
2:117-159.
Wilkinson, C. F. and L. B. Brattsten. 1972.
Drug. Metabol. Rev. 1:153-228.
Williamson, R. L. and M. S. Schecter. 1970.
Biochem. Pharm. 19:1719-1727.
Wilson, B. J. and S. Orrenius. 1972. Biochim.
Biophys. Acta 261:94-101.
Wilson, T. G. and E. Hodgson. 1971a. Insect
Biochem. 1:19-26.
Wilson, T. G. and E. Hodgson. 1971b. Insect
Biochem. 1:171-180.
Yaffe, S. J., A. Rane, F. Sjoqvist, L. O. Boreus
and S. Orrenius. 1970. Life Sci. 9(2):
1189-1200.
Yu, S. J. and L. C. Terriere. 1971. Life Sci.
10(2):1173-1185.
Yu, S. J. and L. C. Terriere. 1972. Pestic.
Biochem. Physiol. 2:184-190.
Yu, S. J. and L. C. Terriere. 1973. Pestic.
Biochem. Physiol. 3:141-148.

1. NIA 16824 is 2-methylpropyl 2-propynyl phenylphosphonate, WL 19255 is 5,6-dichloro-1,2-benzothiadiazole, RO5-8019 is 2-(2,4,5-trichlorophenyl)-propynyl ether and MGK 264 is N-(2-ethylhexyl)-5-norbornene-2,3-dicarboximide.

MAMMALIAN ARYL HYDROCARBON HYDROXYLASES IN CELL CULTURES:
MECHANISM OF INDUCTION AND ROLE IN CARCINOGENESIS

Friedrich J. Wiebel, James P. Whitlock, Jr. and
Harry V. Gelboin

Chemistry Branch
National Cancer Institute
National Institutes of Health

Abstract

Aromatic polycyclic hydrocarbons are ubiquitous environmental pollutants. Several polycyclic hydrocarbons are
carcinogenic in experimental animals and are thought to be
carcinogenic in man. Polycyclic hydrocarbons are primarily
metabolized by microsomal enzyme complexes which belong to
the group of "mixed-function oxygenases". These aryl hydrocarbon hydroxylases are present and inducible in most
mammalian tissues.

The mechanism of hydroxylase induction has been studied
in cells in culture. Induction requires continuous protein
synthesis and transitory RNA synthesis. The synthesis,
transfer, and functioning of induction-specific RNA is independent of concurrent ribosomal RNA synthesis. Enzyme
activity may also be regulated at the post-transcriptional
level. The relative importance of transcriptional and post-
transcriptional control mechanisms varies between different
cell types.

Using the synthetic flavonoid 7,8-benzoflavone as a
probe, at least two forms of aryl hydrocarbon hydroxylase
can be distinguished. The relative activities of these two
forms varies with the age, sex, state of induction, nutrition
and tissue of animals.

Several observations indicate that microsomal oxygenases
convert polycyclic hydrocarbons not only to inactive metabolites, but also to derivatives which are toxic and carcinogenic: 1) The covalent binding of polycyclic hydrocarbons to
DNA is catalyzed by microsomal enzymes 2) Inhibition of
enzyme activity by 7,8-benzoflavone inhibits polycyclic

261

hydrocarbon-induced cytotoxicity. 3) Inhibition of enzyme activity inhibits cutaneous tumorigenesis by 7,12-dimethylbenz[a]anthracene, but not by benzo[a]pyrene. The role which the aryl hydrocarbon hydroxylases play in polycyclic hydrocarbon carcinogenesis may differ for individual hydrocarbons.

Introduction

Man-made pollutants of the environment are ever increasing threats to living organisms. A major mechanism of defense against toxic environmental chemicals in vertebrates and lower organisms is the NADPH-dependent "mixed-function" oxygenase systems. These enzyme systems consist of cytochrome P-450 and electron transporting chain, and lipid component(s) (Lu, et al., 1968; Estabrook, 1974). The microsomal oxygenases are present in most tissues of mammals (Conney, 1967; Gelboin, 1967; Nebert and Gelboin, 1969). They metabolize and are inducible by a wide spectrum of exogenous compounds including pesticides, drugs, and food additives and endogenous substrates such as steroids (Remmer, 1962; Gillette, 1963; Conney, 1967). The inducing compounds have been divided into two major groups, typified by phenobarbital and a polycyclic hydrocarbon, such as 3-methylcholanthrene or benz[a]anthracene, according to their tissue specificity and their selective effect on various oxygenases (Gillette, 1963; Conney, 1967).

The present report is concerned with the microsomal oxygenases metabolizing polycyclic hydrocarbons, the "aryl hydrocarbon hydroxylases" (AHH). Polycyclic hydrocarbons are ubiquitous environmental pollutants produced mainly by incomplete combustion of fuels, wood, and other organic materials. A number of polycyclic hydrocarbons are highly carcinogenic in experimental animals.

The level of oxygenase activity and function depends on a number of variables of which the inducibility and the occurence of different forms are prominent factors. The following describes our studies on the existence and distribution of different forms of aryl hydrocarbon hydroxylases in experimental animals and examines the mechanism of induction in mammalian cells in culture.

Microsomal oxygenases convert chemicals not only to less harmful derivatives, but in the process may form active intermediates which are toxic and carcinogenic. Part of this presentation will be concerned with the role of aryl hydrocarbon hydroxylases in the biological effect of polycyclic

262

hydrocarbons. Our observations suggest that the enzyme system may be responsible for the activation of polycyclic hydrocarbons to cytotoxic and carcinogenic forms.

Microsomal Benzo[a]pyrene Metabolism

Our studies of polycyclic hydrocarbon metabolism have concentrated on benzo[a]pyrene (BP) for several reasons: 1) BP is a major environmental pollutant. 2) BP is carcinogenic in experimental animals and may be carcinogenic in man. 3) BP-hydroxylation is the basis for an extremely sensitive assay of the microsomal mixed-function oxygenase, aryl hydrocarbon(benzo[a]pyrene)-hydroxylase (AHH).

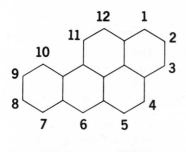

BENZO(a)PYRENE METABOLITES

7, 8 DIHYDRO 7, 8 DIOL

9, 10 DIHYDRO 9, 10 DIOL

4, 5 DIHYDRO 4, 5 DIOL

3 HYDROXY

9 HYDROXY

1, 6 QUINONE

3, 6 QUINONE

Fig. 1. Benzo[a]pyrene metabolites formed by microsomes of rat liver.

Metabolites formed from BP by microsomes of rat liver are listed in Figure 1. They include three dihydrodiols, two phenols, and two quinones (Kinoshita and Gelboin, 1973). Extrapolation from the metabolism of other less complex polycyclic hydrocarbons (Jerina et al., 1970 and 1971; Selkirk et al., 1971) suggests that microsomal enzymes may convert BP to epoxides, which may be either nonenzymatically rearranged to phenols or enzymatically hydrated to dihydrodiols and conjugated, e.g., with glutathione.

Epoxides of BP have not been isolated as products of the microsomal oxidases, and it may be that other species are the reactive intermediates in BP phenol and dihydrodiol formation. The hydroxylated BP products are further metabolized by microsomal oxygenases and/or soluble conjugases (Selkirk, Wiebel, and Gelboin, unpublished).

3-Hydroxy-BP forms a major fraction of the organic-soluble metabolites. The high degree of fluorescence of the phenol and the ease of its extraction by alkali permits the measurement of picomole amounts of BP phenols in biological materials. This sensitive assay provides a tool for studying the characteristics of BP hydroxylases in cells and tissues having low enzyme activities. Since the metabolism of many polycyclic hydrocarbons closely resembles that of BP (Sims, 1970a), hydroxylation of BP is used as an indicator for the presence and inducibility of the aryl hydrocarbon hydroxylases.

Regulation of Aryl Hydrocarbon Hydroxylase (AHH)

We have studied the regulation of AHH activity in cells in culture because such systems permit the observation of regulatory processes under better controlled conditions (Alfred et al., 1967; Nebert and Gelboin, 1968a,b, 1969, 1970; Wiebel et al., 1972a,b).

Table 1 indicates the variety of cells in culture that exhibit AHH activity, reflecting the nearly ubiquitous presence of the enzyme in vivo. Enzyme activity occurs in cells from rodents, man, chick, from adult and embryonic organisms, from hepatic and extrahepatic tissues and in normal and transformed cells. Cell lines devoid of any AHH activity, e.g. HTC-cells or B82-fibroblasts (Table 1) are very rare. The hydroxylase is inducible in those cells having detectable basal enzyme activity (Table 1).

Fig. 2 shows the kinetics of AHH induction at different inducer concentrations. We routinely used benz[a]anthracene (BA) as inducer, since this compound is relatively non-toxic.

The following summarizes what has been learned about the induction of AHH in cells in culture: 1) The inducer is rapidly incorporated into the cell. 2) There is an initial lag period of about 30 min. before enzyme activity increases. 3) Induction requires continuous protein synthesis. 4) Induction requires RNA synthesis initially, but not continuously. 5) This RNA synthesis is independent of protein synthesis. (Nebert and Gelboin, 1968b,1970).

Typical experiments with cultured cells that demonstrate

264

Table 1. Aryl hydrocarbon hydroxylase induction in various
cell cultures*

	Aryl Hydrocarbon Hydroxylase (Specific Activity)*	
Cell cultures	Control	BA-Induced*

Secondaries

Hamster (fetal)[c]	80	600
Mouse (fetal)[a]	8	240
Rat (fetal)[a]	30	100
Chick (fetal)[a]	5	13

Cell lines

BRL, liver (rat)[c]	9	130
HTC, hepatoma (rat)[a]	< 1	< 1
3T3-4C2, fibroblasts (mouse)[b]	10	75
L-A9, fibroblasts (mouse)[b]	< 1	< 1
FIII, fibroblasts (rat)[d]	1	12
HeLa (human)	17	300
JEG-3, choriocarcinoma (human)[b]	4	150
VA-2, SV40-transformed (human)[b]	< 1	1.3
Lymphocytes (human)[c]	< 1	1.5
Lymphocytes, mitogen treated[c]	2	12

* Cell cultures were exposed to BA-containing medium for
18 to 24 hours. AHH activity was determined as described
by Nebert and Gelboin, 1968. Specific activity is given
as $\mu\mu$moles of phenolic product/mg protein/30 min.

a-c Description and references to cell cultures are found
in: a) Nebert and Gelboin, 1968. b) Wiebel et al., 1972.
c) This paper. d) Cells were obtained from
Dr. G. DiMayorca, University of Illinois, Chicago.

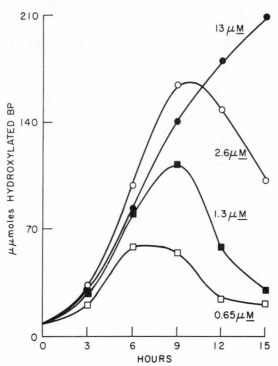

Fig. 2. Kinetics of induction of aryl hydrocarbon hydroxylase
in hamster embryo cells by various levels of benz[a]-
anthracene (BA). Secondaries of monolayer cultures
were exposed to medium containing BA. Collection of
cells, homogenization and assay of aryl hydrocarbon
hydroxylase activity were previously described
(Nebert and Gelboin, 1968).

the requirements for macromolecular synthesis in AHH induction are shown half-schematically in Fig. 3. Cycloheximide
(CY), at a concentration which inhibits protein synthesis
by 95%, completely inhibits AHH induction (BA + CY). Likewise, inhibition of RNA synthesis by actinomycin D (BA +
Act D) prevents the rise in AHH activity. However, there is
an essential temporal difference in the effects of these
inhibitors. Inhibition of protein synthesis at any time
during the induction process halts further increase in enzyme
activity, indicating that induction requires continuous protein synthesis. In contrast, the induction process is not
continuously sensitive to actinomycin D. Thus, when cells
are initially exposed to the inducer plus cycloheximide (BA +
CY to arrow) and the cycloheximide is then removed, actinomycin
D no longer inhibits the increase in enzyme activity (BA +

266

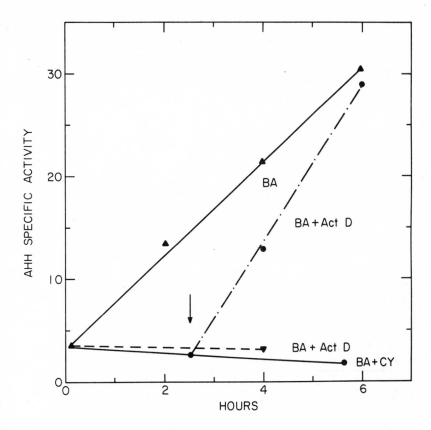

Fig. 3. Requirement for RNA and protein synthesis for aryl hydrocarbon hydroxylase induction. Cultures of the mouse spleen-thymus cell line, JLSV5, were exposed to medium containing 3 ug/ml benz[a]anthracene. Another set of cultures was incubated with medium containing BA and 10 ug/ml of cycloheximide (BA + CY). The medium was removed from some of these cultures (see arrow) and replaced by medium containing BA and 1 ug/ml actinomycin D (BA + Act. D). A third set of cultures was incubated with the BA and Act D containing medium throughout the experimental period. AHH specific activity is given as uu moles of hydroxylated product/mg protein/30 min. Other conditions as described in the text and under Fig. 2.

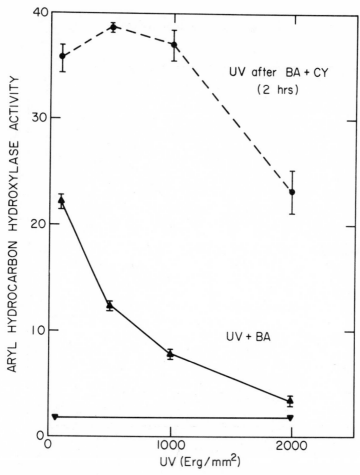

Fig. 4. Effect of UV-irradiation on aryl hydrocarbon hydroxylase induction in JLSV5 cells. Medium was
removed from cultures and cells were UV-irradiated
for various time periods. Immediately after irradiation cells were incubated with medium containing 13 uM BA for 3 hours (▲——————▲ BA + UV).
Another set of cultures was treated identically
except that a 2-hour exposure to medium containing
BA and 10 ug/ml cycloheximide preceded the UV-irradiation (●—————● UV after BA + CY). Control
cultures were grown in medium without addition of
inhibitors or inducers (▼——————▼). AHH activity
is expressed as uu moles of product/mg protein/30
min. Other conditions as described under Fig. 2
and in Wiebel et al., 1972b.

Act D from arrow). This indicates that induction does not require continuous RNA synthesis and that the required transcription can take place in the absence of translation.

The requirement for RNA synthesis can also be demonstrated by the effects of UV-irradiation on cultured cells. UV-irradiation causes damage to DNA (Setlow and Setlow, 1963; Kanazir, 1969) and impairs DNA-template activity. The effects on AHH induction of UV-irradiation (Fig. 4) are similar to those of actinomycin D (compare Fig. 3): a) when UV is applied shortly before the addition of inducer (UV + BA), induction is strongly inhibited with increasing doses of UV, b) when UV is applied after a two-hour exposure to the inducer plus cycloheximide (UV after BA + CY), induction proceeds unimpeded over the subsequent 3-hour period, and some inhibition is observed only at the highest UV-dose, 2000 erg/mm^2. UV-irradiation of 1000 and 2000 erg/mm^2 inhibited the incorporation of ^3H-uridine into RNA over a 3-hour period by 50% and 75% respectively. These data support the conclusions drawn from the studies using actinomycin D, namely that induction requires the synthesis of RNA that accumulates and directs the translation of induction-specific proteins.

Nature of the RNA Species Required for AHH Induction.

Gel electrophoretic analysis of RNA from control and induced cells in culture did not reveal any differences in RNA profiles (Younger et al., 1972).

We have studied the effect of various low doses of actinomycin D on both AHH induction and RNA synthesis (Fig. 5). Actinomycin D at a concentration of 0.03 µg/ml selectively inhibits the appearance of newly-formed ribosomal RNA in the cytoplasm, but has no inhibitory effect on AHH induction. Actinomycin D at low concentrations also selectively supresses the synthesis of nuclear ribosomal RNA precursors (Wiebel et al., 1972b). Several conclusions may be drawn from the findings shown in Fig. 5: a) The essentially complete absence of newly-formed rRNA during enzyme induction indicates that RNA does not specify the synthesis of induction-related protein. b) Since actinomycin D concentrations that inhibit induction do not affect the synthesis of low molecular weight RNA (4-7S), it is unlikely that these species contain the induction-specific RNA. c) The correlation of inhibition of AHH induction with the inhibition of appearance of newly-formed heterogeneous RNA in the cytoplasm suggests that the

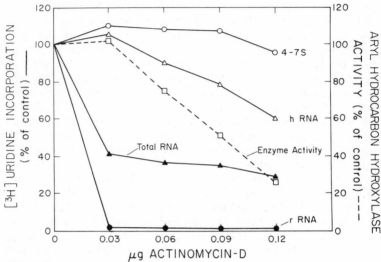

Fig. 5.

Correlation of aryl hydrocarbon hydroxylase induction and [³H]-uridine incorporation into cytoplasmic RNA: effect of low concentrations of actinomycin D. JLSV₅ cultures were exposed to growth medium free of Act. D at various concentrations (0.03-0.12 ug/ml) or growth medium free of Act. D for 90 min. Then BA was added in 0.5 ml of medium to give a final 0.5 ug/ml simultaneously with 250 u Ci of [³H]-uridine, and cultures were incubated for another 180 min. At the end of this period, AHH activity and [³H]-uridine incorporation was measured. Cells were fractionated and cytoplasmic RNA was isolated as described by Wiebel et al., 1972b. Acrylamideagarose gel eletrophoresis of RNA samples was performed following the method of Peacock and Dingman, (1968). "Total RNA" represents trichloroacetic acid precipitable material in the cytoplasmic fraction. The amount of radioactivity in ribosomal RNA (rRNA), low molecular weight RNA (4S-7S), and heterodisperse RNA (h-RNA) was determined from electrophoretograms. The amount of h-RNA was derived by subtraction of counts comprising the peaks of rRNA and 4S-7S RNA from the total counts in the electrophoretic fractions. AHH activity and radioactivity in RNA fractions from Act D treated cultures are expressed as percent of control, i.e., of corresponding activities in cultures not exposed to Act D. Aryl hydrocarbon hydroxylase activity was determined as described previously (Wiebel et al., 1972b).

induction-specific RNA is contained in this fraction, which is usually associated with messenger RNA.

Post-Transcriptional Regulation of AHH Induction.

The preceding data suggest that AHH induction is regulated at the level of transcription. Additional observations (Fig. 6) indicate that the regulation of enzyme activity is more complex.

Enzyme activity decreases rapidly when inducer is removed from preinduced cultures (Fig. 6). The rate of decay is virtually the same in the presence or absence of cycloheximide. This indicates that induction-specific protein synthesis ceases upon removal of the inducer. As shown in Fig. 3, induction-specific RNA accumulates in sufficient amounts and has a sufficiently long half-life to direct protein synthesis for several hours. This is supported by the observation that in fully-induced cultures (22 hr) inhibition of RNA synthesis does not result in a decrease in enzyme activity for at least 3 hr. The cessation of specific protein synthesis while the induction-related RNA is still present suggests that the inducer is essential for the continuous functioning of the induction-specific RNA, i.e., that the inducer also may act at a post-transcriptional level. This might occur by more than one mechanism. Fig. 6 shows that when protein synthesis and enzyme synthesis are inhibited by cycloheximide, the decay of preinduced enzyme activity is slower in the presence of inducer than in its absence. Since most, if not all, of the inducing compounds are also substrates of the enzyme complex, this phenomenon might be due to some form of substrate-stabilization of the enzyme. Examination of the heat sensitivity of the enzyme complex in the presence and absence of its substrates, including benz[a]anthracene, showed that substrates protect partially against heat inactivation (Wiebel and Gelboin, unpublished observations). The relative importance of these post-transcriptional control mechanisms is not yet known. In the cells described above they do not seem to be of major significance.

Induction by Temporary Inhibition of Protein Synthesis.

Observations in other cells in culture indicate that the mode of regulation varies considerably between different cell strains (Whitlock and Gelboin, 1973). Fig. 7 shows the induction of AHH by benz[a]anthracene in Buffalo rat liver cells

271

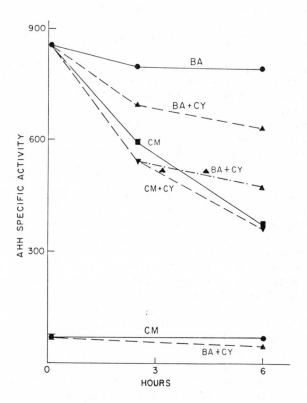

Fig. 6. The decay of aryl hydrocarbon hydroxylase activity
in hamster embryo cell cultures and the stabilization
by benz[a]anthracene. Secondary cultures were exposed to benz[a]anthracene (3 ug/ml medium) for 16
hours. The medium was replaced by conditioned
medium from cell cultures of the same age without
any additions (=CM) or with cycloheximide (=CM + CY),
benz[a]anthracene (=BA) or benz[a]anthracene and
cycloheximide (=BA + CY). The two bottom lines show
the AHH activity in previously untreated cultures
incubated with control medium or medium containing
benz[a]anthracene and cycloheximide (=BA + CY).
Cycloheximide was used at a final concentration of
10 ug/ml medium. Cultures were washed three times
with the appropriate medium prior to the change of
medium.

and the effect of a temporary block of protein synthesis on the enzyme level. Without adding an inducer, protein synthesis was inhibited for 4 hours and then allowed to resume. Following this treatment, AHH activity increases rapidly and to a much greater extent than after exposure to the inducer alone (Fig. 7). Combined induction by benz[a]anthracene and temporary inhibition of protein synthesis causes an increase in enzyme activity that is greater than the sum of the enzyme increases caused by either one alone (Fig. 7). This synergistic effect suggests that two different mechanisms of AHH induction are operative. Induction by temporary inhibition of protein synthesis occurs to lesser degrees in other cell types (Whitlock and Gelboin, 1973). The findings suggest that in these liver cells there are short-lived proteins, which regulate the level of enzyme activity, possibly through a mechanism analogous to that postulated by Tomkins and co-workers (1969) for the regulation of tyrosine aminotransferase. It might be that the repressor-activity of these presumed proteins is counteracted by the inducer, allowing the synthesis of the induction-specific protein (Fig. 6).

Even though our understanding of the mechanism of AHH induction is incomplete, it is apparent that there are various levels of regulation and that their relative importance differs for different cell types and, presumably, for different tissues as well.

Tissue Specific Induction In Vivo.

The diversity of the regulatory mechanisms that we find in tissue culture appears to occur in vivo as well. Mouse strains differ greatly in constitutive levels of hepatic AHH and inducibility (Nebert and Gelboin, 1969; Kodama and Bock, 1970), and it has been postulated that inducibility is an "all-or-none" phenomenon in all tissues of a given mouse strain (Nebert et al., 1972; Gielen et al., 1972). Recent studies have shown that the regulation of inducibility is more complex (Wiebel et al., 1973; Burki et al., 1973). Fig. 8 demonstrates that a single injection of benz[a]anthracene causes a rapid induction of AHH in the liver of C57 BL/6N mice, but has no apparent effect on the hydroxylase of DBA/2N mice. In contrast, AHH activities in lung and kidney from both C57 and DBA mice are induced several-fold after benz[a]-anthracene. This tissue-specific inducibility is also found in other strains of mice and for a number of extrahepatic tissues (Table 2): In four strains of mice, in which hepatic

273

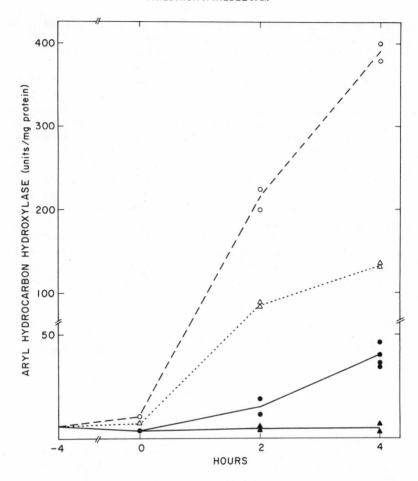

Fig. 7. Aryl hydrocarbon hydroxylase activity in BRL cells exposed to: control medium alone (▲——▲); control medium followed by medium containing benz[a]anthracene (●———●); medium containing cycloheximide, followed by medium containing actinomycin D (△- - - -▲); medium containing benz[a]anthracene plus cycloheximide, followed by medium containing benz-[a]anthracene plus actinomycin D (○— —○). Following initial treatment, each plate received two 15-min washes with the second medium. One unit of AHH corresponds to 1 uu mole of phenolic product/mg protein/30 min. (Whitlock and Gelboin, 1973).

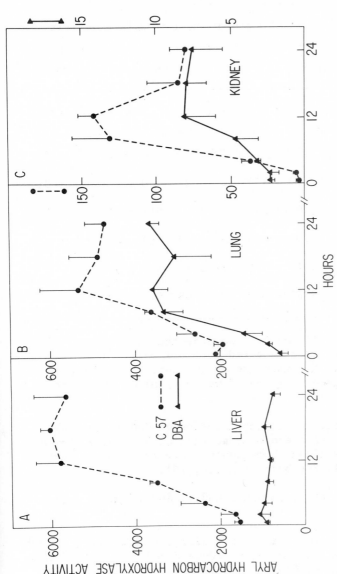

Fig. 8. Aryl hydrocarbon hydroxylase induction in liver, lung, and kidney of C57BL/6N and DBA/2N mice. Benz[a]anthracene (100 mg/kg) was injected intra-peritoneally in 0.2 ml of corn oil. The animals were sacrificed at various times after injection and AHH activity was determined in tissue homogenates as described (Wiebel et al., 1973). AHH activity is expressed as pmoles of phenolic product formed/mg of protein/30 min. The numbers of animals/group were three at 2,4,6 hr and six at 0,12, 18,24 hr. Horizontal bars represent standard deviations. Notice the different scales on the ordinate in C for C57BL/6N (●———●) and DBA/2N (▲———▲).

275

Table 2. Inducibility of aryl hydrocarbon hydroxylase
strains (Wiebel et al., 1973)

	Aryl hydrocarbon hydroxylase activity				
Strain	Liver		Lung		Small
	Control	BA	Control	BA	Control
NZB	3080 ± 1430[c]	2500 ± 470	27 ± 10	300 ± 32	2.0 ± 0.5
NZW	2090 ± 200	2970 ± 153	37 ± 23	460 ± 84	4.7 ± 0.5
AKR	1810 ± 560	2808 ± 241	47 ± 3	514 ± 36	2.7 ± 1.2
SJL	2090 ± 430	1790 ± 370	35 ± 12	260 ± 21	2.5 ± 0.2
DBA	920 ± 90	995 ± 155	56 ± 14	350 ± 30	--
C57	1550 ± 150	5760 ± 500	208 ± 65	540 ± 99	--

[a]Benz[a]anthracene (100 mg/kg) was injected ip in 0.2 ml of
corn oil. Control mice received corn oil only. Animals
were sacrificed 12 hr later and enzyme activities were determined in homogenates (0.5–1.2 mg protein) of the various
tissues.

[b]Sixteen hours after topical application of 300 ug benz[a]-
anthracene in 0.2 ml acetone or acetone alone to the shaven
backs. Cutaneous tissue homogenates were prepared as described previously (Gelboin et al., 1970).

[c]Numbers represent the mean and standard deviation of values
from three animals.

AHH is either not inducible or only slightly inducible, enzyme
activity in lung is induced about 10-fold and 2 to 5-fold in
kidney and small intestine. AHH activity increases also in
skin of all these strains 16 hours after topical application
of 300 ug of benz[a]anthracene (Table 2).

in hepatic and extrahepatic tissues from various mouse

(pmoles of phenolic product/mg protein/30 min)[a]

Intestine		Kidney		Skin[b]	
BA	Control	BA	Control	BA	
8.1 ± 4.4	< 1	6.2 ± 2.5	20 ± 5	79 ± 7	
23.2 ± 2.5	3.2 ± 0.2	13.4 ± 0.3	--	--	
7.9 ± 0.8	< 1	6.1 ± 0.8	8 ± 1	72 ± 28	
17.2 ± 4.8	4.8 ± 1.0	10.8 ± 0.3	25 ± 4	106 ± 4	
--	2.3 ± 0.2	8.2 ± 1.9	36 ± 1	129 ± 13	
--	2.4 ± 0.4	142.0 ± 16.0	63 ± 25	570 ± 190	

All of the mouse strains examined have the genetic and molecular machinery for the induction of the enzyme system. The inducibility appears to be controlled by tissue-specific regulatory mechanisms which are not yet known. It is interesting to note that the consistently inducible tissues, lung, intestine and skin, form the first line of defense against hazardous exogenous substances. The ease of inducibility of the enzyme system and the preponderance of specific forms in these tissues (see below) might help the organism to adapt rapidly to the changing environment.

Different Forms of AHH and Their Distribution.

Earlier observations had indicated that polycyclic hydrocarbons are metabolized by more than one form of microsomal hydroxylases, distinguishable on the basis of their spectral and kinetic properties (Alvares et al., 1967,1968; Hildebrandt et al., 1968; Gurtoo and Campbell, 1969). We previously observed that the synthetic flavonoid, 7,8-benzoflavone, a

277

potent inhibitor of BP hydroxylation, has differential effects on the constitutive and the polycyclic hydrocarbon-induced form of AHH in rat liver (Gelboin et al., 1970). 7,8-Benzoflavone strongly inhibits the polycyclic hydrocarbon-induced AHH, but has a stimulatory effect on the constitutive enzyme and the phenobarbital-induced enzyme (Gelboin et al., 1970; Wiebel et al., 1971). The changes in the relative distribution of the hepatic enzyme forms during the development of rats and between the sexes are shown in Table 3. In newborn rats, constitutive enzyme activity is greatly increased in the presence of 7,8-benzoflavone. In contrast, in young female adult rats, the flavone inhibits the constitutive enzyme by 75% and inhibits slightly the enzyme activity of young adult male rats. 3-Methylcholanthrene (MC) induces the hydroxylase activities to similar, high levels in newborn and adult male and female animals. In contrast to the effect on the constitutive enzyme, 7,8-benzoflavone inhibits the induced enzyme of either sex and either age by 70 to 80%.

In extrahepatic tissues, such as lung or kidney, 7,8-benzoflavone inhibits the enzyme from both MC-treated and untreated animals. However, we have always observed that the inhibition in the untreated animals is somewhat less, suggesting that extrahepatic tissues may also contain a small fraction of the 7,8-benzoflavone-resistent, constitutive form. (Wiebel et al., 1971).

Table 4 gives a summary of the relative distribution of these two forms of AHH in rats. The first type (I) which is stimulated by the flavone, is found in newborn rats and predominates in the liver of male adult rats. This type is induced by phenobarbital. The second type (II), which is inhibited by 7,8-benzoflavone, is found in extrahepatic tissues, comprises a large fraction in liver of female adult rats, and is inducible by polycyclic hydrocarbons in hepatic and extrahepatic tissues. It should be noted that the distribution of types listed in Table 4 indicates the predominance of one type over another and not the exclusive presence of any type in a given tissue.

Aryl Hydrocarbon Hydroxylase and Polycyclic Hydrocarbon Cytotoxicity.

Earlier observations indicated that polycyclic hydrocarbons have little or no cytotoxicity in cells in which AHH is either absent or present in very low amounts (Nebert and Gelboin, 1969; Gelboin et al., 1969).

Table 3. Effect of 7,8-benzoflavone on hepatic aryl hydrocarbon hydroxylase: age and sex dependency

Age and Sex of Rats	AHH Specific Activity*			
	Normal Microsomes		MC-Microsomes	
	In Vitro Addition			
	None	7,8-BF	None	7,8-BF
Newborn (6 days)				
female	0.17	0.64 (+273)	5.45	0.93 (-83)
male	0.17	0.61 (+265)	6.06	1.07 (-82)
Adult (30 days)				
female	0.56	0.14 (-75)	9.19	1.26 (-86)
male	2.09	1.69 (-19)	9.39	2.15 (-77)

*Enzyme activities were determined in the supernatants of liver homogenates from 3-4 rats after centrifugation at 8000 x g for 15 min. Amounts of protein were 0.85 to 1.20 mg per ml of incubation mixture. Incubation period was 10 min. AHH specific activity is expressed as n moles of phenolic products formed/mg of protein/30 min. Other conditions as described by Wiebel et al., 1971. Numbers in parentheses give percent stimulation (+) or inhibition (-) by 7,8-Benzoflavone.

A correlation between AHH activity and the cytotoxicity of polycyclic hydrocarbons is also observed in experiments using 7,8-benzoflavone to inhibit the hydroxylase (Diamond and Gelboin, 1969). The effect of 7,8-benzoflavone on the metabolism of BP in hamster embryo cells in culture is shown in Fig. 9: In the presence of the 7,8-benzoflavone the metabolic conversion of BP to water-soluble products is inhibited more than 70%. 7,8-benzoflavone also inhibits the metabolism of DMBA.

279

Table 4. Occurrence of two forms of aryl hydrocarbon hydroxylases in rats

Form I	Form II
Liver:	Liver:
A) Newborn B) Adult Male	Adult Female
	Extrahepatic Tissues
Phenobarbital	Methylcholanthrene

The effect of 7,8-benzoflavone on the cytotoxicity induced by 1,2-dimethyl-benz[a]anthracene (DMBA) is shown in
Fig. 10. The growth of hamster embryo cells declines rapidly
after addition of 0.1 ug DMBA/ml medium. However, when DMBA
is added in the presence of 1.0 ug/ml of 7,8-benzoflavone
the rate of cell growth is restored to that in control cultures. Inhibition of the metabolism of the polycyclic
hydrocarbons parallels the prevention of polycyclic hydrocarbon cytotoxicity. The observations suggest that the level
of AHH is a major factor in the susceptibility of cells to
polycyclic hydrocarbon cytotoxicity. Also, as shown above,
we do not know what role, if any, the different forms of the
enzyme play in the activation and detoxification of polycyclic hydrocarbons. Preliminary observations indicate that
differences exist in the profile of BP metabolites formed by
the constitutive and MC-induced form of AHH (Kinoshita et al.,
1973). Different ratios of ring - and alkyl-hydroxylation
of 7,12-DMBA upon incubation with normal and induced hydroxylases (Jellinck and Goudy, 1967; Sims, 1970b) are indicative
of the potential significance of the diverse AHH forms.

Aryl Hydrocarbon Hydroxylase and Polycyclic Hydrocarbon
Tumorigenesis.

Evaluation of the role of AHH in polycyclic hydrocarbon
tumorigenesis requires a biological system in which enzyme
activity can be determined in the target tissue and the

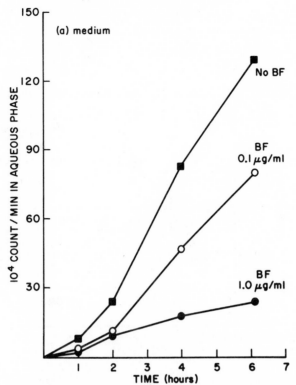

Fig. 9. Effect of 7,8-benzoflavone (BF) on the metabolism of benz[a]pyrene (BP) (Diamond and Gelboin, 1969). Secondary cultures of hamster embryo cells were treated with 7,8-benzoflavone for 18 hours. BP-^{3}H was then added at a final concentration of 0.06 ug/ml. Aliquots of the medium were extracted at times indicated with a mixture of chloroform and methanol (2:1 v/v) and radioactivity in the aqueous phase was assayed.

systemic metabolism of the carcinogen is minimized. The two-stage system of skin tumorigenesis meets these requirements. Topical application of a small dose of DMBA initiates tumorigenesis in mouse skin (Berenblum, 1941; Berenblum and Shubik, 1947). The appearance of visible tumors can be promoted by weekly application of croton oil (Berenblum, 1941; Mottran, 1944). Tumorigenesis can also be induced by repeated doses of DMBA without subsequent croton-oil treatment (Hartwell, 1963).

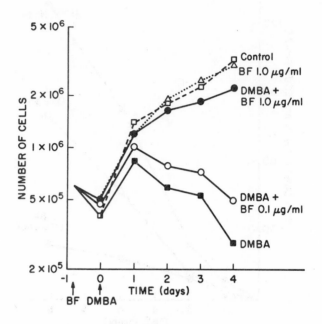

Fig. 10. Effect of 7,8-benzoflavone (BF) on the inhibition
of cell growth by DMBA (Diamond and Gelboin, 1969).
Hamster embryo cultures were treated with 7,8-
benzoflavone for 18 hours before addition of DMBA
at a final concentration of 0.1 ug/ml. Control
cultures received neither 7,8-benzoflavone nor
DMBA.

Inhibition by 7,8-Benzoflavone of Aryl Hydrocarbon
Hydroxylase and Tumorigenesis in Mouse Skin.

Table 5 demonstrates that 7,8-benzoflavone (7,8-BF)
inhibits tumor formation induced by low levels of DMBA.
Topical administration of 7,8-benzoflavone, either in a single application with the carcinogen, followed by weekly
croton oil treatment, or in repeated applications without
croton oil promotion, inhibited the development of papillomata by 70 to 80%. 7,8-Benzoflavone has no inhibitory

effect on tumor formation by a high dose of DMBA (300 ug).
This dose of DMBA is far greater than that required for maximum tumor formation. It is possible that 7,8-benzoflavone
does not sufficiently inhibit the metabolism of high doses of
DMBA to reduce the induction of papillomata. Table 6 shows
that 7,8-benzoflavone does not inhibit tumor formation when
given 12 hours before or 12 hours after the carcinogen, indicating that the early events in tumorigenesis inhibited by
7,8-benzoflavone are completed by 12 hours.

Table 5. Effect of 7,8-benzoflavone, or 1,2-benz[a]anthracene
on DMBA-induced skin tumorigenesis[a]

Group	Treatment	Sur-vivors	Mice w/Tumors	Total Tumors	Tumors Mouse	% Control
	Experiment 1: DMBA 1 X + croton oil weekly			20 weeks		
1	DMBA (25 ug)	25	28	387	13.8	
2	DMBA (25 ug) + 7,8-BF (27 ug)	26	14	61	3.6	26
3	DMBA (25 ug) + BA (23 ug)	28	28	369	13.2	96
	Experiment 2: DMBA 2 X weekly--no croton oil			20 weeks		
1	DMBA (25 ug)	29	29	531	18.3	
2	DMBA (25 ug) + 7,8-BF (27 ug)	21	19	99	4.7	26
3	DMBA (25 ug) + BA (23 ug)	22	22	320	14.5	79

[a]7,8-benzoflavone (7,8-BF) or 1,2-benz[a]anthracene (BA) were
applied simultaneously with 1,2-dimethyl-BA (DMBA) in 0.2 ml
of acetone to shaven backs of mice. After 7 days, 0.2 ml of
croton oil was applied topically as a 1% solution once a week
(Gelboin et al., 1970).

Table 6. Effect of equimolar 7,8-Benzoflavone applied before and after 7,12-DMBA on tumor formation

Time of 7,8-BF	Tumors/Mouse	% Control
	20 weeks	
None	7.45	
- 12 hours	6.04	81
Zero time	1.26	17
+ 12 hours	6.44	86

[a] All groups received DMBA (25 ug) 1 time only + weekly croton oil. (Kinoshita and Gelboin, 1972a) Experimental conditions as given under Table 5.

The presence and inducibility of AHH in mouse skin is shown in Fig. 11. Following a single topical application of benz[a]anthracene enzyme activities increase to various levels, depending on the inducer concentration.

Table 7 shows a comparison of the in vitro effects of 7,8-benzoflavone and benz[a]anthracene on hydroxylase activity in homogenates of mouse skin. Whereas the 7,8-benzoflavone strongly inhibits enzyme activity at concentrations only one-tenth of the substrate, benz[a]anthracene has relatively little effect, even at equimolar concentrations with the substrate, at 10^{-4} M. The inhibition by 7,8-benzoflavone of both the constitutive and the induced activities indicates the similarity to the hydroxylase system of other extrahepatic tissues (Wiebel et al., 1971).

The effect of 7,8-benzoflavone on the cutaneous metabolism of polycyclic hydrocarbons in vivo is demonstrated by the observation that the binding of DMBA to nucleic acids and protein of skin is considerably reduced by simultaneous application of inhibitor of the enzyme (Kinoshita and Gelboin, 1972). Earlier in vitro experiments have indicated that the covalent binding of carcinogenic polycyclic hydrocarbons to cellular macromolecules requires the activation by the NADPH-dependent microsomal enzyme system (Gelboin, 1969; Grover and

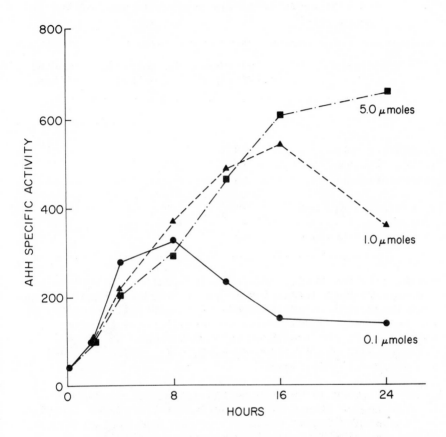

Fig. 11.   Induction of aryl hydrocarbon hydroxylase in mouse
skin by topical application of 1,2-benzanthracene
(BA). Various amounts of BA were applied topically
in 0.2 ml acetone to shaven backs of NIH Swiss
male mice. AHH activity was determined as described
by Gelboin et al., 1970.

Sims, 1969).
    The results described above show that 7,8-benzoflavone
is a strong inhibitor of cutaneous aryl hydrocarbon hydroxylase, whereas benz[a]anthracene, a potent inducer of the
enzyme, is essentially inactive as an inhibitor. The observations suggest that the inhibiton of tumor formation by

Table 7. Effect of 7,8-benzoflavone and benz[a]anthracene
on aryl hydrocarbon hydroxylase in homogenates of
mouse skin[a]

Addition	Concen-tration,M	Control Enzyme	Induced Enzyme
		% Inhibition	
7,8-benzoflavone	10^{-4}	83	91
7,8-benzoflavone	10^{-5}	64	71
7,8-benzoflavone	10^{-6}	10	21
1,2-benz[a]anthracene	10^{-4}	27	21
1,2-benz[a]anthracene	10^{-5}	2	11
1,2-benz[a]anthracene	10^{-6}	0	5

[a]Values give the percent decrease in specific activity of aryl
hydrocarbon hydroxylase (uu moles of product formed/mg protein in 30 min) in the presence of 7,8-benzoflavone or
1,2-benz[a]anthracene. With no additions the specific activity of preparations from control mice was 44, from
1,2-benz[a]anthracene-treated mice, 447. Protein concentration was 1-3 mg/flask.

7,8-benzoflavone is related to the inhibition of enzyme
activity rather than to the induction of the enzyme system.
     Recent studies in cells in culture also suggest that
metabolic activation of polycyclic hydrocarbons is required
for carcinogenicity (Marquardt and Heidelberger, 1972). Increased metabolism of some polycyclic hydrocarbons in cultured
cells caused a higher yield of transformed cells and, correspondingly, inhibition of hydrocarbon metabolism by 7,8-
benzoflavone decreased transformation.
     The reactive intermediate(s) presumed to initiate tumor
formation are unknown. They may be epoxides, which in some
instances are more potent carcinogens than the parent compounds
(Marquardt et al., 1972). The reactive forms of the hydrocarbon have also been postulated to be radical cations (Lesko
et al., 1969; Wilk and Girke, 1969) or carbonium ions (Dipple
et al., 1968). The ultimate carcinogenicity of a polycyclic
hydrocarbon might depend on several enzymatic and non-enzymatic

reactions. Thus, the amount of reactive intermediates, e.g. epoxides, would depend on the relative rates of formation versus inactivation through hydration, conjugation and non-enzymatic rearrangement to phenols. The complexity of the problem is indicated by the observations shown in Table 8. In contrast to its strong inhibitory effect on DMBA-induced tumorigenesis, 7,8-benzoflavone has variable effects on BP-induced tumor formation. In one out of six experiments the flavone reduced the development of tumors by 40%. In all the other experiments there was either a lack of inhibition or even a stimulation of BP-induced tumor formation (Table 8).

Table 8.   Effect of 7,8benzoflavone on benzo[a]pyrene tumorigenesis[a]

	Mice with Tumors	Total Tumors	% Control
Experiment 1:	21 weeks		
BP + BF (ug) (1 X + croton oil weekly)			
BP (50) only	14	40	
BP (50) + 7,8-BF (54)	12	60	150
BP (50) + 7,8-BF (270)	10	25	63
BP (50) + 7,8-BF (540)	15	38	95
Experiment 2:	20 weeks		
BP + BF (ug) (2 X weekly-no croton oil)			
BP (25)	11	15	
BP (25) + 7,8-BF (27)	20	80	533

[a]Experimental conditions as given under Table 6.   (Kinoshita and Gelboin, 1972b)

287

The data indicate that it is difficult to make general-
izations about the activation of polycyclic hydrocarbons to
their carcinogenic form and the manipulation of the activation
process. More likely we have to look at individual polycyclic
hydrocarbons and the unique activating and inactivating pathways for each in order to understand and control their
carcinogenicity.

Aryl Hydrocarbon Hydroxylase and Polycyclic Hydrocarbon Tumorigenesis in Man.

To study the regulation of the enzyme system in man and
its role in carcinogenesis and drug metabolism, methods have
to be developed to determine the enzyme activity and inducibility in readily available human tissues. Circulating
lymphocytes may represent such an easily obtainable tissue
(Whitlock et al., 1972; Busbee et al., 1972).

The properties of AHH in lymphocytes from normal human
subjects is shown in Table 9. The requirement for NADPH,
the inhibition by a carbon monoxide: oxygen mixture and the
inhibition by 7,8-benzoflavone indicate that the enzyme of
lymphocytes is similar to that of rat liver or of rodent
cells in culture (Conney, 1967; Wiebel et al., 1971). The
lymphocytes used in this experiment were cultured in the
presence of phytohemagglutinin for 2 days and were then induced with benz[a]anthrcene for another 18 hrs. The significant effect of this treatment on the enzyme level and
inducibility is demonstrated in Table 10. The constitutive
level and inducibility of lymphocytes cultured in the absence
of mitogens are very low. The presence of mitogens, phytohemagglutinin (PHA) and pokeweed mitogen (PWM) increase both the
constitutive level and the degree of induction by benz[a]an-
thracene.

It has to be determined how closely the enzyme activities
in the mitogen-stimulated cultures reflect those in circulating lymphocytes and, in turn, how indicative these are of
enzyme activities in other human tissues. The potential usefulness of lymphocytes as screening system is suggested by
recent studies on the genetic variation of AHH activity in
these cells from human populations and on the relationship
to the occurance of lung cancer (Kellermann et al., 1973 a,
b). However, before we can begin to understand polycyclic
hydrocarbon carcinogenesis in man and to take appropriate
prophylactic measures, more sensitive methods have to be
developed to a) determine the profile of metabolites and to

Table 9. Requirements for aryl hydrocarbon hydroxylase from
human lymphocytes. (Whitlock et al., 1973)*

Incubation System	AHH Specific activity**
Complete	8.0
No NADPH	1.2
90 percent CO and 10 percent O_2	5.4
7,8-BF $(10^{-4}M)$[+]	4.0
Prior incubation,[++] then complete	8.8
Prior incubation with trypsin (50 ug), then complete	0.9

* Cells were stimulated with phytohemagglutinin for 48 hours
and then exposed to BA for 18 hours. The concentration of
BA in the medium was 25 to 30 uM. Cells were collected,
pooled, homogenized, and treated as described by Whitlock
and Gelboin (1973). Each assay contained 1.6 mg of cellular protein.

**uu moles product/mg protein/30 min.

[+] 7,8-benzoflavone (BF) added in 10 ul of dimethyl sulfoxide.

[++]Prior incubation was for 10 minutes at 37°C in a volume of
0.91 ml, containing 50 umoles of trischloride buffer, pH
7.5, and 3 u moles of $MgCl_2$.

sort out the carcinogenic and non-carcinogenic derivatives,
b) to assay the activity of various enzymes involved, such
as oxidases, epoxide hydrases and conjugases and c) to untangle
the multiple factors which may determine the activity of
various pathways, e.g. age and sex dependency, distribution
of different enzyme types and state of induction.

Table 10. Basal and BA-induced AHH activity in resting and
mitogen-stimulated human lymphocytes. (Whitlock
et al., 1973)*

Mitogen	AHH Specific Activity**
None (2)	
Control	0.8 ± 0.20
BA	1.5 ± 0.27
PHA (4)	
Control	1.8 ± 0.40
BA	5.4 ± 0.50
PWM (2)	
Control	1.8 ± 0.27
BA	11.5 ± 1.7

* Cells were treated with phytohemagglutinin (PHA) or pokeweed mitogen (PWM) for 48 to 72 hours, followed by
exposure to the inducer benz[a]anthracene (BA) for 16 to
18 hours. Concentration of BA in the medium was 25 to 30
uM. Cells were collected and assayed for aryl hydrocarbon
hydroxylase (AHH) activity (Whitlock and Gelboin, 1973).
Values in parentheses indicate the number of different
samples on which each assay was performed.

**uu moles product/mg protein/30 min.

References

Alfred, L. J. and H. V. Gelboin. 1967. Science 157: 75-76.
Alvares, A. P., G. Schilling, W. Levin, and R. Kuntzman.
1967. Biochem. Biophys. Res. Comm. 29: 521-526.
Alvares, A. P., G. R. Schilling, and R. Kuntzman. 1968.
Biochem. Biophys. Res. Comm. 30: 588-593.
Berenblum, I. 1941. Cancer Res. 1: 44-48.
Berenblum, I., and P. Shubik. 1947. Brit. J. Cancer 1:
383-391.
Boyland, E. and K. Williams. 1965. Biochem. J. 94: 190-197.
Burki, K., A. G. Liebelt, and E. Bresnick. 1973. J. Natl.
Cancer Inst. 50: 369-380.

Busbee, D. L., C. R. Shaw, and E. T. Cantrell. 1972. Science 178: 315-316.

Conney, A. H., E. C. Miller, and J. A. Miller. 1957. J. Biol. Chem. 228: 753-766.

Conney, A. H. 1967. Pharmacol. Rev. 19: 317-366.

Diamond, L. and H. V. Gelboin. 1969. Science 166: 1023-1025.

Dipple, A., P. D. Lawley, and P. Brookes. 1968. European J. Cancer 4: 493-506.

Estabrook, R. W. (unpublished data).

Gelboin, H. V. 1967. "Carcinogens, enzyme induction, and gene action." Advances in Cancer Research Vol. 10. Academic Press. New York, N. Y., pp. 1-81.

Gelboin, H. V. 1969. Cancer Res. 29: 1272-1276.

Gelboin, H. V., E. Huberman and L. Sachs. 1969. Proc. Nat. Acad. Sci. U.S.A. 64: 1188-1194.

Gelboin, H. V., F. Wiebel, and L. Diamond. 1970. Science 170: 169-171.

Gielen, J. E., F. M. Goujon, and D. W. Nebert. 1972. J. Biol. Chem. 247: 1125-1137.

Gillette, J. R. 1963. Advances Enzym. Regulat. 1: 215-223.

Grover, P. L. and P. Sims. 1969. Biochem. J. 110: 159-160.

Gurtoo, H. L. and T. C. Campbell. 1969. Biochem. Pharmacol. 19: 1729-1735.

Hartwell, J. L. 1963. Survey of Compounds Which Have Been Tested for Carcinogenic Activity, Ed. 2, Public Health Service Publication No. 149, Washington, D.C.: United States Government Printing Office.

Hildebrandt, A., H. Remmer, and R. W. Estabrook. 1968. Biochem. Biophys. Res. Comm. 30: 607-612.

Jellinck, P. H. and B. Goudy. 1967. Biochem. Pharmacol. 16: 131-141.

Jerina, D. M., J. W. Daly, B. Witkop, P. Zaltzman-Nirenberg, and S. Udenfriend. 1970. Biochemistry 9: 147-156.

Jerina, D. M., N. Kaubisch, and J. W. Daly. Proc. Natl. Acad. Sci. U.S.A. 68: 2545-2548.

Kanazir, D. T. 1969. Progr. Nucl. Acid Res. Mol. Biol. 9: 117-222.

Kellermann, G., M. Luyten-Kellerman, and C. R. Shaw. 1973a. Amer. J. Human Genet. 25: 327-331.

Kellerman, G., C. R. Shaw and M. Luyten-Kellerman. 1973b. New England J. Med. 289: 934-936.

Kinoshita, N. and H. V. Gelboin. 1972a. Cancer Res. 32: 1329-1339.

Kinoshita, N. and H. V. Gelboin. 1972b. Proc. Natl. Acad. Sci. U.S.A. 69: 824-828.

Kinoshita, N., B. Shears, and H. V. Gelboin. 1973. Cancer Res. 33: 1937-1944.

Kodama, Y. and F. G. Bock. 1970. Cancer Res. 30: 1846-1849.

Lesko, S. A., Jr., P. O. P. Ts'o, and R. S. Umans. 1969. Biochemistry 8: 2291-2298.

Marquardt, H. T. Kuroki, E. Huberman, J. K. Selkirk, C. Heidelberger, P.L. Grover, and P. Sims. 1972. Cancer Res. 32: 716-720.

Marquardt, H. and C. Heidelberger. 1972. Cancer Res. 32: 721-725.

Mottram, J. C. 1944. J. Path. Bact. 56: 181-187.

Nebert, D. W. and H. V. Gelboin. 1968a. J. Biol. Chem. 243: 6242-6249.

Nebert, D. W. and H. V. Gelboin. 1968b. J. Biol. Chem. 243:6250-6261.

Nebert, D. W. and H. V. Gelboin. 1969. Arch. Biochem. Biophys. 134: 76-89.

Nebert, D. W. and H. V. Gelboin. 1970. J. Biol. Chem. 245: 160-168.

Nebert, D. W., F. M. Goujon, and J. E. Gielen. 1972. Nature New Biol. 236: 107-110.

Peacock, A. C. and C. W. Dingman. 1968. Biochemistry 7: 668-674.

Remmer, H. 1962. Drugs as activators of drug enzymes, Proc. 1st Intern. Pharmacol. Meeting, Stockholm, Vol. 6, pp. 235-249.

Selkirk, J. K., E. Huberman, and C. Heidelberger. 1971. Biochem. Biophys. Res. Comm. 43: 1010-1016.

Setlow, J.K. and R. B. Setlow. 1963. Nature 197: 560-562.

Sims, P. 1970a. Biochem. Pharmacol. 19: 795-818.

Sims, P. 1970b. Biochem. Pharmacol. 19: 2261-2275.

Tomkins, G. M., T. D. Gelehrter, D. Granner, D. Martin, Jr., H. H. Samuels, and E. B. Thompson. 1969. Science 166: 1474-1480.

Wiebel, F. J., J. C. Leutz, L. Diamond, and H. V. Gelboin. 1971. Arch. Biochem. Biophys. 144: 78-86.

Wiebel, F. J., H. V. Gelboin, and H. G. Coon. 1972a. Proc. Natl. Acad. Sci. U.S.A. 69: 3580-3584.

Wiebel, F. J., E. J. Matthews, and H. V. Gelboin. 1972b. J. Biol. Chem. 247: 4711-4714.

Wiebel, F. J., J. C. Leutz, and H. V. Gelboin. 1973. Arch. Biochem. Biophys. 154: 292-294.

Wilk, M., and Girke, W. 1969. "Radical Cations of Carcinogenic Alternant Hydrocarbons, Amines and Azo Dyes, and Their Reactions with Nucleobases." E. D. Bergmann and

B. Pullman (eds), Physicochemical Mechanisms of Carcinogenesis: The Jerusalem Symposia on Quantum Chemistry and
Biochemistry, Vol. 1, New York: Academic Press, Inc.,
pp. 91-105.

Whitlock, J. P. Jr., H. L. Cooper, and H.V. Gelboin. 1972.
Science 177: 618-619.

Whitlock, J. P., Jr. and H. V. Gelboin. 1973. J. Biol.
Chem. 248: 6114-6121.

Younger, L. R., R. Salomon, R. W. Wilson, A. C. Peacock,
and H. V. Gelboin. 1972. Mol. Pharm. 8: 452-464.

GENETIC REGULATION AND MECHANISMS
OF P-450 OXYGENASE ACTION

I. C. Gunsalus

School of Chemical Sciences
University of Illinois
Urbana, Illinois 61801

and

V. P. Marshall

Fermentation Products
The Upjohn Company
Kalamazoo, Michigan 49001

Abstract

Camphor ring cleavage and chain debranching by Pseudomonas putida are initiated through methylene hydroxylation of the 5-exo-position of camphor. This reaction is catalyzed by a multicomponent monoxygenase of the cytochrome P-450 type. The camphor hydroxylase components function as a short electron transport chain through which electrons derived from DPNH are brought to the level of oxygen, resulting in its cleavage and incorporation into substrate. Hydroxycamphor is then dehydrogenated, forming a 2,5-diketone derivative. Further oxygenation and subsequent ring cleavage yields acetate and iso-butyrate. Isobutyrate undergoes oxidation and chain debranching to become a substrate for the enzymes of central metabolism.

The formation of both the camphor ring cleavage and chain debranching enzymes is under substrate control. Camphor hydroxylase, hydroxycamphor dehydrogenase and ketolactonase I, the early enzymes of camphor metabolism, are induced by camphor and its analogs, while the isobutyrate catabolic enzymes are induced by isobutyrate. The synthesis of both groups of enzymes is repressed by glucose and succinate.

The genetic system coding for the camphor
catabolic enzymes is present as a transmissible
plasmid. This general model appears to account for
the ability of pseudomonads to metabolize a diverse
array of organic molecules found in nature. A
redundancy of the isobutyrate catabolic alleles on
both the chromosome and the plasmid may account
for the plasmid chromosome recognition and pairing.

Introduction

Biological dissimilation of drugs, wastes, pollutants and other toxic substances is frequently
initiated through substrate level oxygen addition.
The most thoroughly investigated and best understood
of these reactions are those catalyzed by the
monoxygenases of the cytochrome P-450 type. These
catalysts are ubiquitous in nature, occurring in
both plants and animals. In mammals, the most
characterized examples are the drug hydroxylases
of liver microsomes (Omura et al., 1965) and the
steroid 11-β hydroxylase of adrenal mitochondria
(Wilson et al., 1965). The role of the microsomal
hydroxylases is associated with the solubilization
of drugs, carcinogens, and other toxic compounds,
rendering them water soluble, and thus manageable
by urinary excretion.

In contrast to mammalian P-450 type monoxygenases, those of microbial origin generally
catalyze initial reactions leading to substrate
dissimilation. Chiefly, the microbial enzymes
attack hydrocarbon derivatives. Specific examples
are the octane hydroxylases of diptheroids (Cardini
and Jurtshuk, 1968) and Candida tropicalis
(Lebeault et al., 1971), and the camphor hydroxylase of P. putida (Katagiri et al., 1968). The
symbiotic bacteroids associated with the rhizosphere
contain cytochromes of the P-450 type whose functions
are so far unknown (Appleby, 1969).

An understanding of the microbial P-450 type
monoxygenases on both the chemical and genetic
levels is particularly important since microorganisms are primarily responsible for dissimilation of organic molecules left in the environment
by natural and synthetic processes. Compounds

metabolized include the plant and insect growth
regulators and inhibitors, and residual hydrocarbons derived from fossil fuels.

The genetic organization of several monoxygenases and their associated pathways in microorganisms includes alleles on transmissible plasmids.
Specific examples include the organization of genes
coding for the octane (Chakrabarty et al., 1973),
naphthalene-salicylate (Dunn and Gunsalus, 1973,
Chakrabarty, 1972), and camphor (Rheinwald et al.,
1973) catabolic enzymes. This genetic array in
organisms with limited chromosomal size appears to
provide a mechanism to code for the large number of
enzymes required for the degradation of the widely
diverse organic molecules found in nature.

Similarities between mammalian and bacterial
P-450 type monoxygenase systems appear despite the
distant evolutionary relationship between these
organisms. An example of this close functional and
structural relationship is seen in the mammalian
steroid 11-β hydroxylase and the pseudomonad camphor hydroxylase. Both monoxygenases catalyze
hydroxylation of terpenes using reducing equivalents
derived from pyridine nucleotide which are transferred to the level of cytochrome P-450 via an electron transport system composed of a flavo-protein
reductase and an iron sulfur protein of ferredoxin
type. The mammalian enzyme is membrane bound and
thus is not available for P-450 model studies, as
is the soluble camphor hydroxylase.

A MICROBIAL EXAMPLE:
Camphor Metabolism by Pseudomonads

Camphor catabolism by the fluorescent pseudomonads has been investigated using P. putida, PpG1
and Ppg5 isolated from soil by camphor enrichment
(Bradshaw et al., 1959). In each case, camphor
metabolism is initiated through methylene hydroxylation and proceeds to the level of isobutyrate
and acetate through a 2,5-diketone intermediate
(Ke5). Specifically, the reaction pathway for
camphor dissimilation in P. putida proceeds by
hydroxylation, dehydrogenation, and two lactoniza-

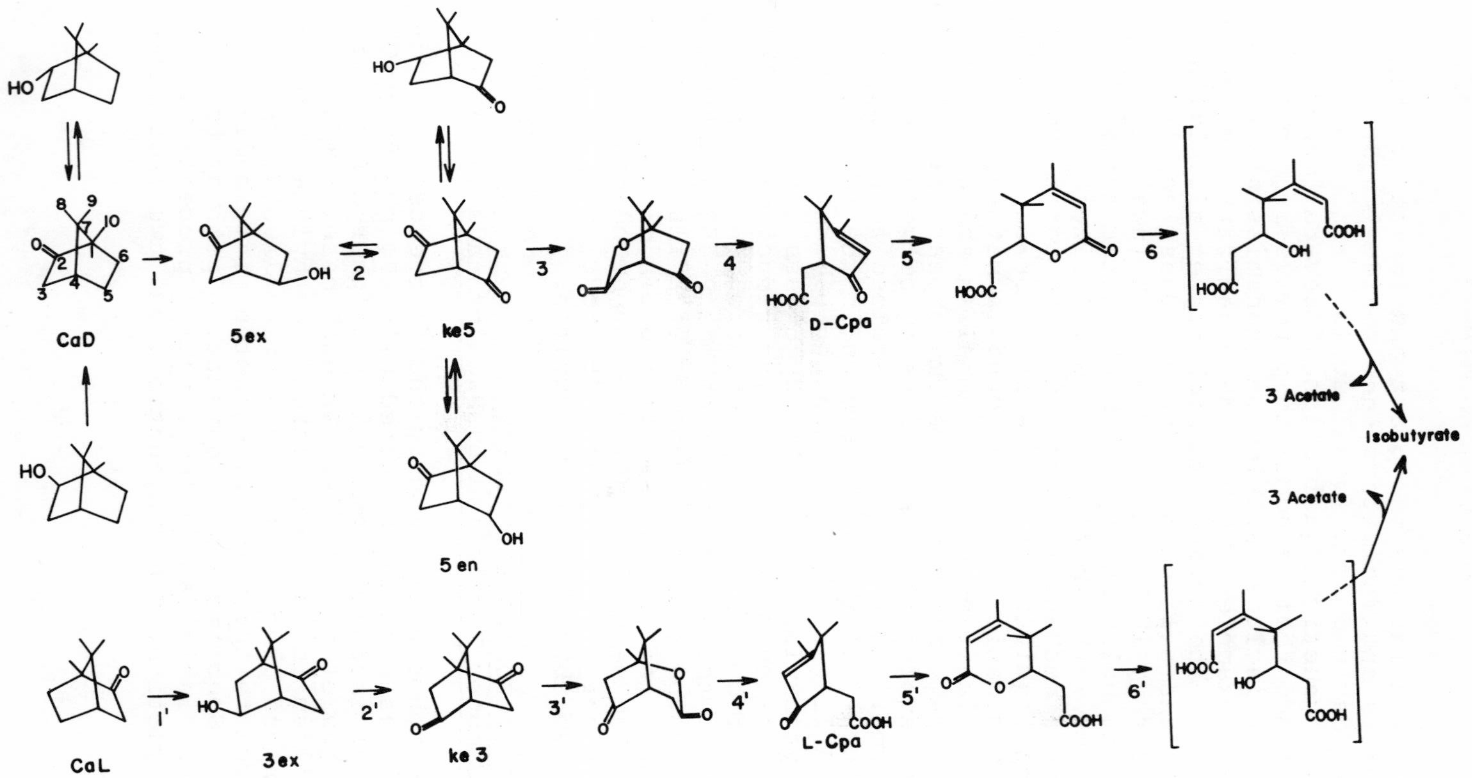

Fig. 1

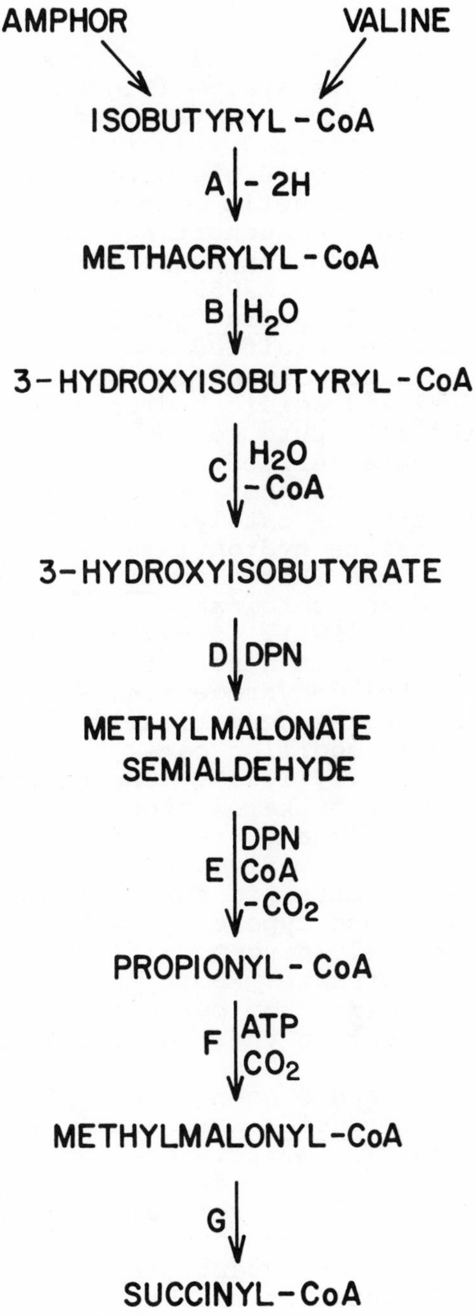

CAMPHOR   VALINE

ISOBUTYRYL – CoA

A $\downarrow$ – 2H

METHACRYLYL – CoA

B $\downarrow$ H_2O

3 – HYDROXYISOBUTYRYL – CoA

C $\downarrow$ H_2O / – CoA

3 – HYDROXYISOBUTYRATE

D $\downarrow$ DPN

METHYLMALONATE
SEMIALDEHYDE

E $\downarrow$ DPN / CoA / – CO_2

PROPIONYL – CoA

F $\downarrow$ ATP / CO_2

METHYLMALONYL – CoA

G $\downarrow$

SUCCINYL – CoA

Fig. 2

tions leading to cleavage of both members of its
bicyclic bornane ring system (Figure 1). The products of ring cleavage, acetate and isobutyrate,
are subsequently oxidized (Figure 2) to enter the
tricarboxylic acid cycle, leading to the production
of energy and biosynthetic intermediates.

Initial evidence supporting the metabolic route
for camphor dissimilation was obtained from experiments (Bradshaw et al., 1959) in which logarithmic
phase cultures of P. putida growing on camphor in
minimal media were acidified and extracted with
halogenated organic solvents. The extracts containing neutral and acidic hydrophobic intermediates
were separated into pure components and were
structurally characterized.

Conversion of camphor (Figure 3) to its 5-exo-
hydroxy derivative is catalyzed by the cytochrome
P-450 type methylene hydroxylase of P. putida termed
camphor hydroxylase (Katagiri et al., 1968), now
highly purified and obtainable in crystalline form
(Yu and Gunsalus, 1970). 5-exo-hydroxycamphor is
then dehydrogenated in a reaction catalyzed by a
DPN-linked alcohol dehydrogenase (Kuo et al., 1964)
forming its 2,5-diketone derivative, (Ke5) a substrate for oxygen addition catalyzed by ketolactonase I (Conrad et al., 1965). The product of the
reaction catalyzed by ketolactonase I, the 1,2-
lactone, is unstable and breaks down to form the
first monocyclic derivative, cyclopentenone acetic
acid (Cpa). The latter is substrate for the second
of the ketolactonase type enzymes, which catalyzes
lactone formation leading to the production of
acetate and isobutyrate. Both ketolactonases are
oxygenases differing from cytochrome P-450 type oxygenase with respect to their noncytochrome catalytic
centers.

Both the L- and D-enantiomers of camphor support growth of P. putida with equal cell yield per
mole (LeGall et al., 1963). Analysis by gas
chromotography yielded evidence for the intermediates of L-camphor growth being identical to
those obtained from D-camphor grown cultures
(Figure 1). Upon subsequent examination, the intermediates were identified as the L- and D-enantiomers
with the configuration of the camphor substrate,

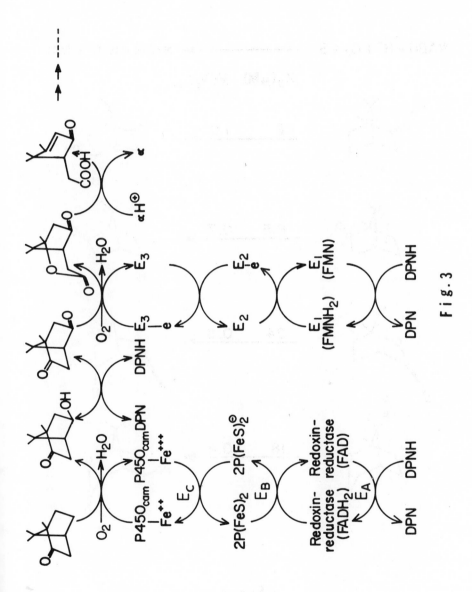

Fig. 3

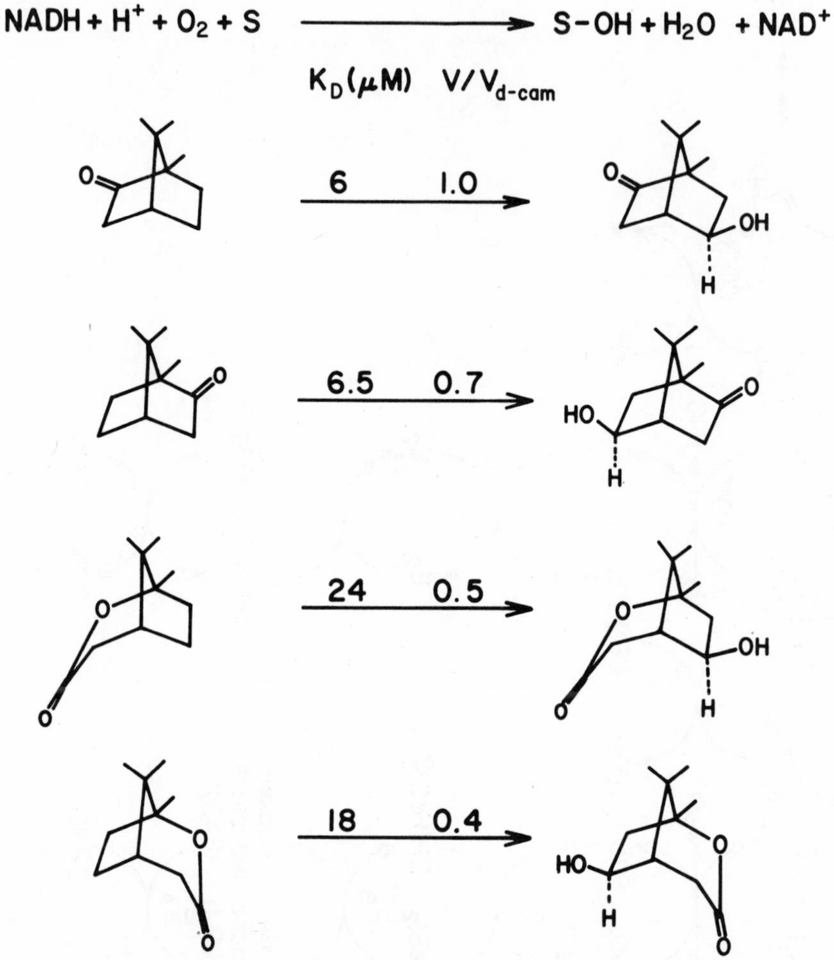

$$NADH + H^+ + O_2 + S \longrightarrow S-OH + H_2O + NAD^+$$

Fig.4

thus introducing the possibility of enantiomer specificity in the camphor degrading enzymes. However, mutant growth responses and purification of a single camphor hydroxylase active on both camphor enantiomers (Figure 4) suggested the induction of a single camphor hydroxylase by both enantiomers. Additionally, mutants unable to grow on either enantiomer of camphor, but able to use all other D-camphor pathway intermediates were isolated (Table 1) (Rheinwald et al., 1973). This phenotype, as well as purification of a single enzyme, suggests a single camphor hydroxylase lacking enantiomer specificity.

Analysis of hydroxycamphor dehydrogenase activity in crude extracts showed the presence of two hydroxycamphor dehydrogenases with overlapping enantiomer specificity. Cells grown on either L- or D-camphor subjected to enzyme purification and kinetic studies were made using the purified hydroxycamphor dehydrogenases with 5-exo- and 3-exo-hydroxycamphor as substrates. In each case, however, the dehydrogenases were most active using the enantiomeric form of hydroxycamphor corresponding to that of the growth substrate.

Ketolactonase I, in contrast, exists in two forms, each showing enantiomer specificity. Mutants of P. putida were isolated which were unable to use D-camphor or the 5-exo hydroxy- and 2,5-diketone derivatives, but were able to grow on L-camphor and the D-enantiomer of cyclopentenone acetic acid (Table 1). These mutants furnish genetic evidence for the L-enantiomer specific form of ketolactonase I.

Enzyme Formation

Formation of the enzymes catalyzing ring cleavage and chain debranching of camphor and its successive lower intermediates is under substrate control. Positive control is exerted through enzyme induction and negative control by catabolite repression. As is often the case with other inducible bacterial catabolic systems (Ornston, 1971), glucose and succinate repress induction of the camphor catabolic enzymes (Gunsalus et al., 1967),

303

Table 1

Growth Response: Cam⁻Mutants *P. putida* PpG1

Carbon Sources

Stock #	Genotype	CaL	CaD	5ex	Ke5	Cpa	Ibu	Prp	Suc	Defect
PpG 1 wt.		+	+	+	+	+	+	+	+	wt.
543	cam-100	−	−	+	+	+	+	+	+	Group I⁻, OH-E$_C^-$
545	cam-102	−	−	+	+	+	+	+	+	Group I⁻, OH-E$_B^-$
544	cam-101	−	−	+	+	+	+	+	+	Group I⁻, OH-E$_A^-$
552	cam-120	−	−	−	+	+	+	+	+	Group I⁻, 5ex DH
553	cam-121	−	−	−	+	+	+	+	+	Group I⁻, 5ex DH
557	cam-133	+	−	−	−	+	+	−	+	Group I⁻, KL-1⁻
554	cam-130	+	−	−	−	+	+	+	+	Group I⁻, KL-1⁻
556	cam-132	−	−	−	−	+	−	−	+	Group I⁻, KL-1⁻
566	cam-206	+	−	−	−	−	+	+	+	Group II⁻
560	cam-200	−	−	−	−	−	+	+	+	Group II⁻
568	cam-208	−	−	−	−	−	+	+	+	Group II⁻
575	ibu-100	−	−	−	−	−	−	+	+	Group III⁻
577	ibu-102	−	−	−	−	−	−	−	+	Group III⁻
571	seg-1	−	−	−	−	−	+	+	+	Del. I, II⁻
572	seg-2	−	−	−	−	−	+	+	+	Del. I, II⁻

Groups I-III - Early, mid and late genes of camphor pathway

PpG571 and 572, Cam⁻mutants spontaneous from penicillin-cycloserine selection--others by nitrosoguanidine treatment.

OH - Methylene hydroxylase; E_A, E_B and E_C - Hydroxylase components (Figure 3); 5ex DH, alcohol dehydrogenase; KL-1, Ketolactonase I.

CaL and CaD, derived respectively from L(-) and D(+) camphor
5ex and Ke5, camphor-5-*exo*-alcohol and 2,5-bornanedione
Cpa, Cyclopentenone acetic acid from D-camphor
Ibu - Isobutyrate; Prp - Propionate; Suc - Succinate
Wt. - Wild type

while camphor, its intermediates and analogs
(Gunsalus et al., 1965) cause increased rates of
enzyme synthesis. L-Glutamate and citrate show
little effect as catabolite repressors, and have
no influence on the induction of the camphor
catabolic enzymes (Jacobson, 1967); thus they have
been effective tools in studies of metabolic
regulation.

Formation of the early camphor enzymes catalyzing bornane ring cleavage apparently occurs in
response to camphor. Mutants unable to grow on
camphor, but able to utilize hydroxycamphor and
lower intermediates, were isolated (Rheinwald, 1970)
(Table 1). Extracts of these mutants grown on
L-glutamate and induced with D-camphor were used
to determine the role of camphor in the induction
process. Since camphor is metabolically inert in
these mutant strains and enzyme induction occurs,
it can be concluded that camphor itself acts as the
physiological inducer of camphor hydroxylase, hydroxycamphor dehydrogenase, and ketolactonase I
(Table 2).

The enzymes catalyzing chain debranching and
other reactions of isobutyrate catabolism appear
to be induced by isobutyrate, and repressed by
succinate and glucose (Marshall and Sokatch, 1972).
Two of these enzymes, 3-hydroxyisobutyrate dehydrogenase and methylmalonate semialdehyde dehydrogenase are synthesized under coordinate control (Schmidt, 1967).

Genetic Organization

Recent studies emanating from earlier investigations of Rheinwald and Chakrabarty give evidence
of the presence of plasmid alleles encoding peripheral pathway enzymes. The camphor system (Rheinwald
et al., 1973) appears to be forming as a general
model for the genetic organization of these pathways, including the genes for octane (Chakrabarty
et al., 1973) and naphthalene-salicylate (Dunn and
Gunsalus, 1973; Chakrabarty, 1972) catabolism.

The linkage found between the camphor genes
by transduction and conjugation has highlighted
one difference. A very close genetic linkage of

305

Table 2

Induction of the Early Camphor Enzymes by Camphor in *P. putida*

Organism	Carbon Sources Utilized	Hydroxylase			Alcohol Dehydrogenase	Ketolactonase I	
		E_A	E_B	E_C		E_1	$E_{2,3}$
					(n moles per min per mg protein)		
PpG1 (wt)	CaD^+, $5ex^+$	40	40	450	180	750	90
PpG543	CaD^-, $5ex^+$	30	30	0	140	630	90
PpG544	CaD^-, $5ex^+$	0	40	440	140	570	70
PpG545	CaD^-, $5ex^+$	40	0	300	100	670	80

1. CaD, D-camphor
2. 5ex, 5-exo-hydroxycamphor
3. E_A, E_B, and E_C, hydroxylase components
4. E_1, E_2, and E_3, ketolactonase I components
5. wt, wild type

From Rheinwald, J.G., MS Thesis, University of Illinois, 1970

the camphor hydroxylase and the hydroxycamphor
dehydrogenase is shown by transduction. Conjugation experiments indicate that the hydroxycamphor
dehydrogenase genes are transferred late in the
transfer sequence, while the camphor hydroxylase
genes are transferred early. These observations
suggest closed circularity of the camphor plasmid
(Chakrabarty and Gunsalus, 1971).

High frequencies of cotransduction of camphor
gene markers among mutants of P. putida, (PpGl)
indicate two clusters of closely linked genes
specifying the reactions of early and midpathway
enzymes. These genes, listed as Groups I and II
are plasmid borne, while those of Group III which
specify isobutyrate (Ibu) to propionate enzymes
are chromosomal.

More recent experiments indicate a redundancy
of several early isobutyrate (Ibu) alleles (Group
III) on the Cam plasmid in addition to the full
chromosomal complement (Dunn, personal communication). This observation has led to the hypothesis
of possible homology to account for recognition
and pairing between plasmid and chromosome. Mitomycin C was used to prepare Cam$^-$, Ibu$^+$ strains since
mitomycin increases the rate of curing or segrega-
tion of the plasmid borne genes from a spontaneous
rate of about 10^{-4} to approximately 10^{-1}. Muta-
genesis of these segregants followed by selection
for isobutyrate nonutilizing strains resulted in
Cam$^-$, Ibu$^-$ organisms. However, on introduction of
the plasmid by conjugation, some mutants regenerated
the ability to grow on isobutyrate, thus indicating
a redundancy of isobutyrate catabolic alleles.
Studies of chromosome mobilization (Shaham et al.,
1973) will allow further and more complete investigation of the redundancy phenomenon and its relationship to recognition and pairing.

Oxygenation Cycles and Components

Of the cytochrome P-450 type hydroxylase systems
available for study, the camphor hydroxylase presents
itself as a representative model amenable to study
by classical biochemical means (Gunsalus et al.,
1972). The hydroxylase occurs as an electron

307

transport system composed of a DPNH reduced FAD linked flavoprotein termed redoxin reductase (E_A), and a ferredoxin type iron sulfur protein, putidaredoxin (E_B), linked to cytochrome P-450 (E_C), the oxygen-substrate binding catalytic center (Figure 5). The compositions, molecular weights, and prosthetic groups of the hydroxylase components (Tsai et al, 1971) are outlined in Table 3. The reaction catalyzed by the complete hydroxylase system is:

$$\text{D-camphor} + \text{DPNH} + \text{H}^+ + \text{O}_2 \rightarrow \text{5-}\underline{\text{exo}}\text{-hydroxy-}$$
$$\text{camphor} + \text{DPN}^+ + \text{H}_2\text{O}$$

The cytochrome P-450 oxygenase cycle based on observed spectral entities (Figure 5) is presented in Figure 6 (Gunsalus et al., 1971). Initially, camphor binds the ferric form of the cytochrome, causing a blue shift of the Soret absorption maximum from 417 to 391 nm. The ferric cytochrome-camphor complex next receives a single reducing equivalent derived from DPNH via the flavoprotein, E_A, and the iron sulfur protein, E_B, resulting in a red shift in the Soret maximum to 408 nm. The ferrous cytochrome-camphor complex can bind oxygen in its catalytic cycle, which results in formation of an oxygen adduct displaying maximal Soret absorption at 418 nm, or the reduced cytochrome can react with carbon monoxide to form a chromophore with a Soret maximum at 446 nm. This far-red shifted Soret absorption of the cytochrome-CO complex is the basis for the P-450 nomenclature. The reduced camphor oxy-P-450 apparently occurs in a low spin ferric state (Sharrock et al., 1973) with its electron associated with oxygen, possibly forming a superoxide radical. Upon reduction by the second electron, the Soret absorption maximum of the cytochrome at 418 nm rapidly disappears resulting in formation of 5-exo-hydroxycamphor and water, and a return of the 391 nm Soret pigment absorption maximum. This indicates a return of the cytochrome to the initial stage of the hydroxylation cycle.

Ketolactonases I and II, which lack cytochrome P-450 are responsible for cleavage of camphor's bicyclic bornane ring system (Figure 3). Ketolac-

Table 3

Methylene Hydroxylase Components

	Camphor-*exo*-5			Steroid-11-β
Amino Acid	Cyto-chrome E_C	Reductase E_A	Putida-redoxin E_B	Adreno-doxin
Asp	27	25	10 $\atop$ 4 $\Big\}$ 14	25
Asn	9	15		
Thr	19	20	5	10
Ser	21	18	7	7
Glu	42	16	9 $\atop$ 3 $\Big\}$ 12	12
Gln	13	24		
Pro	27	18	4	1
Gly	26	33	9	8
Ala	34	48	10	7
Val	24	34	15	7
Met	9	6	3	3
Ile	24	24	6	8
Leu	40	42	7	13
Tyr	9	6	3	1
Phe	17	10	2	4
His	12	6	2	3
Lys	13	13	3	5
Trp	1	3	1	0
Arg	24	24	5	4
CyS/2	6	6	6	5
Total	397	393	114	118
Free SH	6	6	4	5
N-terminus	Asx	Ser	Ser	Ser
C-terminus	Val	Ala	Trp	Ala
Mol. wt.	45,000	43,500	12,500	13,100
Prosthetic Group	Ferri-heme	1 FAD CHO	$(FeS)_2$	$(FeS)_2$

Tsai, R.L., Gunsalus, I.C. and Dus, K., *Biochem. Biophys. Res. Commun.*, 45, 1302, 1971.

309

tonase I (Yu and Gunsalus, 1969) catalyzes the
following reaction:

2,5-bornanedione (ke5) + DPNH + H$^+$ + O$_2$ →
    5-keto-1,2-campholide + DPN$^+$ + H$_2$O

Despite the absence of cytochrome P-450 in ketolactonase I, many features of this system (Figure 3)
resemble camphor hydroxylase. Both enzymes are
monoxygenases initially reduced by DPNH at the
flavoprotein level (i.e. E_1 vs E_A). The flavo-
proteins of each system catalyze the reduction of
iron containing proteins (i.e. E_2 vs E_B), which in
turn reduce the oxygenase active centers (i.e. E_3
vs E_C) causing oxygen activation and the addition
of one atom into a terpene substrate.

Unfortunately, these physiologically important
monoxygenases lacking cytochrome P-450 present themselves as extremely difficult subjects for structural and mechanistic analyses since there is an
absence of optical spectra sensitive to different
states of their catalytic cycles.

Concluding Remarks

More sophisticated experiments concerning the
chemical regulation of enzyme synthesis and activity
are required to clarify the interaction of two
aspects of peripheral metabolism. Two of them are
the flow of intermediates from peripheral substrates in the presence of excess carbon and energy
and the regulation of plasmid expression when multiple copies are present in a single cell. A
beginning has been made on the former and some
aspects of the latter are presently under investigation.

A basis has been laid for the elucidation of
mechanistic and structural aspects of the cytochrome P-450 type oxygenases. Key questions yet to
be answered deal with the physical nature of electron transport and oxygen activation (including its
incorporation into substrate). Presently, the
cytochrome P-450 type oxygenase of camphor hydroxylase is in crystalline form. Hopefully, X-ray
analysis of the hydroxylase will lead to an under-

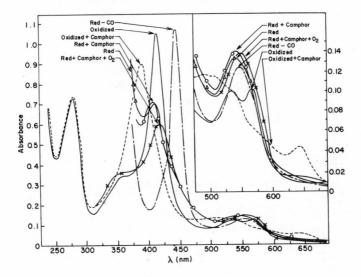

Fig.5

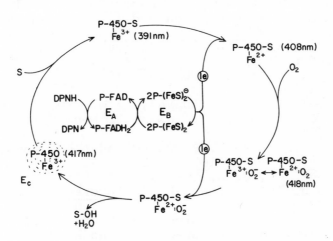

P-450 Cytochrome Oxygenation and Reduction Cycle
28/7/70 Gunsalus, Tyson, Tsai

Fig.6

311

standing of structure-function relationships as has been the case in the investigation of cytochrome c.

Acknowledgements

This work was supported in part by the Department of Health, Education and Welfare, Public Health Service Grants 5F02HD41376-03 and AM00562 in addition to U.S. National Science Foundation Grant GB33962X.

References

Appleby, C. A. 1969. Biochim. Biophys, Acta. 172: 71-87.

Bradshaw, W. H., H. E. Conrad, E. J. Corey, I. C. Gunsalus and D. Lednicer. 1959. J. Am. Chem. Soc. 81:5507.

Cardini, G. and P. Jurtshuk. 1968. J. Biol. Chem. 243:6070-6072.

Chakrabarty, A. M. and I. C. Gunsalus. 1971. Bacteriol. Proc. 46.

Chakrabarty, A. M. 1972. J. Bacteriol. 112:815-823.

Chakrabarty, A. M., G. Chou and I. C. Gunsalus. 1973. Proc. Nat. Acad. Sci., U.S.A. 70:1137-1140.

Conrad, H. E., R. Dubus, M. J. Namtvedt and I. C. Gunsalus. 1965. J. Biol. Chem. 240:495-503.

Dunn, N. W. and I. C. Gunsalus. 1973. J. Bacteriol. 114:974-979.

Gunsalus, I. C., H. E. Conrad, P. W. Trudgill and L. A. Jacobson. 1965. Isreal J. Med. Sci. 1:1099-1119.

Gunsalus, I. C., A. U. Bertland and L. A. Jacobson. 1967. Arch. Mikrobiol. 59:113-122.

Gunsalus, I. C., C. A. Tyson, R. Tsai and J. D. Lipscomb. 1971. Chem.-Biol. Interactions. 4:75-78.

Gunsalus, I. C., J. D. Lipscomb, V. Marshall, H. Frauenfelder, E. Greenbaum and E. Munck. 1972. In: Biological hydroxylation mechanisms. (G. S. Boyd and R. M. S. Smellie, eds.). Acad. Press. pp. 135-157.

Jacobson, L. A. 1967. Enzyme induction and repression in the catabolism of (≠) - camphor by Pseudomonas putida. Ph.D. Dissertation, Univ.

of Ill.

Katagiri, M., B. N. Ganguli and I. C. Gunsalus. 1968. J. Biol. Chem. 243:3543-3545.

Kuo, J-F., R. Prairie and I. C. Gunsalus. 1964. 6th Int. Cong. Bioch., Abstracts.

Lebeault, J-M., E. T. Lode and M. J. Coon. 1971. Biochem. Biophys. Res. Commun. 42:413-419.

LeGall, J., A. U. Bertland, M. J. Namtvedt and H. E. Conrad. 1963. Fed. Proc. 22:295.

Marshall, V. deP. and J. R. Sokatch. 1972. J. Bacteriol. 110:1073-1081.

Omura, T., R. Sato, D. Y. Cooper, O. Rosenthal and R. W. Estabrook. 1965. Fed. Proc. 24:1181-1189.

Ornston, L. N. 1971. Bacteriol. Rev. 35:87-116.

Rheinwald, J. G. 1970. The genetic organization of peripheral metabolism: a transmissible plasmid controlling camphor oxidation in Pseudomonas putida. M. S. Thesis, Univ. of Ill.

Rheinwald, J. G., A. M. Chakrabarty and I. C. Gunsalus. 1973. Proc. Nat. Acad. Sci., U.S.A. 70:885-889.

Schmidt. G. L. 1967. B. S. Thesis, Univ. of Ill.

Shaham, M., A. M. Chakrabarty and I. C. Gunsalus. 1973. J. Bacteriol. 116:944-949.

Sharrock, M., E. Munck, P. G. Debrunner, V. Marshall, J. D. Lipscomb and I. C. Gunsalus. 1973. Biochemistry. 12:258-265.

Tsai, R. L., I. C. Gunsalus and K. Dus. 1971. Biochem. Biophys. Res. Commun. 45:1300-1306.

Wilson, L. D., D. H. Nelson and B. W. Harding. 1965. Biochim. Biophys. Acta. 99:391-393.

Yu, C-A. and I. C. Gunsalus. 1969. J. Biol. Chem. 244:6149-6152.

Yu, C-A. and I. C. Gunsalus. 1970. Biochem. Biophys. Res. Commun. 40:1423-1430.

313

GENETICS OF DETOXICATION SYSTEMS IN INSECTS

Frederick W. Plapp, Jr.

Department of Entomology
Texas A&M University

Synopsis

A number of insecticide detoxication systems are known
in insects. Higher than normal levels occur in many resistant populations and are frequently the cause of resistance.
Resistance genes associated with increases in insecticide
detoxication are usually inherited in a semidominant manner.
Their activity can frequently be blocked by synergists and
conversely, can be induced by a wide variety of chemical inducers including many of the insecticides themselves.

Introduction

We know that insects have the ability to detoxify most
insecticides with which they come into contact. This fact
was first understood and dealt with in the 1930's when the
antioxidant synergist piperonyl butoxide was combined with
pyrethrins insecticide to increase the effectiveness of the
latter by interfering with its detoxication. Since the introduction of many new types of insecticides in the inter-
vening years, the study of insecticide detoxication has been
of great importance, both from the standpoint of the fate
of such chemicals in non-target organisms, i.e. man, as well
as in target organisms, i.e. pest insects.

Resistant insects usually detoxify more insecticide
than susceptible insects. Indeed, combined genetic and
biochemical studies have shown that an increased rate of
detoxication is frequently, although not always, the cause
of resistance. Because of the close relationship between
detoxication and resistance, the genetics of the two factors
are usually studied together. In practice, there would seem
to be no valid reason for measuring insecticide detoxication
in insects were it not a component of resistance.

315

With cyclodiene insecticides and sometimes with
chlorinated hydrocarbons and pyrethrins, detoxication is not
apparently a major component of resistance. This fact is
known from genetic studies which have allowed the isolation
and characterization of non-metabolic resistance mechanisms.
As will be discussed later, the nature of inheritance of
non-metabolic resistance factors is distinctly different from
that of detoxication-dependent mechanisms. An understanding
of the interaction between the two types is necessary for a
comprehension of the total phenomenon of resistance as well
as of the role detoxication plays in it.

Overall, the development of resistance and the selective
processes that have brought it about are, as described by
Tsukamoto (1969), an outstanding example of rapid microevolu-
tion caused by artificial selection. The situation has progressed to the point where insects are sometimes resistant
to new chemicals or even whole classes of chemicals when
these agents are first introduced as insect control agents.
This adaptability represents a striking example of the ability
of organisms to survive in toxic environments.

Role of Genetic Studies

Considerable progress has been made in identifying the
genetic factors responsible for insecticide resistance.
Further, we have learned something of the biochemistry of
these genes, particularly in cases where resistance is associated with detoxication. Most progress has been made with
the house fly, Musca domestica, probably the most studied
insect in terms of insecticide work. Pertinent recent reviews of the subject have been by Tsukamoto (1969), Brown
(1971), Brown and Pal (1971), Georghiou (1972), Oppenoorth
(1972), and Wilkinson and Brattsten (1972).

Rapid progress occurred in research on the biochemistry
and genetics of resistance when visible genetic mutants mark-
ing chromosomes of the house fly became available. These
mutations enable entomologists to identify the various
chromosomes containing resistance genes and to make tentative
determinations of the loci of different resistance genes.
More importantly, availability of mutants made it possible
to prepare insect populations containing single resistance
genes. When these populations were prepared it was possible
to make biochemical comparisons between resistant and susceptible strains and thus, to elucidate the nature of resistance.

Research in genetics as it relates to resistance in the

316

house fly was greatly facilitated by the formal genetic
studies of Hiroyoshi (1960, 1961), Sullivan (1961), Tsukamoto
et al. (1961), and Hoyer (1966). These workers identified
the linkage groups in the house fly and, along with other
researchers, reported more than 100 visible mutations.
Actual identification of the karyotype of the house fly
(which linkage group is which chromosome) was accomplished
by Wagoner (1967).

Most methods widely used in performing genetic analyses
of resistance in the house fly were developed by Tsukamoto
(1963, 1964, 1965). Typical test cross procedures have
involved crossing resistant strain females with males
of a susceptible multi-mutant strain. Since only 4 of
the 5 autosomes in the house fly are known to bear resistance
genes, marker strains with either 3 or 4 mutants have proved
adequate. Resistance levels and/or detoxication activity
can be measured in F_1 populations and compared with those of
parent strains. Additional crosses can then be performed to
gain more information.

To estimate all resistance mechanisms present, F_1
populations can be selfed and resistance and detoxication
measured in the F_2. This procedure is necessary to identify
the occurrence of recessive resistance genes.

A more typical and useful assay is the F_1 male backcross
in which F_1 males are backcrossed to the mutant parent.
Crosses of this type yield populations composed of approximately equal numbers of all possible phenotypes. Assay
of these can accurately determine the contribution of each
chromosome to both resistance and detoxication activity.
This assay makes use of the fact that in the house fly, as
in Drosophila, no crossing-over occurs in male flies, thus
allowing accurate determinations of the total contribution
of each chromosome to resistance.

The reverse assay, crossing F_1-females with susceptible
mutant males, will, under ideal conditions, allow the
determination of the loci of individual resistance and detoxication genes, or at least the distance in crossing-over
units that intervenes between the genes and the mutant. The
F_1-female assay allows a determination of the coidentity
of detoxication and resistance genes. Where the F_1-male assay allows only a determination of linkage, the F_1-female
assay allows a far more accurate estimation of the relationship between detoxication and resistance by determining if
both factors are introduced simultaneously into mutant
strains by crossing-over.

317

As discussed by Tsukamoto (1969) the F_1-female crossing procedure is best done as a three-point cross, i.e., when one resistance gene and two visible mutants are used. This procedure has not been frequently carried out, due in part to a lack of appropriate mutant characters. Other limiting factors include the necessity of producing monogenetic resistant strains before undertaking the test crosses, a procedure necessary to eliminate the effect of additional major resistance genes and of modifiers which can confuse test results. A second limitation is the lack of detailed knowledge of the karyotype of the house fly and the possible effects of chromosomal inversions and translocations.

Major Resistance Genes:

A. Hydrocarbon Insecticides

More than 100 different chemicals are presently used as insecticides. Logically, one might expect an insect to possess one or more genes conferring resistance to each chemical. In practice this is not true. The best available evidence indicates that not more than 10 distinct genetic loci in the house fly confer resistance to insecticides. The same is true for other insect species whose resistance biochemistry has been studied. Different alleles of some of the major resistance genes confer greater or lesser resistance to individual chemicals. This allelism, plus the interaction of various combinations of resistance genes, is responsible for most known types of resistance.

The following discussion will briefly review the major known types of resistance genes and their relationship to detoxication. Major emphasis will be placed on house fly studies with some reference to similar work in other insect species.

DDT dehydrochlorinase - (Deh)

DDT and related chlorinated hydrocarbons such as DDD (TDE) and Methoxychlor comprise the first major class of synthetic insecticides to be introduced on a wide scale. Predictably, resistance developed first to these insecticides. Three major genes, 2 of which involve detoxication, confer resistance to DDT in the house fly. Evidence from studies with other insects indicates that similar genes are widespread.

318

The first major resistance gene characterized and known to involve detoxication was DDT dehydrochlorinase, mutant symbol Deh. This is a semidominant chromosome II resistance factor involving an increased ability to detoxify DDT by dehydrochlorinating it to yield DDE. DDD is similarly converted to DDMU. This mechanism confers only slight resistance to analogs such as Methoxychlor or o-chloro DDT which can be dehydrochlorinated only with extreme difficulty. DDT dehydrochlorinase can be blocked by the use of synergists such as DMC or WARF. These chemicals evidently act as competitive substrates for the enzyme.

Initially, entomologists assumed that ability of resistant insects to dehydrochlorinate DDT represented a qualitative change to high enzyme level from having none at all. It is now known that most insects can convert some DDT to DDE and the nature of the change involved in resistance is quantitative, not qualitative. Susceptible house flies have been shown via GLC analysis to dehydrochlorinate DDT (Khan and Terriere, 1968) as do susceptible and resistant strains of Culex tarsalis (Plapp et al., 1965). Insects normally tolerant to DDT such as the Mexican bean beetle, Epilachna varivesta, readily dehydrochlorinate DDT and may owe their tolerance to this ability.

Resistance depending on DDT dehydrochlorinase is apparently not common. In addition to house flies, only Aedes mosquitoes and possibly some DDT-resistant lepidoptera possess resistance mechanisms depending on this detoxication mechanism.

The most important recent studies on DDT dehydrochlorinase have been those of Dinamarca et al. (1969, 1971). These researchers purified the enzyme from resistant house flies and found that it consisted of 4 subunits with a molecular weight of 30,000 each. The trimer possessed only about 10% of the activity of the tetramer while the monomer and dimer were inactive. Glutathione, not a cofactor in the reaction, was required to maintain the enzyme in the active form. Unfortunately, no comparable studies have yet been performed with susceptible house flies.

Microsomal detoxication - (DDTmd)

A second major DDT resistance gene involving detoxication was reported from the Danish house fly strain F_c (Oppenoorth and Houx, 1968). This chromosome V gene, known as DDTmd (for microsomal detoxication) involves an increased ability to

319

detoxify DDT via NADPH-dependent processes. Biological verification has come from demonstrations of the ability of antioxidant synergists such as piperonyl butoxide and sesamex to effectively block DDT resistance in F_c and similar strains (Oppenoorth, 1967).

Surprisingly, the identity of the metabolites of DDT produced in strains possessing the gene DDTmd remains unknown. The major metabolites are highly polar, more polar than dicofol (DDT alcohol) which may be an intermediate in their formation (Gil et al., 1968).

Additional studies on strains F_c have shown that DDTmd also confers an increased ability to detoxify numerous organophosphate and carbamate insecticides and thus allowing for resistance to them (Plapp and Casida, 1969). The presence of similar DDT resistance mechanisms in other insects has not been definitively demonstrated, but Lloyd (1969) has presented evidence for a sesamex-suppressible DDT resistance in Sitophilus granarius which is probably very similar to that occurring in house flies.

Knockdown resistance - (Kdr)

A third mechanism of resistance to DDT, and probably the most common cause of resistance to this insecticide is associated with a recessive gene known as knockdown resistance (kdr). Resistance associated with kdr is broad in spectrum, extending to all DDT analogs (Hoyer and Plapp, 1968). This gene also confers resistance to pyrethroid insecticides and even to pyrethrins-synergist combinations. Several genetic studies in house flies (Farnham, 1971) and mosquitoes (Plapp et al., 1965) have confirmed this relationship.

Resistance associated with the gene kdr apparently does not involve insecticide detoxication and may, as suggested by Tsukamoto et al. (1965), relate to a decreased sensitivity of nervous tissue to effects of the insecticides. Further evidence that detoxication is not involved is the failure to demonstrate synergists which block resistance to DDT in kdr strains.

Widespread occurrence of kdr-type resistance in Culex and Anopheles mosquitoes has seriously hampered many public health programs based on the use of DDT for interrupting transmission of mosquito-borne diseases.

Cyclodiene insecticides have proven to be very refractory to detoxication in all biological systems. While resistance to this class of compounds occurs widely, it is apparently independent of detoxication. Resistant insects do not degrade appreciably more insecticide than susceptible insects. Rather they are less susceptible to effects of the insecticides and frequently carry body burdens of many times a lethal dose to susceptible insects.

One metabolic difference has been observed that may prove of significance in terms of resistance. According to Telford and Matsumura (1970, 1971) nervous tissue of dieldrin-resistant cockroaches accumulates less dieldrin than comparable tissue from susceptible insects. Similar decreases in the binding of endrin in larvae of cyclodiene-resistant tobacco budworms, Heliothis virescens, have been reported (Polles and Vinson, 1972).

Shankland and Schroeder (1973) indicate that cyclodienes may owe their toxicity to an ability to cause release of acetylcholine from presynaptic vesicles. This finding raises the possibility that resistance may relate to a change in release rate of acetylcholine rather than to any increased detoxication activity.

B. Organophosphate and Carbamate

Insecticides

With organophosphate and carbamate insecticides, the relationship between detoxication and resistance is more clearcut. Insecticides of these types are metabolized by a variety of enzymatic processes. Evidence indicates that increases in ability to detoxify by several of these pathways characterize many resistant strains. Selection for resistance to a particular organophosphate or carbamate insecticide usually results in an insect strain with a high ability to detoxify that compound. Such strains usually have a high ability to detoxify many more-or-less closely related insecticides as well. This means that broad-spectrum cross resistance to organophosphates and carbamates occurs in many resistant strains.

Ali-esterase

The first discovered major genetic factor for resistance to organophosphates involved a hydrolytic enzyme, one that normally metabolizes aliphatic esters such as methyl n-butyrate, and is known, therefore, as an ali-esterase.

Enzymes of this type are susceptible to inhibition by organophosphate insecticides. Work by Van Asperen and Oppenoorth
(1959), confirmed independently by Bigley and Plapp (1960),
demonstrated an apparent decline in level of the enzyme in
several organophosphate resistant house fly populations.

As reviewed by Oppenoorth (1972) the missing enzyme has
been replaced by a mutant form that slowly degrades the oxygen
analogs of phosphorothioates to which the strain is resistant.
The mutation involves a change in substrate specificity of
the enzyme. It loses the ability to hydrolyze carboxylic
acid esters and acquires an ability to slowly hydrolyze phosphate esters. A number of allelic forms may exist. The
allelism is considered an explanation for some of the different
resistance spectra that occur in various fly strains.

Changes in esterase activity in insects are frequently
a factor in organophosphate and possibly in carbamate resistance as well. Evidence for involvement of carbamates with
esterase activity comes from the finding (Plapp and Bigley,
1961) that carbamates, like organophosphates, inhibit ali-
esterase activity. Further, carbamate resistant house flies
may possess altered ali-esterase levels (Plapp et al., 1964)
and finally, synergists that block esterase-associated resistance in organophosphate-resistant flies also act as synergists
for carbamate resistant flies (Plapp and Velega, 1967).

In addition to the house fly, decreased ali-esterase
activity has been shown in malathion-resistant populations
of the blow fly, Chrysomya putoria (Townsend and Busvine,
1969).

The opposite phenomenon, increased ali-esterase activity,
occurs in some resistant insects. Ozaki and Kasai (1970)
reported increased ali-esterase activity in a malathion
resistant planthopper, Laodelphus striatellus. Whitten and
Bull (1970) reported a similar increase in activity occurs
in methyl parathion-resistant tobacco budworms, Heliothis
virescens. The relationship between increased ali-esterase
activity and organophosphate resistance has not been shown.
It may be that increased esterase activity is available to
react with insecticides and thus, make less available to
react with target enzymes such as acetylcholinesterase.

Alkyl transferase

A second pathway of organophosphate detoxication involves
a glutathione-dependent transferase reaction which cleaves
O-alkyl ester linkages. Evidence for occurrence of this

322

reaction, first reported by Plapp and Casida (1958), was
provided by Fukami and Shishido (1963, 1966). High levels
of glutathione transferase in resistant house flies were
first reported by Lewis (1969) and confirmed by Motoyama and
Dauterman (1972). Earlier, Motoyama et al. (1971) reported
similar high levels of alkyl transferase in an organophosphate-resistant predaceous mite, Neoseiulis fallacis.

Further studies on alkyl transferase in house flies
were reported by Oppenoorth et al. (1972). These authors
demonstrated that several resistant strains possessed high
levels of enzyme activity. Genetic studies revealed semidominant inheritance controlled by a chromosome II gene,
mutant symbol g. Similar studies on the fly strain studied
by Motoyama have confirmed these genetic findings (Plapp,
unpublished results).

Available evidence clearly indicates that alkyl transferase is an important detoxication mechanism for organophosphate insecticides. How important the system is in overall
detoxication and in comparison to other resistance mechanisms
remains to be fully evaluated.

Microsomal mixed-function oxidase (ox)

Recently research on detoxication and resistance in
insects has centered on the microsomal mixed function oxidase
system. This enzyme system has proven particularly important
in organophosphate and carbamate resistance and is discussed
in detail elsewhere in this symposium volume (Hodgson, 1974).

Evidence that increased levels of oxidative detoxifying
enzymes characterize organophosphate and carbamate resistant
fly strains has frequently been reported (Schonbrod et al.,
1968; Tsukamoto and Casida, 1967; Tsukamoto et al., 1968;
Oppenoorth and Houx, 1968; Plapp and Casida, 1969; Sawicki
et al., 1966). In the case of strains F_c and SKA, chromosome
V factors conferring resistance to DDT also confer resistance
to organophosphates and carbamates as well as increased
detoxifying activity for all 3 insecticide types. In all
other strains that have been subjected to biochemical and
genetic study, chromosome II genes confer oxidative resistance.
The latter have been named Oxidase, mutant symbol ox.

Data from metabolic studies with a variety of insecticide
and non-insecticide substrates (see review by Wilkinson and
Brattsten, 1972) indicate that only one enzyme system is involved in metabolizing an extremely wide range of chemicals.
How one enzyme system can serve to metabolize such a wide

range of chemicals remains unexplained. Nevertheless, existence of the system and widespread evidence for its occurrence at high levels in resistant house flies are evidence of its importance as a mechanism of detoxication and resistance.

Although only limited evidence is presently available, it seems likely that high levels of microsomal oxidase characterize other resistant insect species. Several good studies (Williamson and Schecter, 1971; Bull and Whitten, 1972; Plapp, 1973) have shown the occurrence of high levels of oxidase activity in methyl parathion resistant tobacco budworms. Kuhr (1971) has shown a similar occurrence in parathion resistant cabbage loopers, Trichoplusia ni.

Questions concerning the genetic and biochemical nature of the relationship of high oxidase activity to resistance and detoxication are presently under investigation. Resistant house flies frequently have more cytochrome P-450 than susceptible house flies (Philpot and Hodgson, 1972; Tate et al., 1973). The CO difference spectra of resistant strains have a peak at 448 or 449 nanometers as compared to 450 or 451 for susceptible insects (Morello et al., 1971; Philpot and Hodgson, 1972). Additional differences in Type I, II, and III difference spectra also occur (Tate et al., 1973). Genetic studies followed by biochemical assays of appropriate substrains have shown (Tate et al., 1974) that in the diazinon resistant Rutgers strain, both quantitative and qualitative differences in cytochrome P-450 are controlled by genes on chromosome II. In contrast, in strain F_c with a major chromosome V resistance gene, both chromosome II and chromosome V are involved in controlling changes in cytochrome P-450. Genetic studies (Tate et al., 1974) suggest that at least in the Rutgers strain all the variations appear to be inherited together as a single genetic unit. The nature of the interrelationships among these quantitative and qualitative changes remains unclear.

In the house fly the 3 resistance mechanisms described above have much in common. All involve increased detoxication, all are inherited in a semidominant manner, and all are controlled by genes on chromosome II. It is tempting to speculate that there may be further interrelationships among these apparently independent genetic factors, but as yet there is no evidence in this area.

Discussion

At least 2 resistance mechanisms, altered ali-esterase

and high oxidase, can be blocked by synergists which inter-
fere with insecticide detoxication. Antioxidant synergists
which have long been known to block carbamate resistance can
also block oxidative resistance to organophosphates (Plapp,
1970). Noninsecticidal organophosphates such as triphenyl
phosphate and S,S,S-tributylphosphorotrithioate which block
resistance associated with altered ali-esterases can also
synergize carbamates (Plapp and Valega, 1967) which is
evidence that they block oxidative resistance as well.

Pyrethroid insecticides are rapidly detoxified in insects. In practice, this rapid detoxication is blocked by
antioxidant synergists. In spite of this, the major resistance mechanism for pyrethrins in house flies, the chromosome
III gene kdr, does not appear to involve detoxication. This
is true because levels of resistance associated with this
gene are similar for pyrethrins only and for pyrethrins:pip-
eronyl butoxide combinations (Plapp and Hoyer, 1968a).

Farnham (1973) characterized some additional pyrethrins
resistance genes in house flies. At least 2 of these, py
ses and py ex, probably involve increased oxidative detoxication and may very well be identical with DDTmd and ox.
Their total contribution to resistance proved to be less
than that associated with kdr, further evidence for the
relatively minor role of detoxication in resistance to these
insecticides.

Pyrethrins resistance in several other insects is apparently similar to that in the house fly in that it is related to broad spectrum resistance to chlorinated hydrocarbons.
This is true for Culex tarsalis (Plapp and Hoyer, 1968a) and
for Sitophilus granarius (Lloyd, 1969). If the above
described relationship is general in insects, it would appear
that increases in detoxication rate are not of great significance in resistance to these insecticides.

The newest class of insect control agents is insect
growth regulators or juvenile hormone analogs. These chemicals are subject to metabolism in insects via both oxidative
and hydrolytic processes (Slade and Zibbitt, 1972).

Recently several reports of resistance to juvenile
hormone analogs have appeared. Two of these (Cerf and
Georghiou, 1972; and Plapp and Vinson, 1973) have been in
organophosphate-resistant house flies. The third report
(Dyte, 1972) involved a strain of Tribolium castaneum resistant to many insecticides. Genetic studies (Vinson and
Plapp, 1974) indicate that resistance to juvenile hormone
analogs in the house fly is semidominant and controlled by a

325

factor on chromosome II. In all probability, the gene conferring resistance to these chemicals is identical to the oxidative gene conferring resistance to organophosphates and carbamates. This hypothesis has not yet been verified by appropriate biochemical studies.

One additional resistance gene which relates to insecticide detoxication is known. In the house fly this is a chromosome III gene which acts to decrease the rate of absorption of insecticides. Such a mechanism increases the effectiveness of other resistance mechanisms by allowing them more time in which to act. Decreased absorption rate as a resistance mechanism in the house fly has been known since the work of Forgash et al., (1962) and Farnham et al., (1965). As reviewed by Georghiou,(1972) similar factors occur in other resistant insect species including Aedes aegypti, Culex fatigans, Euxesta notata, and Heliothis virescens.

The first genetic determinations of genes for decreased rates of absorption of insecticides in house flies were reported by Hoyer and Plapp (1968) and Sawicki and Farnham (1968). In the former case the gene was named tin for organotin-R as it was first shown to confer resistance to these insecticides. Sawicki and Farnham named it pen for reduced penetration.

When the tin gene was combined with other genes conferring resistance to insecticides it acted to increase their effectiveness. Increases were from 1.5 to 25 times with detoxication genes for resistance to DDT and malathion and even greater in combination with nonmetabolic genes for resistance to DDT or dieldrin (Hoyer and Plapp, 1971). Similar increases in resistance were reported by Sawicki (1973) when the pen gene was combined with major resistance genes from the SKA strain of house flies. A test cross performed by Sawicki indicated that pen and tin are alleles.

Interaction of Resistance Genes

The previous discussion dealt primarily with resistance genes and/or detoxication mechanisms studied alone. Such tests are necessary to gain an understanding of the biochemistry and resistance spectrum associated with each resistance gene.

In practice, resistance genes usually occur in combinations. When they do, resistance levels frequently increase greatly. The effect of combining two genes (Plapp, 1970) is multiplicative rather than additive.

An important study (Khan, et al., 1973) dealt with the biochemistry of chromosome II and chromosome V oxidative resistance genes in the house fly. When the genes were combined in the same strain, total enzyme activity as measured by an aldrin epoxidase assay was additive. Total resistance was not reported, but was probably more than additive since a doubling of detoxifying activity usually produces far more than a doubling of resistance.

Inheritance of Resistance

Another consistent finding from resistance studies deserves comment. Genetic factors involving increases in ability to detoxify insecticides are inherited semidominant or rarely, as dominant genes. Conversely, non-metabolic resistance genes such as kdr and pen are inherited in a manner recessive to susceptibility. Why detoxication genes are dominant and non-detoxication genes are recessive is not known, however, the pattern is remarkably consistent from all reported studies. It suggests that the two types of resistance are controlled by different mechanisms.

Induction of Detoxication

The ability of insects to detoxify insecticides is not fixed. Activity varies greatly with age and sex as well as with resistance or susceptibility. In addition, many insecticide detoxication mechanisms are inducible. That is, exposure of insects to appropriate chemicals can "induce" or "derepress" synthesis of enzymes involved in detoxication.

Initial research in this area was done by Agosin and coworkers in connection with their research on DDT metabolism and resistance in Triatoma infestans. They demonstrated (Ilevicky et al., 1964) induction of NAD-kinase in DDT-treated insects and also (Agosin et al., 1965) enhanced protein synthesis in DDT-treated Triatoma. Later (Gil et al., 1968), induction of microsomal oxidative enzymes in house flies treated with DDT was demonstrated.

Findings of the Agosin group were confirmed (Plapp and Casida, 1970; Walker and Terriere, 1970) in experiments with DDT and dieldrin as inducers of insecticide detoxication by microsomal oxidases in house flies. Increased activity was shown for napthalene hydroxylation as well as for metabolism of a wide variety of insecticide chemical substrates. A direct effect on insecticide toxicity was shown by Walker and

FREDERICK W. PLAPP, Jr.

Terriere (1970) when they protected flies against carbaryl
by prior treatment with dieldrin. The presumed effect was
to increase carbaryl detoxifying enzymes by dieldrin pre-
treatment.

It is now evident that other detoxication mechanisms can
be induced in addition to microsomal oxidase. Yu and
Terriere (1972) induced DDT dehydrochlorinase by treatment
of flies with cyclodienes. Other experiments (Terriere and
Yu, 1973) demonstrated microsomal induction in house flies
treated with a juvenile hormone analog. Rhee and Plapp (1974)
have obtained evidence that most types of insecticides can
induce oxidative metabolism. This includes organophosphates,
carbamates and pyrethroids, in addition to the chlorinated
insecticides which are known inducers.

The role of induction in insecticide detoxication and
resistance is not yet well understood. It is obvious that
induction is useful in enabling insects to detoxify insecticides. High detoxifying activity strains act sometimes as
if they are permanently induced (Hodgson and Plapp, 1970).
Other experiments (Terriere et al., 1971) have shown that
additional induction can occur in high oxidase as well as in
low oxidase house fly strains.

Conclusion

Material presented here demonstrates that our knowledge
of biochemistry and genetics of detoxication mechanisms in
insects has expanded greatly in recent years. It is well to
point out that most of our knowledge applies only to house
flies. We know much less about many major pest species which
are resistant to insecticides. There is no certainty that
these insects will respond as house flies do.

Another major unknown is the actual nature of the
genetic changes taking place in connection with the increased
ability to detoxify insecticides that characterizes resistance.
Are the mutations changed structural genes or do they represent changes in regulator genes? Evidence from studies
with microsomal oxidases indicates that both possible types
of changes--qualitative and quantitative--occur.

Since virtually nothing is known of the nature of
genetic regulation in eukaryotes, the question as to the
nature of genes involved in resistance is not presently
answerable. It is, however, my hypothesis that most genetic
changes associated with resistance, at least with detoxication, act like operator constitutive mutants, mutants which

328

render more difficult repression of the synthesis of
structural detoxifying genes. Mutations of this type would
be inherited as incomplete dominants as are the resistance
genes. Finally, it is worth noting that the genetics and
biochemistry of resistance in insects should provide good
biologic material for research on the nature of genetic control mechanisms in higher animals.

References

Agosin, M., L. Aravena, and A. Neghme. 1965. Exp. Parasitol.
16:318-324.
Bigley, W. S., and F. W. Plapp, Jr. 1960. Ann. Entomol. Soc.
Amer. 53:360-364.
Brown, A. W. A. 1971. "Pesticides in the Environment," v. 1.
White-Stevens (ed.), Marcel Dekker, New York, pp. 457-552.
Brown, A. W. A., and R. Pal. 1971. Insecticide Resistance in
Arthropods. WHO, Geneva, Monograph Ser. No. 38. 491 p.
Bull, D. L., and C. J. Whitten. 1972. J. Agr. Food Chem. 20:
561-564.
Cerf, D. C., and G. P. Georghiou. 1972. Nature 239:401-402.
Dinamarca, M. L., I. Saavedra and E. Valdes. 1969. Comp.
Biochem. Physiol. 31:269-282.
Dinamarca, M. L., L. Levenbook, and E. Valdes. 1971. Arch.
Biochem. Biophys. 147:374-383.
Dyte, C. E. 1972. Nature 238:48-49.
Farnham, A. W. 1971. Pest. Sci. 2:138-143.
Farnham, A. W., K. A. Lord, and R. M. Sawicki. 1965. J. Ins.
Physiol. 11:1475-1488.
Forgash, A. J., B. J. Cook and R. C. Riley. 1962. J. Econ.
Entomol. 55:545-551.
Fukami, J., and T. Shishido. 1963. Botyu-Kagaku 28:77-81.
Fukami, J., and T. Shishido. 1966. J. Econ. Entomol. 59:
1338-1346.
Georghiou, G. P. 1972. Ann. Rev. Ecol. Systematics 3:133-168.
Gil, L., B. C. Fine, M. L. Dinamarca, I. Balazs, J. R.
Busvine, and M. Agosin. 1968. Entomol. Exp. Appl. 11:15-29.
Hiroyoshi, T. 1960. J. Econ. Entomol. 53:985-990.
Hiroyoshi, T. 1961. Genetics 46:1373-80.
Hodgson, E. 1974. Amer. Zoologist. In press.
Hodgson, E. and F. W. Plapp, Jr. 1970. J. Agr. Food Chem.
18:1048-1055.
Hoyer, R. F. 1966. J. Econ. Entomol. 59:133-136.
Hoyer, R. F. and F. W. Plapp, Jr. 1968. J. Econ. Entomol.
61:1269-1276.

Ilivicky, J., M. L. Dinamarca, and M. Agosin. 1964. Comp. Biochem. Physiol. 11:291-301.

Khan, M. A. Q. and L. C. Terriere. 1968. J. Econ. Entomol. 61:732-736.

Khan, M. A. Q., R. I. Morimoto, J. T. Bederka, Jr., and J. M. Runnels. 1973. Biochem. Genetics 10:243-252.

Kuhr, R. J. 1971. J. Econ. Entomol. 64:1373-1381.

Lewis, J. B. 1969. Nature. 224:917-198.

Lloyd, C. J. 1969. J. Stored Prod. Res. 5:357-363.

Morello, A., W. Bleecker, and M. Agosin. 1971. Biochem. J. 124:199-205.

Motoyama, N., G. C. Rock, and W. C. Dauterman. 1971. Pest. Biochem. Physiol. 1:205-215.

Motoyama, N. and W. C. Dauterman. 1972. Pest. Biochem. Physiol. 2:113-122.

Oppenoorth, F. J. 1967. Entomol. Exp. Appl. 10:75-86.

Oppenoorth, F. J. 1972. "Toxicology, Biodegradation and Efficacy of Livestock Pesticides." M. A. Khan and W. O. Haufe, (ed.), Swets & Zeitlinger, Amsterdam, pp. 73-92.

Oppenoorth, F. J., and N. W. H. Houx. 1968. Entomol. Exp. Appl. 11:81-93.

Oppenoorth, F. J., V. Rupes, S. ElBashir, N. W. H. Houx, and S. Voerman. 1972. Pest. Biochem. Physiol. 2:262-269.

Ozaki, K. and T. Kassai. 1970. Entomol. Exp. Appl. 13:162-172.

Philpot, R. M. and E. Hodgson. 1971. Chem.-Biol. Interactions 4:399-408.

Plapp, F. W., Jr. 1970. "Biochemical Toxicology of Insecticides." R. D. O'Brien, and I. Yamamoto (eds.), Academic Press, New York, pp. 119-192.

Plapp, F. W., Jr. 1973. Pest. Biochem. Physiol. 2:447-453.

Plapp, F. W., Jr. and J. E. Casida. 1958. J. Econ. Entomol. 51:800-803.

Plapp, F. W., Jr. and W. S. Bigley. 1961. J. Econ. Entomol. 54:793-796.

Plapp, F. W., Jr., G. A. Chapman and W. S. Bigley. 1964. J. Econ. Entomol. 57:692-695.

Plapp, F. W., Jr., G. A. Chapman and J. W. Morgan. 1965. J. Econ. Entomol. 58:1064-1069.

Plapp, F. W., Jr. and T. M. Valega. 1967. J. Econ. Entomol. 60:1095-1102.

Plapp, F. W., Jr. and R. F. Hoyer. 1968a. J. Econ. Entomol. 61:761-765.

Plapp, F. W., Jr. and R. F. Hoyer, 1968b. J. Econ. Entomol. 61:1298-1303.

Plapp, F. W., Jr. and J. E. Casida. 1969. J. Econ. Entomol.

62:1174-1179.

Plapp, F. W., Jr. and J. E. Casida. 1970. J. Econ. Entomol. 63:1091-1092.

Plapp, F. W., Jr. and S. B. Vinson. 1973. Pest. Biochem. Physiol. 3:131-136.

Polles, S. G. and S. B. Vinson. 1972. J. Agr. Food Chem. 20: 38-41.

Rhee, K. S. and F. W. Plapp, Jr. 1974. Chem.-Biol. Interactions.

Sawicki, R. M. 1973. Pestic. Sci. 4:171-180.

Sawicki, R. M., M. G. Franco and R. Milani. 1966. Bull. Wld. Hlth. Org. 35:893-903.

Sawicki, R. M. and A. W. Farnham. 1968. Bull. Entomol. Res. 59:409-421.

Schonbrod, R. D., M. A. Q. Khan, L. C. Terriere, and F. W. Plapp, Jr. 1968. Life Sci. 7:681-688.

Shankland, D. L. and M. E. Schroeder. 1973. Pest. Biochem. Physiol. 3:77-86.

Slade, M. and C. H. Zibbitt. 1972. "Insect Juvenile Hormones." J. J. Menn and M. Beroza (ed.), Academic Press, New York, pp. 155-176.

Sullivan, R. L. 1961. J. Heredity 52:282-289.

Tate, L. G., F. W. Plapp, Jr., and E. Hodgson. 1973. Chem.- Biol. Interactions 6:237-247.

Tate, L. G., F. W. Plapp, Jr. and E. Hodgson. 1974. Biochem. Genetics. In press.

Telford, J. N. and F. Matsumura. 1970. J. Econ. Entomol.63: 795-800.

Telfor, J. N. and F. Matsumura. 1971. J. Econ. Entomol. 64: 230-238.

Terriere, L. C., S. J. Yu and R. F. Hoyer. 1971. Science 171:581-583.

Terriere, L. C. and S. J. Yu. 1973. Pest. Biochem. Physiol. 3:96-107.

Townsend, M. G. and J. R. Busvine. 1969. Entomol. Exp. Appl. 12:243-249.

Tsukamoto, M. 1963. Botyu-Kagaku 28:91-5.

Tsukamoto, M. 1964. Botyu-Kagaku 29:51-59.

Tsukamoto, M. 1965. Japan. J. Genetics 36:168-75.

Tsukamoto, M. 1969. Residue Rev. 25:289-314.

Tsukamoto, M., Y. Baba and S. Hiraga. 1961. Japan. J. Genet. 36:168-178.

Tsukamoto, M., T. Narahashi and T. Yamsaki. 1965. Botyu- Kagaku 30:128-132.

Tsukamoto, M. and J. E. Casida. 1967. Nature 213:49-50.

Tsukamoto, M., S. P. Shrivastava, and J. E. Casida. 1968. J. Econ. Entomol. 61:50–55.

Van Asperen, K. and F. J. Oppenoorth. 1959. Entomol. Exp. Appl. 2:48–57.

Vinson, S. B. and F. W. Plapp, Jr. 1974. J. Agr. Food Chem. In press.

Wagoner, D. E. 1967. Genetics 57:729–737.

Walker, C. R. and L. C. Terriere. 1970. Entomol. Exp. Appl. 13:260–274.

Whitten, C. J. and D. L. Bull. 1970. J. Econ. Entomol. 63: 1492–1495.

Wilkinson, C. F. and L. B. Brattsten. 1972. Drug Metabolism Reviews 1:153–228.

Williamson, R. L. and M. S. Schechter. 1970. Biochem. Pharmacol. 19:1719–1727.

Yu, S. J. and L. C. Terriere. 1972. Pest. Biochem. Physiol. 2:184–190.

Acknowledgments

Approved for publication as Technical Paper 10980 by the Director, Texas Agricultural Experiment Station. I thank R. R. Fleet for helpful discussions and critical review of the manuscript.

ECOLOGICAL AND HEALTH EFFECTS OF THE PHOTOLYSIS OF INSECTICIDES

M. A. Q. Khan and H. M. Khan
University of Illinois at Chicago Circle
Chicago

D. J. Sutherland
Rutgers-The State University of New Jersey
New Brunswick, N. J.

Introduction

A chemical released into the environment is subject to physical and biological processes which determine its fate and effectiveness. The former includes chemical reactions brought about by environmental factors such as light, heat, air, etc., in atmosphere, and on soil, water and plant surfaces. Since solar radiation in the form of light is the main source of energy for earth, which is transformed to other forms of energy, its direct effects on chemicals, e.g. pesticides[1], in the environment, have become a subject of increasing scientific investigations.

The solar radiations reaching earth's surface is devoid of high energy waves below 2860 Å because of the absorption of the latter by ozone layer of the atmosphere.

In the primary process, each quantum of light[2]

---

[1] For chemical formulae see Kenaga (1966).

[2] If E (kcal/Einstein) is the energy of a single quantum (or particle) of light, ν the frequency of light (= velocity of light (c)/wave length) and h the Planck's constant, then $E = h\nu$ or $hc/\lambda = 2.8591 \times 10^5$/wave length in Angstroms. The einstein is a mole of quanta; absorption of one einstein of light of 3000 Å will impart 94.6 kcal/mole to the molecule.

absorbed excites one molecule electronically. Excited molecules may lose their excess energy by
dissociation (oxidations, reductions), isomerization, fluorescence, phosphorescence, eliminations,
radiationless transitions or by other deactivation
routes. Dissociation of a co-valent bond by solar
energy often produces a pair of free radicals,
which then react chemically and may initiate chain
reactions. The light absorbing molecule (A*) may
not react chemically but can transfer the energy
to a second species (D) that does not absorb light
in the region of the exciting wave length. 'A'
thus acts as a "sensitizer".

$$A + h\nu \rightarrow A^* \text{ (donor)}$$

$$A^* + D \text{ (acceptor)} \rightarrow A + D^*$$

$$D^* \rightarrow \text{products}$$

The acceptor molecule may undergo photolysis.
The products of photochemical reaction by sensi-
tized energy transfer may differ from the products
of direct photolysis. The 'donor' or initiator
may also undergo facile homolysis (dissociation of
co-valent bonds forming a pair of free radicals)
which can initiate chain reactions that will result in oxygenated products from otherwise photochemically inert substrates.

Oxygen is highly electronegative and a di-
radical; it interacts with other substances and
light (only through a chromophore) by several
important mechanisms, including direct free-radical reactions, energy transfer to oxidizable substrates, and the excitation of the ground state
(triplet) oxygen itself. Free radicals generated
by light and other initiators can react with
ordinary triplet oxygen to form peroxy radicals,
which are capable of further reactions including
the abstraction of hydrogen from organic substrates and the generation of radical chains.
In such chain processes the initial reaction of a
single molecule eventually can form many molecules
of product with correspondingly high yield of products per quantum of light originally absorbed.

The conversion of triplet oxygen by light to
singlet molecular oxygen may cause many dye-sen-

sitized photooxidations. There are two singlet
states of oxygen = O_2 ($^1\Delta g$) with 37.4 kcal/mole
and O_2 ($\Sigma + g$) with 22.4 kcal/mole) The excited
singlet oxygen no longer shows the free radical
character, rather, it exhibits the properties and
reactions expected of a true oxygen-oxygen double
bond ($\ddot{O}=\ddot{O}$), such as combination with dienes.

Singlet oxygen sensitizers are Biphenyl (65
kcal/mole); Naphthalene (60.8 kcal/mole); Pyrene
(48 kcal/mole); Anthracene, Eosin and Rose Bengal
(42 kcal/mole); Tetracene (29.4 kcal/mole), as
well as chlorophyll, riboflavin, hematoporphyrins.
    The photolysis of pesticide chemicals can
take place on surface or in solution either by
direct electronic excitation following light absorption or through sensitizers. It can be mediated through singlet oxygen, e.g. photodechlorina-
tion of chlorinated aromatic herbicides (McGuire
et al., 1970), or through a triplet sensitizer e.g.
carbon-carbon bridge formation of cyclodienes
(Rosen, 1972), or hydrogen-abstraction by hydro-
carbon-free radical in a suitable solvent as in
the case of DDT (Plimmer et al., 1970).
    The most commonly used insecticides which
have been studied in the field and laboratory
for photolysis are: DDT, methoxychlor, dieldrin,
aldrin, isodrin, endrin, heptachlor, chlordane,
chlordene, heptachlor epoxide, carbaryl
parathion, Abate, pyrethroids and rotenoids.
    A brief description of the photolysis of
some of these insecticides will be dealt here.

DDT and Its Analogues:

Slow photodecomposition of DDT from surfaces
has been observed in the field (Dachauer, 1962,
Harrison et al., 1967). In vitro photooxidation
of DDT and DDE has been studied by Crosby (1969)
and Plimmer et al., (1970). Photolytic (2600 Å)
generation of free radicals that may abstract
hydrogen from solvent (methanol) react with oxygen,

or abstract hydrogen from unreacted substrate.
Further decomposition of short-lived intermediates

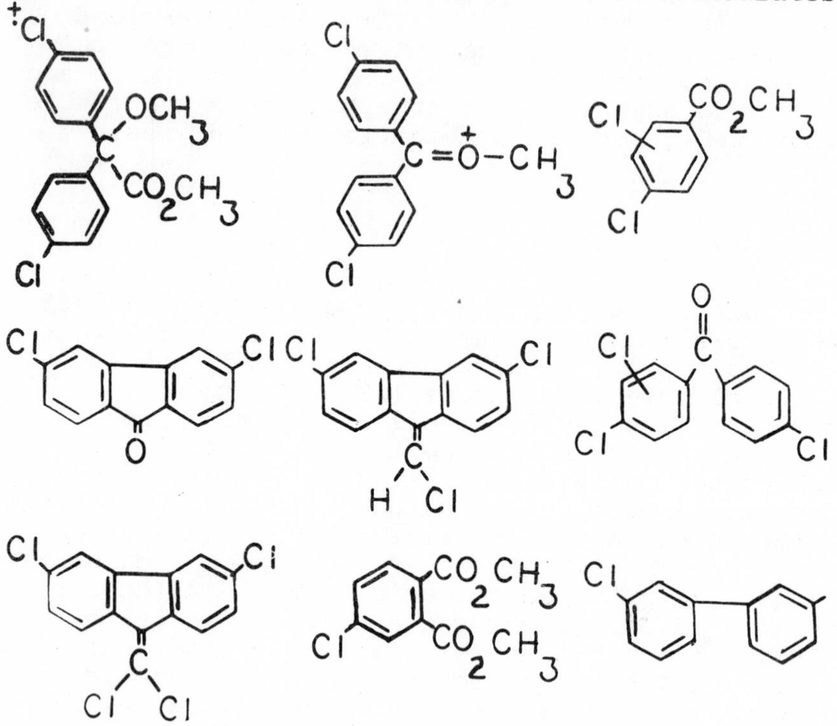

Figure 1. Some of the photolysis products of DDT
and DDE (Plimmer et al., 1970).

yields many compounds. Oxidative products include
benzoic acids, aromatic ketones, and chlorinated
phenols. DDE, in addition, undergoes photocycliza-
tion to form dichlorofluorene derivatives. In the
presence of excess oxygen, photochemically generated free radicals from DDT and DDE add oxygen. Rearrangement and reaction of unstable intermediates account for the formation of the photooxidation products (Fig. 1).

The major products from DDT were: DDE,
$(C_6H_4Cl)_2$, $(C_6H_4Cl)_2CO$ in oxygen and DDD,
$C_6H_5.C_6H_4Cl.CH.CH.CH.Cl_2$, $(C_6H_4Cl)_2.CH.COO.CH_3$ and
$C_6H_5.C_6H_4Cl.CH.COOCH_3$ under nitrogen.

The major products from DDE were: $C_6H_5.COO.CH_3$,

$(C_6H_5)_2CO$, $(C_6H_5)_2C=CHCl$ under nitrogen and $C_6H_5.COOCH_3$, $(C_6H_5)_2.C(OCH_3).COOCH_3$, and (III) in oxygen (Fig. 1).

Compounds of high molecular weight are probably present in small quantity. Certain aromatic amines induce photolysis of DDT in cyclohexane by UV light (Miller and Narang, 1970). The products in the presence of diethylaniline include DDE, DDD, dichlorobenzophenone, and two other unidentified products. These reactions involve charge transfer from amine to DDT.

Methoxychlor undergoes rapid facile photooxidation involving a free-radical pathway to give primarily a mixture of 4,4'-dimethoxybenzophenone, p-methoxybenzoic acid, and p-methoxyphenol (Fig. 2) (Crosby, 1969; Li and Bradley, 1969).

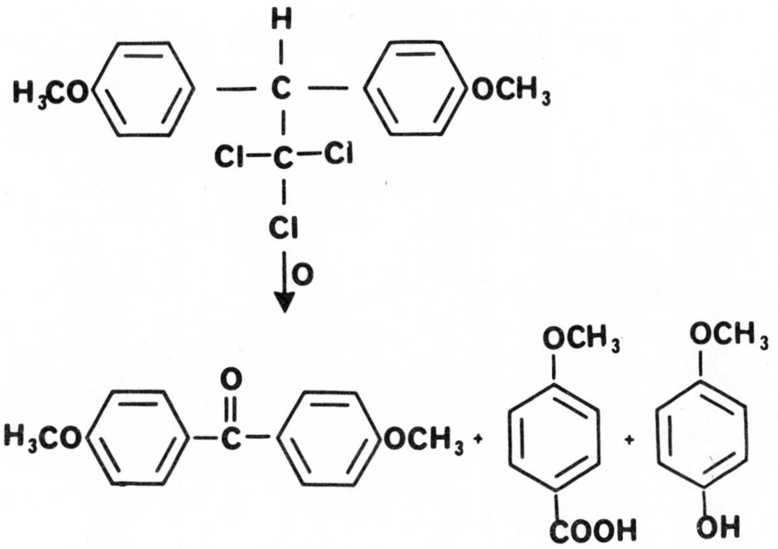

Figure 2. Photolytic oxidation products of Methoxychlor (Li and Bradley, 1969).

337

Table 1. Toxicity of certain cyclodienes and their photoisomers to houseflies and four freshwater animals (Khan et al., 1973).

Animal[b]	LC_{50} : p.p.b.[a]									
	A	PA	D	PD	H	PH	I	PI	C	PC
Bluegill	260	90	170	30	-	-	12	25	218	346
Minnow	-	-	24	10	13	8	6	10	-	-
Asellus	80	40	-	-	100	60	-	-	-	-
Aedes	3	0.5	6	3	5	2	19	19	130	150
Musca	14	6.9	9.8	8.3	11	5.6	54	113	158	179

[a] 24-hour mortality; for flies the LD_{50} is in µg/fly

[b] 2-month old fish fry, late 3rd instar Aedes aegypti (susceptible) larvae, 3-day old female houseflies.

338

Table 2. Toxicity ratios of certain cyclodienes and their photoisomers to various freshwater animals (Khan et al., 1973).

Animal	Toxicity ratios:[a]				
	A/PA	D/PD	H/PH	I/PI	C/PC
Crustacea:					
Daphnia (Water Flea) pulex	1.425	1.27	1.24	0.45	0.91
Gammarus (amphipod) spp.	1.83	12.22	1.45	0.43	–
Asellus (isopod) spp.	2.13(2.0)	1.60(1.7)	–	0.64	0
Insects:					
Aedes aegypti larvae (mosquito)	5.68(6.0)	2.30(2.0)	2.80(2.5)	0.30(.33)	–
Fish:					
Gambia affinis (Guppy)	2.41	2.57	–	0.45	–
Pimephalus promelas (Bass)	1.42	1.11(2.4)	1.23(1.63)	0.3(.60)	–
Lepomis macrochirus (Bluegill)	3.60(2.9)	5.14(5.7)	–	0.75(.48)	0.72(.63)

[a] Ratios calculated from LT_{50} values (Georgacakis and Khan, 1971) and from LC_{50} values (Table 1), the ratios in parenthesis are from the latter.

Aldrin, Dieldrin and Other Cyclodienes

On exposure to UV-light (2537 Å) aldrin (A) undergoes epoxidation to dieldrin, (D), dechlorination to pentachloroaldrin and cage-isomerization to photoaldrin (PA) - the latter may undergo further epoxidation to yield photodieldrin (PD) (Rosen, 1967; Henderson and Crosby, 1967; Rosen and Sutherland, 1967). Dieldrin is readily isomerized to photodieldrin (Parsons and Moore, 1966; Henderson and Crosby, 1967; Harrison et al., 1967; Rosen and Carey, 1968; Benson, 1971) and two other products (Benson, 1971). Under intense illumination dieldrin can also yield pentachlorodieldrin (Henderson and Crosby, 1967) (Fig. 3).

These photolytic reactions can occur on films deposited on glass plate, silica gel, and cellulose paper as well as in solutions (ethyl acetate, benzene or hexanes) (Benson, 1971). The photoisomerization is rapid in the presence of sensitizers such as benzophenone, rotenone, acetone, chlorophyll, etc. (see Lykken, 1972). Some high molecular weight polymers can also result after photooxidation (Rosen, 1972).

On grass and crops at least three photoconversion products of dieldrin are reported (Roburn, 1963). On bean leaves about 70% of the dieldrin is converted to PD in 1 hr in the presence of sunlight and rotenone (Ivie and Casida, 1970). On corn leaves, photodieldrin was formed after 4 hrs of exposure of aldrin to sunlight (unpublished data: Reddy and Khan). On bean leaves rotenone is most effective 'sensitizer' for aldrin and dieldrin (and also endrin). Xanthone, tetradifon, triphenylamine, and flavone are also effective sensitizers (Ivie and Casida, 1971).

The UV irradiation of isodrin (I), heptachlor (H), chlordene (C), and chlordanes results in the formation of their corresponding cage isomers (Rosen et al., 1969; Khan et al., 1969; Benson et al., 1971).

Exposure of solid heptachlor epoxide to sunlight and UV light produces a semicage ketone and

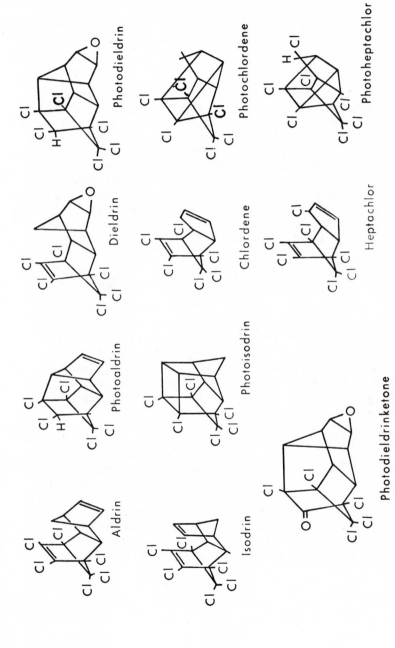

Figure 3. Cyclodienes and their photoisomerization products and the meta-bolite of PA and PD, the photodieldrin ketone.

341

an intermediate which may be converted to an enantiomorph semicage ketone (Graham et al., 1973).

The photolysis of endrin on bean leaves produces ketone and aldehyde semicaged isomers without epoxide (Ivie and Casida, 1971a).

Organophosphate esters:

Several types of organosulfur compounds are readily photooxidized under environmental conditions. Thioethers such as demeton form sulfoxides. P=S is converted to P=O under a variety of conditions. Light and air are known to accomplish this in the case of parathion and in other instances a sulfoxide-like intermediate may be involved.

Photolysis of parathion in aqueous ethanol or tetrahydrofuran forms O, O, S-triethylthiophosphate as major and O, O, O-triethylthiophosphate, paraoxon and triethyl phosphate as minor products. Photolysis of paraoxan is responsible for the last compound (Grunwell and Erickson, 1973) (Fig. 4).

Abate in methanol is rapidly decomposed by sunlight. The major product, sulfoxide, is further photolyzed rapidly to at least 6 other products. Sulfone can be formed either directly from Abate or from its sulfoxide (Rosen, 1972).

Rotenone can enhance photolysis of certain organophosphates such as diazinon, malathion, imidan and dyfonate. Anthraquinone can enhance photodecomposition of dyfonate and malathion (Ivie and Casida, 1971a).

Carbamates:

According to Ivie and Casida (1971), carbaryl, mesurol, primicarb, zectran and SD-8530 (Landrin) are photolyzed on silica gel plates which can be enhanced by rotenone. They also showed that aqueous suspensions of spinach chloroplasts are effective in accelerating the photodecomposition of N-methylcarbamates, mesurol and zectran.

342

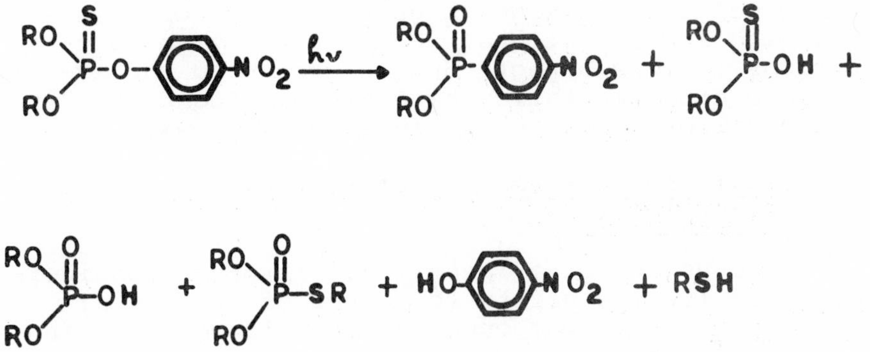

Figure 4. Photolysis of parathion and related esters.

Other insecticides:

Sunlight, especially in the presence of 'sensitizers', can cause decomposition of dinitrophenol derivatives, dinobutan and insecticide synergist, piperonyl butoxide (Ivie and Casida, 1971).
Pyrethroids are rapidly oxidized and degraded in sunlight and air, undergoing structural changes in the acid moiety (Chen and Casida, 1969). SBP-1382 (a pyrethroid) and its alcohol decompose very rapidly in sunlight (Rosen, 1972). Rotenone is also rapidly degraded in sunlight and air (see Lykken, 1972).

General considerations:

Most of the photolytic reactions have been studied in vitro under simulated conditions. The application of some of this data to field condi-

tions should be carried with care in cases
where photolysis is initiated by short wave
radiations. However, some of the commonly used
insecticides such as dieldrin, parathion,
carbaryl, methoxychlor, are photolyzed in the
field. The toxicology of photoconversion products
in target and nontarget organisms therefore needs
thorough investigations. Unfortunately investigations on this aspect, due to prolonged and extensive experimentation have not been conducted.
The available data is presented as follows.

Toxicological Aspects of Photoconversion of
Insecticides:

The usuage of a 'pesticide' involves consideration of (i) its safety to nontarget organisms;
and (ii) how the compound is metabolized by living
organisms and by environmental factors. The photoconversion of insecticides during and after their
application may alter their chemical structure
which can altogether affect their persistance and
biological activity. Such conversions whether
occurring on surfaces or in the atmosphere (directly applied or those volatilized from surfaces) may
produce products which may be either as toxic or
less or more toxic than the original parent compound to target and nontarget organisms. This has
serious implications regarding the effectiveness
and the ecological aspects of a particular
pesticide.

Some of the safest and most useful compounds
have limited use due to their photodecomposition.
Methoxychlor, a biodegradable analogue of DDT,
has not been able to replace DDT because of its
photodecomposition. Pyrethrins and rotenone,
safer to humans, are used only indoors because of
their photolysis to less toxic products which thus
reduces their post-application hazards. In order
to use these and other safer and biodegradable
insecticides in the field, it will be necessary,
according to Crosby (1972a), to add chemicals
which can act as "sun screens" to prevent their
photodecomposition. Since the oxidizing species
is strongly electrophilic (singlet oxygen) the

344

particular insecticide molecule should have the
ability to resist its action.

The end products as well as transient intermediates in case of photodegradable insecticides
may serve as sensitizers to bring about photodecomposition and biodegradation of other chemicals
in the environment and may thus have ecological
significance.

The most significant aspect of photolysis of
insecticides is that some of the most commonly
used insecticides, aldrin, dieldrin, parathion,
for example, are converted to more toxic products.

The cases of parathion poisoning among farm
workers occur after its application when the
residues reach a "safe level" (Quinby and Lemon,
1958; Milby et al., 1964). This is apparently due
to its photooxidation to its oxygen analogue.
Paraoxon (Milby et al., 1964) may be synergized by
another photoconversion product, O, O, S-triethylthiophosphate as it happens with malathion by O, O,
S-trimethylthiophsophate (Pellegrini and Santi,
1972; Grunwell and Ericksen, 1973).

The photoconversion products of aldrin, dieldrin and heptachlor have been reported to be
generally more toxic to mammals, fish and other
vertebrates and invertebrates ((Khan et al., 1973).
Table I shows LC_{50} values of various cyclodienes
and their photoisomers to houseflies and aquatic
animals. Photoaldrin (PA) becomes 2 to 6 times
more toxic; Photodieldrin (PD) becomes 1 1/2 to
6 times and Photoheptachlor (PH) 1 1/2 to 2 1/2
times more toxic than the parent compound.
Photoisodrin (PI) and photochlordene (PC) become
less toxic. Table 2 shows the toxicity ratios,
obtained from LT_{50} values of the parent cyclodiene
and its photoisomer. As seen, the mosquito larvae
and the blue gill fry are most sensitive to PA. A
similar increase in sensitivity is seen with PD,
Gammarus becomes highly susceptible to PD as
compared with other aquatic animals (Khan et al.,
1973).

Photodieldrin is also 5-10 times more toxic
to mammals (dogs, pigs, mice), birds (pigeons),
and some other fish (FAO, 1968; Brown et al., 1968;
Henderson and Crosby, 1967; Rosen et al., 1966).

Since photodieldrin can be the "terminal residue" of aldrin, dieldrin and of photoaldrin, its fate in the environment is being investigated in this laboratory. Some of these results are presented (Khan and Khan, 1974).

Aquatic food chain organisms, although more sensitive to PD than D (Table 1), absorb PD at a slower rate than dieldrin as seen with mosquito larvae (Fig. 5). There are species differences among invertebrates; those with thick exoskeleton absorb much less PD than soft-bodied invertebrates (Fig. 5). But all these animals keep absorbing PD and a steady state probably reaches after 6 days of exposure. Daphnia absorbs at a much faster rate than any other invertebrate; Gammarus and Simocephalus appear intermediate between Daphnia and other invertebrates, such as shrimp, clam and crayfish.

Freshwater fishes generally show maximum absorption within 24 hours of continuous exposure (Fig. 6). A steady state is apparently reached during this period. There is a slow decline of PD residues in these fishes after this period. However, the livebearing fish, Guppy, behaves differently than other fishes. It keeps absorbing PD during the continuous exposure. A steady state is probably reached some time after 6 days.

Absorption of dieldrin and PD from aqueous suspensions by freshwater alga, Ankistrodesmus spiralis, shows maximum levels during 4 hours (Tables 3 & 4).

Table 3. Elimination of ^{14}C-dieldrin by Daphnia after a 24-hr exposure to this insecticide in the presence or absence of food (yeast algae, 1000 cells/ml) (Rio, unpublished data).

	D.P.M. Daphnia pre-fed on:		
sample	no food	yeast	algae
Water	1750	1690(1130)	4340(1550)
Filter (1μ)	1%	1%	1%
Filter (34μ)	NIL	580(240)	830(270)
Daphnia	410	3970(2560)	4960(2460)
Total	2160	6240(3930)	10100(4280)
% in Daphnia	19.2	63.7(65.1)	48.9(57.4)

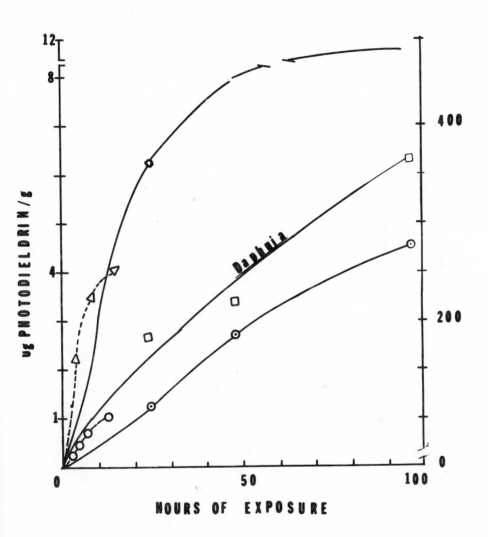

Figure 5.   Absorption of PD by mosquito larvae
o—o, <u>Gammarus</u> o—o, <u>Simocephalus</u>,◻ --◻ <u>Daphnia</u>.
The values on the left apply only to <u>Daphnia</u>. A-
mount of dieldrin absorbed by mosquito larvae
(△·-△) is also shown (Khan and Khan, 1974).

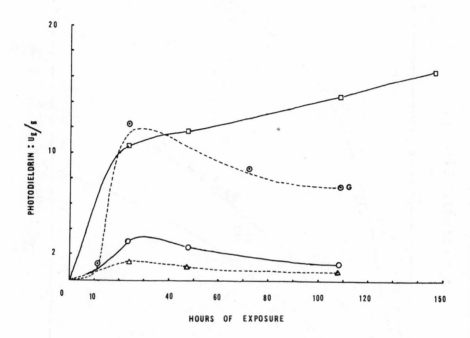

Figure 6. Absorption of PD by freshwater fishes, Bluegill (B), Minnows (M), Goldfish (g) and Guppys (G).

Table 4. Absorption of ^{14}C-Photodieldrin by freshwater alga, <u>Ankistrodesmus spiralis</u> (Khan and Khan, 1974).

Exposure time hr	Photodieldrin in algae* total: ng	conc.: ng/g	Biological magnification**
0.5	23.30	932	280
1.0	29.94	1197	360
2.0	47.20	1888	567
3.0	53.30	2132	640
4.0	53.69	2147	660

* 21,000 cells, 25 mg fresh wt/ml exposed to 3.33 ppb Photodieldrin
**Concentration of PD in algae/conc. of PD in water.

Transfer of algae, <u>Daphnia</u> and <u>Goldfish</u>, after exposure to D or PD, to clean water results in rapid elimination of D by <u>Daphnia</u> (Table 3) (Rio, unpublished data, this lab.) but slow elimination of PD is observed by Goldfish (Khan and Khan, 1974a).

The biological magnification ratios (concentration of PD in the fish/concn of PD in water) are: 63,000 for <u>Daphnia</u>; about 1,000 for <u>Simocephalus</u> and <u>Gammarus</u> and about 700 for <u>Aedes</u> larvae (Table 5). Such ratios for clam, crayfish and shrimp are, respectively, 4, 8 and 30 (Khan and Khan, 1974). For fishes, bluegill, minnow and goldfish, the maximum ratios, respectively, are 133, 150 and 609. For guppy, a ratio of 820 is seen (Table 6).

Table 5. Biological magnification of Photodieldrin by freshwater invertebrates (Khan and Khan, 1974).

Hours of Exposure	Biological Magnification Ratio* Daphnia	Simocephalus	Gammarus	Aedes
4	----	----	----	366
8	----	----	----	583
12	----	----	----	666
24	27,300	200	626	Dead
48	34,160	----	802	
72	----	400	----	
96	63,300	1020	1172	

*Concentration of insecticide in the animal/conc. of the insecticide in water.

Table 6. Biological magnification of Photodieldrin by freshwater fishes (Khan and Khan, 1974).

| Days of Exposure | Biological Magnification Ratio | | | |
	Bluegill	Minnow	Goldfish	Guppy
12 hrs	57	45	51	400
1 day	133	150	609	517
2 days	118	125	495	568
3 days	---	115	440	577
4 days	78	70	381	718
6 days	---	60	325	820

The magnification ratios obtained for PD are quite comparable with those reported by other investigators for other cyclodienes using these and other aquatic animals (Table 7).

In spite of slower absorption of PD as compared with that of D, biological magnification ratios of D and PD are comparable. As PD is more toxic than D to aquatic animals, such an absorption of PD may have more drastic long-term effects on food chains. Thus the fate of PD, the terminal residue of A, PA and D, in animals becomes very important. Both PA and PD are found to be metabolized in some animals to a more toxic and more lipophilic ketone, the Klein's metabolite. House fly, Musca domestica L., and the yellow fever mosquito, Aedes aegypti L., rapidly dehydrochlorinate PA and PD, a metabolism that can be blocked by the antioxidant Sesamex (Khan et al., 1970). The onset of toxic symptoms of PA and PD are apparently related with the appearance of the toxic photodieldrin ketone in the mosquito larvae (Fig. 7) and housefly adults. In fact this ketone is more toxic to houseflies than D or PA (Khan et al., 1973).

Such a ketone has also been produced from PD and is excreted in the urine of male rats (Klein et al., 1970). However, in most other organisms including female rats, algae, aquatic invertebrates

Table 7. Biological magnification of cyclodiene insecticides by aquatic animals.

Animal	Cyclodiene	Conc.	Magnification	Reference
Eastern Oyster	Endrin & Dieldrin	1 ppb/10 days	1,000	Wilson (1965)
Oyster[a]	Heptachlor	10 ppb/10 days	17,000	Wilson (1965)
Bluegill	Heptachlor	50 ppb	300	Cope (1966)
Trout	Dieldrin	2.8 ppb	3,300	Holden (1966)
Minnow	Dieldrin	15 ppt	10,000	Mount & Putnicki (1966)
Daphnia[b]	Aldrin	167 ppt/3 days	141,000	Johnson et al. (1971)
Mayfly (nymphs)[b]	Aldrin	21.3 ppt/3 days	31,000	Johnson et al. (1971)
Chironomus (larvae)[b]	Aldrin	21.3 ppt/3 days	23,000	Johnson et al. (1971)

[a]in running water.
[b]values expressed on dry wt. basis.

351

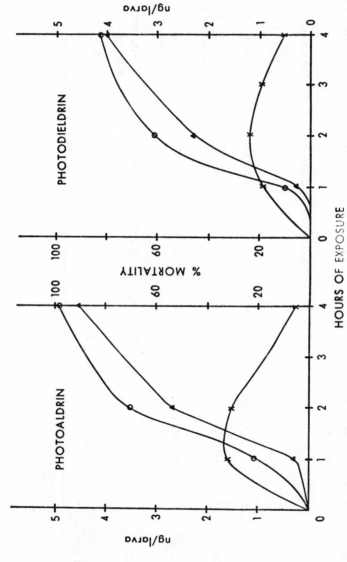

Figure 7. Relationship between the toxicity of photoaldrin or photodieldrin (% mortality, O——O), the degree of absorption of these photoproducts (ng/larva, ▲——▲), and their metabolism to photodieldrin ketone (ng/larva, X——X), and hours of exposure of mosquito larvae to 70 ppb of photoaldrin or photodieldrin (Khan et al., 1973).

and plants, PD is either not metabolized at all or converted in low amounts to hydrophilic metabolite (Klein et al., 1970; Reddy and Khan, unpublished data; Khan and Khan, 1974). The toxicity and biological magnification data presented here show that the terminal residue of A, PA and D, the photodieldrin, can create more harm than aldrin, photoaldrin and dieldrin to aquatic and terrestrial animals.

Thus the effects and fate in the environment of the photoconversion products of these and other extensively used insecticides must be investigated thoroughly if the use of pesticides has to continue.

Acknowledgements

Partial support from a research grant, ES-00808, from National Institute of Environmental Health Sciences is acknowledged. Thanks are due to Dr. G. Reddy for assistance in proofing the manuscript.

References Cited

Benson, W. R. 1971. J. Agri. Food Chem. 19: 66.

Benson, W. R., P. Lombardo, I. J. Egry, R. D. Ross, Jr., R. P. Barron, D. W. Mastbrook and E. A. Hansen 1971. J. Agr. Food Chem. 19: 857.

Brown, V. K. H., J. Robinson and A. Richardson. 1967. Food Cosmet. Toxicol. 5: 771.

Chen, Y. L. and J. E. Casida 1969. J. Agri. Food Chem. 17: 208.

Cope, O. S. 1966. J. Appl. Ecol. 3: 33 (Supplement on Pesticides in environment and their effects on wildlife).

Crosby, D. G. 1969. Residue Rev. 25: 1.

Crosby, D. G. 1972. In "Degradation of synthetic molecules in the biosphere". National Academy of Sciences: Washington, D.C. 260 pp.

Crosby, D. G. 1972a. In: Environmental Toxicology of Pesticides. (F. Matsumura, G. M. Boush and T. Misato, editors). Acad. Press, 637 pp.

Dachauer, A. C. 1962. The deuterium isotope rate effect in free radical reactions of t-carbon

deuterated DDT and its analogs. Ph.D. thesis.
Fordham University, New York.

Food and Agricultural organization of the United
Nations, World Health Organization. "1967.
Evaluations of Some Pesticide Residues in
Food". FAO/PL; 1967/M/11/1, WHO/Food Add.
68-30, Rome, 1968, 104 pp.

Georgacakis, E. and M. A. Q. Khan 1971. Nature
233: 120.

Graham, R. E., K. K. Burson, C. F. Hammer, L. B.
Hansen and C. T. Kenner. 1973. J. Agri. Food
Chem. 21: 824.

Grunwell, J. R. and Erickson, R. H. 1973. J.
Agri. Food Chem. 21: 929.

Harrison, R. B., D. C. Holmes, J. Roburn, J. O.
G. Tatton 1967. J. Sci. Food Agri. 18: 10.

Henderson, G. L. and D. G. Crosby 1967. J. Agri.
Food Chem. 15: 888.

Holden, A. V. 1966. J. Appl. Ecol. 3: 45 (Supplement on Pesticides in the environment and
their effects on wildlife).

Ivie, G. W. and J. E. Casida. 1970. Science 167:
1620.

Ivie, G. W. and J. E. Casida 1971. J. Agri Food
Chem. 19: 405.

Ivie, G. W. and J. E. Casida. 1971a. J. Agri.
Food Chem. 19: 410.

Johnson, T. J., C. R. Saunders, H. O. Saunders, and
R. S. Campbell 1971. J. Fish. Res. Board
Canada 28: 705.

Kenaga, E. E. 1966. Bull. Entomol. Soc. Amer.
12: 161.

Khan, H. M. and M. A. Q. Khan 1974. Archiv.
Environ. Contam. Toxicol. (in press).

Khan, M. A. Q., R. H. Stanton, D. J. Sutherland,
J. D. Rosen, and N. Maitra 1973. Archiv.
Environ. Contam. Toxicol. 1: 159.

Khan, M. A. Q., D. J. Sutherland, J. D. Rosen and
W. F. Carey 1970. J. Econ. Ent. 63: 470.

Khan, M. A. Q., J. D. Rosen and D. J. Sutherland.
1969. Science 168: 318.

Klein, A. K., R. E. Dailey, M. S. Walton, V. Beck,
J. D. Link 1970. J. Agr. Food Chem. 18:
705.

Li, C. F., and R. L. Bradley 1969. J. Dairy Sci.
52: 27.

Lykken, L. 1972. In: "Environmental Toxicology of Pesticides." (Matsumura, F., G. M. Boush and T. Misato, Eds.). Academic Press, New York and London. 449 pp.

McGuire, R. R., M. J. Zabik, R. D. Schetz and R. D. Flotard. 1970. J. Agr. Food Chem. 18: 319.

Milby, T. H., F. Ottoleoni and H. W. Mitchell 1964. J. Amer. Med. Assn. 189: 351.

Miller, L. L. and R. S. Narang. 1970. Science 169: 368.

Mount, D. I. and G. J. Putnicki 1966. Trans. N. Amer. Wildlife Natur. Resources Conf. 31: 177.

Parsons, A. M. and D. J. Moore 1966. J. Chem. Soc. (C) 2026.

Pellegrini, G. and Santi, R. 1972. J. Agr. Food Chem. 20: 944.

Plimmer, J. R., U. I. Klingebed and B. E. Hummer. 1970. Science 167: 67.

Quinby, G. E. and Lemon, A. B. 1958. J. Amer. Med. Assn. 166: 740.

Reddy, G. and M. A. Q. Khan, unpublished data, this laboratory.

Rio, D. F., unpublished data, this laboratory.

Roburn, J. 1963. Chem. Ind. 41: 1555A.

Robinson, J., A. Richardson, B. Bush and K. E. Edgar. 1966. Bull. Environ. Contam. Toxicol. 1: 127.

Rosen, J. D. 1972. in: Environmental Toxicology of pesticides. (Matsumura, F., G. M. Boush, and T. Misato, Eds.). Academic Press, New York and London. 435 pp.

Rosen, J. D. 1967. Chem. Commun. p 189.

Rosen, J. D., D. J. Sutherland, G. R. Lipton 1966. Bull. Environ. Contam. Toxicol. 1: 133.

Rosen, J. D., D. J. Sutherland, M. A. Q. Khan 1969. J. Agr. Food Chem. 17: 404.

Rosen, J. D. and D. J. Sutherland 1967. Bull. Environ. Contam. Toxicol. 1: 127.

Rosen, D. J. and W. F. Carey 1968. J. Agr. Food Chem. 16: 536.

Wilson, A. J. 1965. In: Annu. Rep. Bur. Commer. Fisher. Biol. Lab., Gulf Breeze, Fla., the fiscal year ending June 1965. W. S. Bur. Commer. Fish. Cir. 247.

FACTORS AFFECTING THE BEHAVIOR OF CHEMICALS IN THE ENVIRONMENT

R. Haque and N. Ash*

Department of Agricultural Chemistry
Environmental Health Sciences Center
Oregon State University

Introduction

Chemicals in one form or the other have been used since the beginning of civilization, although their use has increased phenomenally with the industrialization of our society. Some of the major uses of chemicals include pesticides, fertilizers, drugs and detergents. It would not be an exaggeration to say that living with chemicals is our way of life. This huge consumption of chemicals has resulted in a wide range of environmental contamination. Some well known examples are the world wide distribution of DDT-type insecticides, polychlorinated biphenyls (PCBs) and mercury compounds. In spite of the environmental contamination due to a few persistent ones, chemicals in general have provided immense benefits in regard to the comfort and welfare of human populations. Thus, at this stage, it is impossible to abandon the use of chemicals. However, the danger to ecosystems may be greatly reduced if we have a better understanding of the factors involved in predicting the behavior of chemicals in the environment. In this presentation we shall describe how physical-chemical properties may be helpful in describing the transport, persistence and mode of action of toxic chemicals in the environment. Although most of the examples are concerned with pesticides, the discussion may be extended to other organic chemicals. Indeed, this approach could aid in understanding some of the mechanisms of survival in a toxic environment.

Once a chemical is introduced into the environment its behavior to a large degree will depend upon two factors;

*Department of Biological Sciences, University of Illinois at Chicago Circle, Chicago.

the surrounding environment and the physical-chemical properties of the chemical. The chemical will be transported in
the hydrosphere, lithosphere, atmosphere and biota. Such
characteristics as the water solubility, vapor pressure, soil
adsorption, leaching in soils, degradation and binding with
biological macromolecules (proteins, phospholipids and membranes) will be important in explaining the behavior of a
chemical. Now we shall discuss some of these characteristics
in the light of the transport of chemicals in the environment.

Water Solubility and Behavior in the Hydrosphere

Water solubility and heat of solution are the two important properties controlling the transport of a chemical
in the hydrosphere. A rough estimate of the water solubility
could be made from the molecular formula and chemical structure of the compound. Inorganic salts and salts of organic
acids possess higher water solubility. Most pesticides being
relatively non-polar organic compounds are sparingly soluble
in water and show solubility values in the range of parts per
million to parts per billion. Water solubility of a few
typical environmental chemicals are given in Table 1.

Chemical	Water Solubility $\sim 25^\circ C$	Vapor Pressure
2,4-dichlorphenoxy acetic acid	600-700 ppm	0.4 mm 160°C
p,p'-DDT	1.2 ppb	1.9×10^{-7} mm (20°C)
Polychlorinated biphenyls Aroclor 1254 (PCBs)	53 ppb	0.3 mm (150°C)
Dichlorvos	~ 1000 ppm	1.2×10^{-2} mm (20°C)
Dieldrin	110 ppb	7.78×10^{-7} mm (25°C)
Lindane	10 ppm	9.4×10^{-6} mm (20°C)

Table 1. Water Solubility and Vapor Pressure of Selected
Environmental Chemicals

The water solubility of chlorinated hydrocarbons, DDT,
polychlorinated biphenyls (Aroclor 1254), dieldrin and lindane is in the parts per billion range. The extremely low
water solubility of these compounds plays an important role
in the widespread environmental contamination due to these
chemicals. Such low water solubility means in general high
lipid affinity. In other words once a chemical is transported in a living system it will be stored in the fatty

tissue. This has been observed for the high affinity of DDT-type compounds, polychlorinated cyclodienes and polychlorinated biphenyls. An extremely low water solubility indicates that the compound would also have a strong tendency to accumulate at the lipid-water interface. This has been demonstrated by Bowman et al. (1960) and Bigger et al. (1967) who observed that DDT-type compounds form clusters of varying particle size.

Many environmentally important chemicals contain chlorine atoms. Solubility sometimes shows dependence on the number of chlorine atoms present in the molecule with the polychlorinated biphenyls presenting a good example (Haque and Schmedding, 1973). Polychlorinated biphenyls result from the chlorination of biphenyl and may be represented by the general formula given below: Thus many isomers of PCB's are possible. Aroclor 1254 is a commercial product containing 54% of chlorine in the biphenyl. A typical gas chromatogram of the compound is shown in Fig. 1. The numbers in the chromatogram represent the peaks, corresponding to the number of chlorine atoms present in the isomer. It is interesting to note that the intensities of peaks in the Aroclor 1254 standard show significant differences when compared with the chromatogram of the corresponding aqueous extract. The intensities of the peaks in the aqueous extract decrease with increasing number of chlorine atoms in the isomers. The total solubility of Aroclor 1254 was found to be 53 ppb. The solubility of pure PCB isomers has been found to be highly dependent upon the number of chlorine atoms present in the molecule. The solubilities of five PCB isomers (Haque and Schmedding, 1973) are given in Table 2. In general, addition of a chlorine atom in an organic molecule decreases its water solubility.

Biphenyl Isomer	Solubility at 25°C (ppb)
2,4'-dichlor-	773
2,5,2'-trichloro-	307
2,5,2'5'-tetrachloro-	38.5
2,4,5,2',5-pentachloro-	11.7
2,4,5,2',4',5'-hexachloro-	1.3

Table 2. Water Solubilities of Polychlorinated Biphenyl Isomers

The partition coefficient of a chemical in an octanol/water system is another important property of biologically

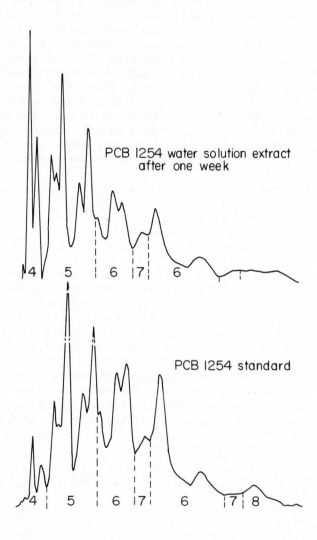

Fig. 1. Typical gas-chromatogram of standard and a water extract of Aroclor 1254 in hexane.

active chemicals. It has been found that partition coefficient values may be correlated with the biological activity of a particular toxicant (Hansch and Fujita, 1964). Thus, although the concentrations of DDT and other chemicals in water may be quite low, many organisms are able to concentrate them in their body tissues. Eastern oysters can concentrate ambient DDT levels of 0.1 ppb by a factor of 70,000 (Butler, 1964). Further biological concentration typically occurs in the food chain with carnivorous birds carrying residues at a concentration which is more than a million times greater than that of their environment (Woodwell et al., 1967).

Vapor Pressure and Behavior in the Atmosphere

The vapor pressure of a compound will primarily determine its transport into air. The vapor pressure values of some environmentally important chemicals are given in Table 1. It is apparent that vapor pressures vary over a wide range. Organophosphates and some carbamates possess appreciable vapor pressures whereas DDT, dieldrin, lindane, etc. are low vapor pressure compounds. The vapor pressure value can give a good estimate of the transport of the chemical as long as it is in the free state or evaporating from an inert surface. The loss of the polychlorinated biphenyl Aroclor 1254 from a planchet surface has been reported to be significant (Fig. 2) especially at higher temperatures (Haque et al., 1973). From a poorly sorbing sand surface the loss was also found to be substantial (Fig. 3) and was dependent upon the number of chlorine atoms present in the isomer. As expected (Fig. 3), the higher chlorine containing isomers show the least loss and vice-versa. In similar experiments, the loss from soil surfaces was found to be small (Haque et al., 1973). This supports the earlier findings of Guenzi and Beard (1970) who reported small losses of the chlorinated hydrocarbon DDT from soil surface. The vapor loss will depend strongly on the adsorption of the chemical on the surfaces of soil constituents. The vapor loss of a number of chemicals in terms of relative behavior from soil surface (Haque and Freed, 1974) is shown in Table 3.

Behavior in the Lithosphere

Most toxic chemicals come in contact with a surface material when they are released into the environment. The interaction of herbicides and plant growth regulators with

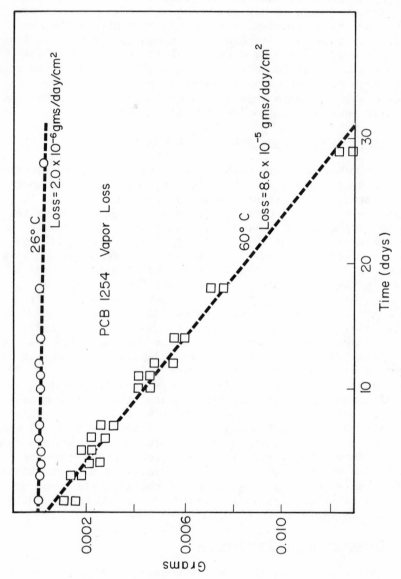

Fig. 2. Loss of Aroclor 1254 from itself as a function of time.

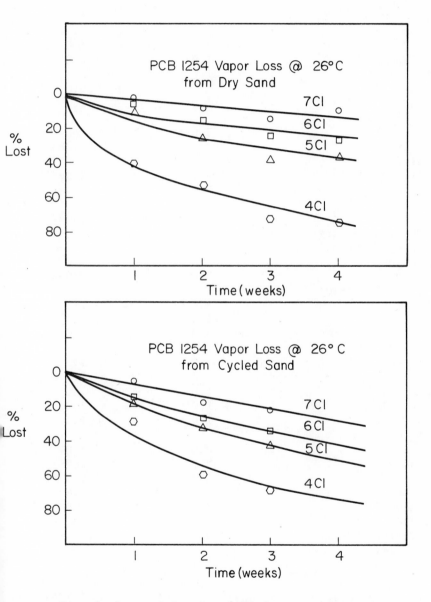

Fig. 3. Loss of Aroclor 1254 from an ottawa sand.

Compound	Vaporization[2] Index (from soil)	Leaching[3] Index
Herbicides		
Alchlor	3.0	1.0-2.0
Propanil	2.0	1.0-2.0
Trifluralin	2.0	1.0-2.0
Dalapon-Na	1.0	4.0
MCPA (Acid)	1.0	2.0
2,4-D (Acid)	1.0	2.0
2,4,5-T (Acid)	1.0	2.0
Insecticides		
Carbaryl	3.0-4.0	2.0
Malathion	2.0	2.0-3.0
Naled	4.0	3.0
Dimethoate	2.0	2.0-3.0
Fenthion	2.0	2.0
Diazinon	3.0	2.0
Ethion	1.0-2.0	1.0-2.0
Oxydemeton-methyl	3.0	3.0-4.0
Azinophos-methyl	---	1.0-2.0
Phosphamidon	2.0-3.0	3.0-4.0
Mevinophos	3.0-4.0	3.0-4.0
Methyl Parathion	4.0	2.0
Parathion	3.0	2.0
DDT	1.0	1.0
BHC	3.0	1.0
Chlordane	2.0	1.0
Hepatchlor	3.0	1.0
Toxaphene	4.0	1.0
Aldrin	1.0	1.0
Dieldrin	1.0	1.0
Endrin	1.0	1.0
Fungicides		
Captan	2.0	1.0
Benomyl	3.0	2.0-3.0
Zineb	1.0	2.0
Maneb	1.0	2.0
Mancozeb	1.0	1.0
Fumigant		
Methylbromide	N.A.	
Rodenticide		
Zinc Phosphide	N.A.	

Table 3. Comparative Environmental Behavior[1] of Pesticides in Soil

soils is a good example. The adsorption characteristics will be important in determining the biological activity, fate, and behavior in soils (Freed and Haque, 1973). Soils, being a heterogeneous mixture of clays, sand, and inorganic salts, provide active sorbing sites for the interaction of chemicals. Thus, whenever a chemical reaches the soil it gets adsorbed to some degree depending on the number of active sites present on the surfaces. The amount of chemical adsorbed is usually represented by an isotherm. The most common isotherm used in pesticide-adsorption is the Freundlich type isotherm represented by the following equation:

Where x is the amount of chemical

$$\frac{x}{m} = KC^n \qquad (1)$$

sorbed, m the mass of soil surface, C the equilibrium concentration of chemical and K and n are constants. To represent the adsorption data $\log \frac{x}{m}$ is usually plotted against $\log C$. The intercept and slope of the plot give the value of $\log K$ and n respectively. The values of n and K for the adsorption of 2,4-dichlorophenoxy acetic acid on various surfaces (Haque and Sexton, 1968) are given in Table 4. The constant K is a measure of the extent of the adsorption, whereas n tells something about the mechanism of adsorption. A high value of K means higher adsorption capacity of the surface. For a poorly adsorbing surface K is small and vice-versa. It is interesting to note that K for a poorly adsorbing sand surface is smaller than for humic acid. The high K value for humic acid is attributed to the larger surface area and the presence of more functional groups and active sites on this surface.

The adsorption of chemicals usually increases with organic matter present in the soil. Thus a soil rich in organic matter adsorbs more than sandy soil. Solubility of the chemical in water is generally inversely proportional to the amount of chemical sorbed. Thus, DDT-type compounds and PCBs possessing solubilities in the parts per billion range are

Footnotes for Table 3:

[1]Estimated from best available information for loam soil at 25°C under annual rainfall of 150 cm.

[2]A vaporization index number of 1 = vapor loss of less than 0.1 Kg/hectare/year, 2 = from 0.2 to 3.0 Kg/ha/yr or more, 3 = 3.5 to 6.5 Kg/ha/yr or more, 4 = 7 to 14 Kg/ha/yr or more.

[3]A leaching index number indicates the approximate number of centimeters moved through the soil profile with an annual rainfall of 150 cm. Thus, an index of 1 = < 10 cm, 2 = < 20 cm, 3 = > 35 and 4 = > 50 cm.

Surface	Temp ($^{\circ}$C)	n	Log K
Illite	0	0.658	1.11
	25	0.719	1.02
Montmorillonite	0	0.925	−0.63
	25	1.004	−0.186
Sand	0	0.671	−0.984
	25	0.827	−1.45
Humic Acid	0	0.86	0.931
	25	2.01	1.9
Alumina	0	0.97	−0.06
	25	1.01	−0.08
Silica-gel	0	1.0	0.58
	25	1.0	0.31

Table 4. Freundlich Isotherm Constants K and n for the
Adsorption of 2,4-dichlorophenoxy acetic acid
(2,4-D) on Surfaces

readily adsorbed on the soil surfaces. Adsorption of such
compounds on particulate matter represents an important factor
for the transport of chlorinated hydrocarbons in the biosphere.

The Langmuir isotherm, as noted above, is another
important equation which is used to represent adsorption data.
This equation is described as follows:
Here a and b are constants while x,
m and C are defined in equation (1).
The constant b represents the capacity

$$\frac{x}{m} = \frac{abC}{1+aC} \tag{2}$$

of the adsorbant for a particular adsorbate. This equation
rarely holds true for adsorption of organic chemicals on
soils. The adsorption of cadmium metal on soils has, however,
been represented by this isotherm (Matt, 1972).

The temperature dependence of adsorption gives an estimate of the heat of adsorption ΔH. A value of ΔH in the
range of 10 or more KCal/mole is indicative of chemisorption,
or actual bond formation, whereas ΔH in the range of 1 KCal/
mole or less represents a physical-type adsorption. For the
majority of pesticide-soil interactions the value of ΔH falls
somewhere in the range of 1 KCal/mole. The value of ΔH
usually decreases with an increasing amount of chemical
sorbed (Haque and Coshow, 1971). Further insight into the
mechanism of adsorption is usually obtained by observing the
changes in the infra-red spectrum of the pesticide or chemical
in the adsorbed state as compared to the free state (Haque
et al., 1970).

Leaching and diffusion of chemicals are two other

important factors in controlling the behavior of chemicals in soils. The adsorption characteristics, water solubility, moisture, temperature and nature of the soil are important factors affecting the leaching and diffusion of chemicals in soils. The diffusion constant of chemicals decreases with increasing adsorption. The values of diffusion constants of most organic chemicals in soils are in the range of .05 to 5×10^{-7} cm^2/sec (Hamaker, 1972). The relative leaching tendency of a series of chemicals in soils is given in Table 3.

Degradation of Chemicals

The degradation of a chemical in the environment could be accomplished in three ways; chemical, biological and photochemical. Chemical decomposition is most common in air and water, whereas the biological (microbial) degradation is important in water and soils. Well known examples of chemical degradation may include the hydrolysis of many environmental chemicals such as acid decomposition of s triazine herbicides and alkaline dehydrochlorination of DDT.

In general the decomposition of chemicals may be represented by a first or second order rate law: where C is the concentration of the chemical, k the rate constant, and n = 1 or 2 de-

$$-\frac{dc}{dt} = KC^n \quad (n = 1 \text{ or } 2) \quad (3)$$

pending on whether the reaction is of first or second order. The reaction rate could also be represented by the well known Michaelis-Menton equation for enzyme kinetics (4), where Vm is the velocity, E the enzyme concentration, Km the Michaelis constant and k_1 and k_2 the two rate constants.

$$\frac{dc}{dt} = \frac{Vm\ EC}{Km+C} = \frac{k_1 C}{k_2+C} \quad (4)$$

The decomposition of chemicals in soils is more complex than a simple first order rate mechanism. This is especially true for microbial degradation. For microbial degradation there is a lag period before breakdown occurs when a chemical reaches the soil. This lag period is probably the time required for the build up of appropriate microbes. A rough estimate of the half life of herbicides in soils could, however, be obtained using simple first order kinetics. Nash and Woolson (1967) have estimated the half life of chlorinated hydrocarbons in sandy soils to be in the order of several years.

Micro-organisms alter environmental chemicals in many cases by converting them into new chemical entities. For example, it has been observed that certain organisms methylate

the inorganic mercury species to methyl mercury in aquatic
environments (Jensen and Jernelov, 1969). This new chemical
can be readily taken up by fish and may explain the uptake and
dispersion of mercury in the biota of lakes.

The photochemical reactions of chemicals in the environment represent important mechanisms of degradation. Most well
known is the photochemical reaction of hydrocarbons and gases
in the atmosphere to form smog. The radiation from sun light
provides enough photons to cause a photo-chemical reaction.
Unfortunately many photochemical products are more toxic than
the parent reactants and thus are more harmful. The photochemical reactions of organic chemicals and pesticides take
place in water as well as in air (Crosby, 1969).

Interaction with Biota

Most of the environmental chemicals interact with the
macromolecules present in the biota. Organophosphate type
insecticides interact with acetylcholinesterase enzymes;
chlorinated hydrocarbons interact with phospholipids; whereas
metals form complexes with the amino group, sulfhydryl group
or other electronegative groups. Thus, a knowledge of how
chemicals interact with important constituents of biological
polymers may disclose the possible site for the accumulation
of chemicals in the living system.

The structure and physical-chemical properties of a
chemical may throw much light on the possible binding site in
the biological system. It is generally accepted that organophosphates and carbamates inhibit the activity of cholinesterase enzymes (O'Brien, 1967). The inhibition involves the
formation of a complex between the insecticide and the enzyme
which is followed by the phosphorylation or carbamylation of
the enzyme. The reaction may be represented in two steps:
E $\cdot$ OH represents a func-
tional group in the enzyme,

$$E\text{—}OH + AX \underset{k_{-1}}{\overset{k_1}{\rightleftharpoons}} EOH \cdot AX \qquad (5)$$

AX the insecticide. A is
the acetyl group or the
dialkylphosphoryl group.

$$EOH \cdot AX \xrightarrow{k_2} E\text{—}OA + H^+ + X^- \qquad (6)$$

The chlorinated hy-
drocarbon insecticides, owing to their high hydrophobic nature, are usually stored in the lipids of living organisms.
Depending upon the functional groups availability in the
insecticide and the phospholipid, one may expect an interaction. The binding of the insecticide with cockroach nerve
was reported by O'Brien and Matsumura (1964). Recent studies

of Haque et al. (1972) have established that DDT-type compounds bind with the phosphatide, lecithin. The binding
characteristics also have some correlation with the toxicity.
The benzylic proton of DDT-type insecticides and the phos-
phatidyl group of the lecithin was involved in the binding.
The relatively non-toxic DDE, not possessing the benzylic
proton, did not bind with lecithin. Other similer compounds
(DDD, methoxychlor, DDA, dicofol, etc.) did bind with lecithin to varying degrees. One may picture the distribution of
DDT-type compounds as distributing at a lipid-protein interface. In such a spatial distribution the benzylic proton of
DDT would be in an appropriate position to bind to the phospholipid. The distribution model picture is based on the
earlier findings of Holan (1971) and Mullins (1955).

The presence of metal compounds such as lead, cadmium
and mercury in a living system may be a serious health concern. Such metals compete with the nutritionally important
metals which are associated with enzymes. The environmentally
toxic metal would thus compete for binding sites with essential metals. Depending upon the stability constant (see pp.
), the foreign metal may displace the essential metal from
some of the enzymes and macromolecules and change the function-
ality of the enzyme. A study of the stability constants of
metals with different ligands may tell how various metals compete for binding sites. The relative binding constants of different metals with a variety of ligands are given Table 5.
It is clear that mercury binds with some of the ligands much
more strongly than the others. This is especially true for
the binding of mercury compounds with the sulfhydryl group.

| Metal | Stability Constant (Log K) | | | | |
	Oxalate	Glycine	Ethylene-diamine	Mercapto-acetate	Mercapto-ethylamine
Mn^{++}	3.9	3.44	2.73	4.38	--
Fe^{++}	3.05	4.3	4.34	--	--
Co^{++}	4.69	5.23	5.9	5.84	7.7
Ni^{++}	5.3	6.18	7.12	6.98	9.23
Cu^{++}	5.5	8.62	10.72	--	∼16
Zn^{++}	4.9	5.52	5.9	7.8	8.07
Cd^{++}	3.2	4.27	5.69	--	9.4
Hg^{++}	--	10.3	14.3	∼24	--
Pb^{++}	--	5.47	--	8.5	9.9

Table 5. Stability Constants of Metal-Ligand Complexes

The binding characteristics and lipid/water partition coefficient data have been found to be very useful in correlating biological activities with chemical structure. Hansch (1969) has developed a relationship between the activity of biologically active compounds and the partition coefficients between 1-octanol and water. The Hansch relationship may be represented as:

$$\log \text{Activity} = k_1 \log P + k_2 \text{(electronic)} + k_3 \text{(steric)} + k_4$$

where P is the partition coefficient of the compound and k_1, k_2, k_3, and k_4 are constants. This equation has found widespread use in biological activity-structural correlations (Van Valkenburg, 1972).

References

Bigger, J. W., G. R. Dutt and R. L. Riggs. 1967. Bull. Environ. Contam. Toxicol. 2:90.

Bowman, M. C., F. Acree and M. K. Corbett. 1960. Ag. Food Chem. 8:406.

Butler, P. A. 1964. U. S. Fish Wildlife Serv. Circ. 226:65.

Crosby, D. G 1969. Res. Rev. 25:1.

Freed, V. H. and R. Haque. 1973. "Pesticide Formulations", W. Van Valkenburd, (ed.). Marcell-Dekker, New York.

Guenzi, W. D. and W. E. Beard. 1970. Soil Sci. Soc. Amer. Proc. 34:44.

Hansch, C. 1969. Accounts of Chem. Res. 2:232.

Hansch, C. and T. Fujita. 1964. J. Am. Chem. Soc. 86:1616.

Hamaker, J. W. 1972. "Organic Chemicals in the Environment", C. A. I. Goring and J. W. Hamaker, (eds.). Vol I, Marcell-Dekker, New York.

Haque, R. and D. Schmedding. To be published.

Haque, R., D. Schmedding and V. H. Freed. Environ. Sci. Technol. 8:139. (1974)

Haque, R. and V. H. Freed, Res. Rev., in press.

Haque, R., I. J. Tinsley and D. Schmedding. 1973. Mol. Pharm. 9:17.

Haque, R. and W. R. Coshow. 1971. Env. Sci. Technol. 5:139.

Haque, R., S. Lilley and W. R. Coshow. 1970. J. Coll. Inter. Sci. 33:185.

Haque, R. and R. Sexton. 1968. J. Coll. Inter. Sci. 27:88.

Holan, G. 1971. Nature 232:644.

Jensen, S. and A. Jernelov. 1969. Nature 233:753.

Matt, J. K. 1972. Can. J. Soil Sci. 52:343.

Mullins, L. J. 1955. Science 122:118.
Nash, R. G. and E. A. Woolson. 1967. Science 157:924.
O'Brien, R. D. 1967. "Insecticides: Action and Metabolism",
Academic Press, New York.
O'Brien, R. D. and F. Matsumura. 1964. Science 146:657.
Van Valkenburg, W. 1972. "Biological Correlations: The Hansch
Approach", Adv. Chem. Ser.:114.
Wood ell, G. M., C. F. Wurster, and P. A. Isaacson. 1967.
Science 156:821.

Acknowledgments

Research supported in part from N.I.H. Grants No.
ES 00040 and ES 00210 and EPA Grant No. R802250.

INSECTICIDE RESISTANCE IN VERTEBRATES

James D. Yarbrough

Department of Zoology
Mississippi State University

Abstract

Although vertebrate insecticide resistance is
probably related to a number of factors, the studies
in this report have been directed at only one aspect
of the phenomenon, that is, the membrane and its
involvement in resistance. The evidence presented
demonstrates an effective cell membrane and brain
barrier in the insecticide-resistant mosquitofish
population that is less effective in the susceptible
population. In conjunction with the brain barrier,
there is an apparent insensitivity to organochlorine
insecticides at the site of action which is more
effective in R fish than S fish. In addition,
physical factors such as increased tissue and body
fat and apparent structural membrane changes
(myelin) in R fish are contributory to resistance.

Introduction

Insecticide resistance may be defined as "a
population's ability to tolerate levels of a toxicant which would provide lethal to the majority of
individuals in another population of the same
species." Although resistance is an expression of
the genetic change in the susceptibility of a population there are individuals with varying degrees
of tolerance just as there are in the susceptible
population. Therefore, the expression of toxicity
(LC_{50} value) is based on a concentration of a

toxicant that will kill 50% of a test population within a given time paeriod (48-96 hr). Comparison of the LC_{50} values between two populations of the same species is used to express the magnitude of resistance.

Although insecticide resistance is widely reported in insects and the mechanism of that resistance has been extensively studied, the reports of naturally occurring vertebrate insecticide resistance are limited. In 1963, Vinson et al. reported DDT resistance in a Mississippi delta population of mosquitofish (Gambusia affinis). Later this popula- was shown to have a cross-resistance to cyclodiene insecticides (Boyd and Ferguson, 1964a), and evidence indicated that resistance and cross-resistance were genetically based (Boyd and Ferguson, 1964b). The extent of this resistance encompassed a wide spectrum of organochlorine insecticides (Culley and Ferguson, 1969), and included organophosphorus insecticides (Ferguson and Boyd, 1964).

Based on comparisons of LC_{50} values between resistance (R) and susceptible (S) mosquitofish populations, organochlorine insecticide resistance ranges from about a 5-fold resistance for DDT to about a 500-fold resistance for endrin (Table 1).

Other fish from the same collecting areas as the R mosquitofish have been shown to be organochlorine insecticide resistant (Ferguson et al., 1964). These species include golden shiners (Notemigonus crysoleucas), bluegill sunfish (Lepomis macrochirus) and green sunfish (Lepomis cyanellus). These populations are resistant to toxaphene, aldrin, dieldrin and endrin, but are not resistant to DDT. In addition, mosquitofish popualtions in Texas have been shown to be resistant to at least three organochlorine insecticides. The resistance pattern appears to be different from that found in the Mississippi population (Dziuk and Plapp, 1973).

The Mississippi delta is a rich agricultural area and represents a region of high insecticide use. Residues in resistant fish show seasonal fluctuations, with the highest levels appearing in the winter. In a 12-month study from April 1968 –

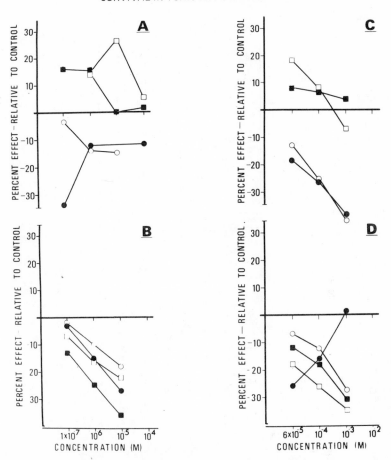

Figure 1. The percent effect of endrin and dieldrin on succinic dehydrogenase activity in mitochondrial preparations from liver and brain of insecticide-resistant (R) and susceptible (S) mosquitofish. (●——● S-Brain; ◐——◌ S-Liver; ◼——◼ R-Brain; and ◻——◻ R-Liver).

A. Intact mitochondrial preparation treated with endrin.

B. Disrupted mitochondrial preparation treated with endrin.

C. Intact mitochondrial preparation treated with dieldrin.

D. Disrupted mitochondrial preparation treated with dieldrin.

375

Table 1. Comparative 48 hr LC50 values (ppb) and 95% confidence intervals of susceptible and resistant mosquitofish populations for selected organo-chlorine insecticies.a

Insecticide	Susceptible			Resistant			Fold Difference
	LOWER LIMIT	LC_{50}	UPPER LIMIT	LOWER LIMIT	LC_{50}	UPPER LIMIT	
DDT	15.45	18.92	22.31	16.59	96.16	113.47	5.1+
Methoxychlor	104.64	109.15	113.67	173.34	186.21	208.55	1.7+
Endrin	0.59	0.63	0.69	129.22	314.06	529.26	498.5+
Aldrin	33.22	36.17	39.16	2366.62	2558.12	2734.99	90.7+
Dieldrin	7.22	8.02	9.81	355.30	433.60	502.34	54.1+
Toxaphene	10.40	11.63	12.91	3284.43	4518.66	8934.35	388.5+
Heptachlor	23.78	34.96	46.01	8990.33	125000.12	20961.04	357.6+

a Culley and Fergson (1969).

+ Significant difference between susceptible and resistant at $P < 0.05$ as determined by t-test.

376

April 1969, Finley (1970) reported residues in whole body R mosquitofish in excess of 80 ppm total DDT in January-February, to a low of less than 10 ppm in June 1969. The same pattern was seen for toxaphene. In recent residue analysis, the DDT residue levels have dropped considerably.

The mechanism of insecticide resistance is probably the result of many factors: degradative activity and metabolic turn-over, changes in whole body uptake, membrane barriers, storage or compartmentalization in fat, decreases in sensitivity to the toxicant, and even behavior. Although degradation has been shown to be the major factor in insect resistance to DDT, no clear mechanism of resistance to the other organochlorine insecticides has been reported, nor has the mode of action of the organochlorine insecticides been effectively demonstrated.

The work presented in this paper directly or indirectly relates to the role that membranes may play in the resistance phenomenon demonstrated by mosquitofish to organochlorine insecticides.

In vitro Mitochondrial Studies

The first indication of a membrane difference between resistant (R) and susceptible (S) mosquitofish appeared in studies in the in vitro effects of endrin on succinic dehydrogenase activity, in which the mitochondrion was used as a model membrane system (Yarbrough and Wells, 1971). These studies involved the enzyme succinic dehydrogenase, which is related to cellular energy metabolism and is an inseparable part of the inner membrane of the mitochondrion. When intact mitochondria, isolated from liver and brain of R fish, where exposed to endrin concentrations of from 10^{-7} to 10^{-4}M, there was no effect on succinic dehydrogenase activity. However, when mitchondrinal preparations from S fish were exposed to the same endrin concentrations, there was inhibition of succinic dehydrogenase activity at all levels (Fig. 1-A). When mitochondrial preparations from both populations were disrupted by repeated freezing and thawing and exposed to the same endrin concentrations, there

was inhibition in all cases (Fig. 1-B). These data
suggested a membrane barrier to endrin in R fish.

In studies using DDT, toxaphene and dieldrin
similar effects were obtained (Moffett and Yarbrough,
1972). The enzymatic activity in intact mitochondria
from R fish was either stimulated or not affected
by dieldrin or DDT (Fig. 1-C, Fig. 2-A). Toxaphene
slightly inhibited succinic dehydrogenase activity
from intact mitochondrial preparations from R brain
tissue, but the effect did not appear to be significant (Fig. 2-C). The enzymatic activity of intact
mitochondrial preparations from S fish was inhibited
by all three insecticides.

These studies clearly demonstrated that enzyme
activity in intact mitochondrial preparations from
R fish is not affected by the same concentrations
of insecticide that inhibit activity in intact
preparations from S fish. Further, when the mitochondrial membrane from S and R fish preparations
is disrupted, the insecticide effect is the same
in mitochondrial preparations from both populations.
This simplies a membrane barrier in the R fish that
is either less effective or absent in S fish (Fig.
1-D, Fig. 2-B, 2-D).

It is obvious that the "membrane barrier" is
not total, nor can it withstand infinite concentrations. It is reasonable to suggest that at 10^{-4}M
endrin we may be nearing the limits of the ability
of the membrane to function as a barrier (Fig. 1-A).
For dieldrin this limit may be between 10^{-4} and
10^{-3}M (Fig. 2-C), for DDT between 10^{-8} to 10^{-7}M
(Fig. 2-A) and for toxaphene probably 10^{-8}M
(Fig. 2-C).

Stimulation of succinic dehydrogenase activity
in intact preparations from R fish is of interest
and might be used as a basis for questioning the
membrane barrier concept. It should be emphasized
that the insecticide does not have to penetrate the
mitochondria to cause an effect in the enzyme assay.
One very simple and highly plausible explanation
involves an increase in substrate concentration.
In mitochondrial preparations from R fish the
insecticide is prevented from penetrating the
membrane, but binds to it, thereby altering the

378

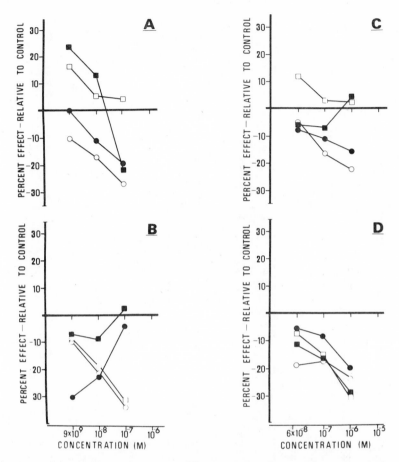

Figure 2. The percent effect of DDT and toxaphene on succinic dehydrogenase activity in mitochondrial preparations from liver and brain of insecticide-resistant (R) and susceptible (S) mosquitofish. (●—● S-Brain; O—O S-Liver; ▨—▨ R-Brain; and ◻—◻ R-Liver)

A. Intact mitochondrial preparation treated with DDT.

B. Disrupted mitochondrial preparation treated with DDT.

C. Intact mitochondrial preparation treated with toxaphene.

D. Disrupted mitochondrial preparation treated with toxaphene.

Table 2. Effect of endrin on succinic dehydrogenase activity in mitochondrial preparations from insecticide-resistant (R) and susceptible (S) green sunfish (Lepomis cyanellus).

Mitochondrial	Intact[b]			Disrupted[c]		
	Control	10^{-4} M endrin treatment	% effect	Control	10^{-4} M endrin treatment	% effect
R - brain	44.58±1.01	34.33±1.02	-23	41.63±2.72	31.64±1.93	-24
R - liver	41.42±1.59	39.76±1.67	- 4	40.27±1.20	39.88±1.30	- 1
S - brain	57.30±0.60	49.85±0.84	-13	57.63±2.28	50.71±0.60	-12
S - liver	49.80±3.00	37.35±0.66	-25	49.08±2.71	53.01±0.50	+ 8

[a] Sample size is three replicates each in triplicate. Mean values are expressed in μl O_2/30 min/mg protein ± SE.

[b] Enzyme assayed immediately after mitochondrial preparation.

[c] Enzyme assayed following repeated freezing and thawing of mitochondrial preparation.

Table 3. In vivo organochlorine insecticide retention ratios of insecticide-susceptible (S) to insecticide-resistant (R) mosquitofish brain and liver subcell fractions.

Fraction	S/R[a]			
	^{14}C-DDT	^{14}C-Endrin++	^{14}C-Aldrin	^{14}C-Dieldrin
Cell Membrane[b]	1.35(0.96)	1.65(1.11++)	2.68++(0.48)	4.78++(1.66++)
Nuclei[c]	--	--	3.97++(1.04)	2.44++(0.97)
Myelin[d]	--	--	3.24++	4.50++
Mitochondria[e]	2.05++(1.04)	3.41(1.32++)	2.40++(1.09)	4.52++(0.79)
H-microsomes[f]	2.17++(0.67+)	3.63(1.80++)	2.33++(1.09)	3.23++(1.27)
L-microsomes[g]	2.79++(1.43)	1.91(0.49++)	4.23++(0.83+)	4.72++(1.23)
Total homogenate	2.34++(0.84)	2.92(1.16++)	2.74++(0.98)	3.54++(1.03)

[a]The open values are for brain and those in parentheses for liver. Significant difference between S and R at $P < 0.05$ (+) or $P < 0.01$ (++) as determined by t test. [b]600 g/10 min. pellet. [c]Prepared by the method of Matsumura and Hayashi (1969). [d]Prepared by the method of Cuzner et al. (1965). [e]600 g supernatant sedimented at 54,000 g for 10 min. [f]5,000 g supernatant sedimented at 54,000 g for 60 min. [g]54,000 g supernatant sedimented at 100,00 g for 15 hr.

permeability of the membrane to the substrate. More
substrate enters the mitochondria and this causes
an increase in enzyme activity.

The possibility exists that the mosquitofish
response we have reported is unique and is not
related to insecticide resistance in other vertebrate species. The green sunfish (Lepomis cyanellus)
has been shown to be endrin resistant (Ferguson
et al., 1964). It would appear that the response
we have reported for R mosquitofish tissue is not
the same for R green sunfish preparations (Table 2).
It may be that 10^{-4}M endrin is beyond the membrane's
ability to function as an effective barrier. Lower
endrin concentrations could well reveal the limits
of the membrane barrier. The level of endrin
toxicity to mosquitofish as compared to the sunfish
is quite different. The 36 hr LC_{50} value of endrin
for S green sunfish is 3.4 ppb and for R green sunfish is 16 ppb, whereas the 48 hr LC_{50} value for S
mosquitofish is 0.6 ppb and for R mosquitofish is
314 ppb (Table 1). Therefore, R sunfish would be
expected to have a less effective membrane barrier
than R mosquitofish.

The in vitro concentrations used are much
greater than those that would normally be
encountered in an environmental situation. Therefore, using the mitochondrion as a model membrane
system, we can conclude that the R mosquitofish
membrane systems are a very effective barrier to
many organochlorine insecticides and may be a major
contributory factor to vertebrate insecticide
resistance.

Organochlorine Insecticide Retention
by Cellular Fractions

The nature of organochlorine compound binding
to membranes is unclear. It may possibly involve
attachment to specific sites or moieties on the
membrane surface, or a hydrophobic interaction/
solubilization of the organochlorine compound in
the membrane lipid bilayer. Mullins (1965) suggested that chlorinated hydrocarbon toxicity is

related to a precise fit into the intermolecular lattices of membranes by these compounds. It has been suggested that a charge-transfer complex occurs between molecules of the membrane and organochlorine insecticides (O'Brien and Matsumura, 1964). This charge-transfer complex between DDT and an axonic component would result in destabilization of the axon and disruption of normal axonic function.

Previous data indicate that cell membrane preparations bind the greatest amount of organochlorine insecticides (Matsumura and Hayashi, 1969; Telford and Matsumura, 1970). These in vitro studies involved DDT and dieldrin binding in insect and mammal central nervous system particulate fractions.

Comparisons of organochlorine insecticide retention patterns between cellular fractions of resistant (R) and (S) mosquitofish nervous tissue is useful in providing information on the extent of membrane involvement in resistance. (The terms binding and retention as used in this paper refer to the insecticide present in tissue preparations after a stated treatment. No distinction is made between these terms.) Both in vivo and in vitro binding experiments have been performed on R and S mosquitofish using DDT (Wells and Yarbrough, 1972a), endrin (Wells and Yarbrough, 1972b), and aldrin and dieldrin (Wells and Yarbrough, 1973).

In in vivo binding studies the brain fractions from S fish consistently retained more insecticide than the corresponding brain fractions from R fish (Table 3). The in vivo treatments consisted of: 75 ppb DDT (5 hr); 2 ppb ^{14}C-endrin (6 hr); 150 ppb ^{14}C-aldrin (4 hr); and 25 ppb ^{14}C-dieldrin (4 hr).

Expressed as ratios of the organochlorine insecticide retained by brain fractions of S fish to R fish, comparisons for all in vivo organochlorine insecticide treatments were significantly different ($P < 0.01$), with the exception of the DDT treated cell membrane preparation (Table 3). The differences between insecticide retention in livers of S fish and that of R fish were not as great as for the brain. All liver fractions from the in vivo endrin treatments exhibited significant

Table 4. In vitro organochlorine insecticide retention ratios of insecticide-susceptible (S) to insecticide-resistant (R) mosquitofish brain and liver subcell fractions.

Fraction	S/R [a]			
	^{14}C-DDT	^{14}C-Endrin	^{14}C-Aldrin	^{14}C-Dieldrin
Cell membrane[b]	1.17(1.31)	2.23++(1.34++)	1.00(0.83)	2.83++(1.67++)
Mitochondria[c]	1.35+ (1.90+)	1.77++(1.33++)	0.89(1.11)	1.77+ (3.03++)
H-microsomes[d]	1.17++(2.79++)	2.45++(1.87++)	0.63(1.12)	1.63++(1.47)
L-microsomes[e]	2.31++(3.08++)	1.37 (1.82++)	1.49(1.58)	1.71+ (1.44)
Total homogenate	1.42++(1.96++)	1.73++(1.53++)	1.10(1.12)	2.14+ (1.98)

[a]The open values are for brain and those in parentheses for liver. Significant difference between S and R at $P < 0.05$ (+) or $P < 0.01$ (++) as determined by t test. [b]600 g/10 min. pellet. [c]Prepared by the method of Matsumura and Hayashi (1969). [d]Prepared by the method of Cuzner et al. (1965). [e]600 g supernatant sedimented at 54,000 g for 10 min. [f]5,000 g supernatant sedimented at 54,000 g for 60 min. [g]54,000 g supernatant sedimented at 100,00 g for 15 hr.

differences ($\underline{P}$ < 0.01) when comparisons of endrin retention were made between S fish and R fish preparations. For the DDT treatment, only the heavy microsome fraction was significantly different ($\underline{P}$ < 0.05 in comparisons of S fish and R fish preparations. For aldrin, only the cell membrane fraction ($\underline{P}$ < 0.01) and the light microsome fraction ($\underline{P}$ < $\overline{0}$.05) from S fish were significantly different from the R fish fractions. In the dieldrin treatment only the cell membrane fractions of S fish and R fish were different (P < 0.01).

In parallel in vitro binding studies of whole brain and liver, the patterns were somewhat different from those in the in vivo studies (Table 4). For endrin, there was significantly more retention in the brain and liver preparations of S fish than in the brain and liver preparations of R fish. This same pattern was essentially true for the DDT treatment. For the aldrin treatments, there were no significant differences between the brain and liver preparations of S fish as compared to R fish. For the dieldrin treatment, the brain preparations from S fish were consistently higher ($\underline{P}$ < 0.01) than comparable preparations from R fish. In general, the in vitro liver results were similar to the in vivo liver data. The brain in vivo and in vitro results were similar for DDT, endrin and dieldrin, but there was a real difference in the S/R comparisons between the aldrin in vivo and in vitro treatments.

If we look at binding based on percent, that is the retention by each fraction of a preparation relative to the total insecticide retained by that preparation, a comparison of insecticide distribution within the cells of S fish and R fish is possible (Fig. 3-A; Fig. 4-A). The distribution pattern of endrin throughout the brain cell fractions in R fish and S fish preparations show some interesting differences. The cell membrane from brain and liver of S fish retains less endrin than the cell membrane from brain and liver of R fish. This pattern is reversed for the mitochondrial preparations. There was much less total endrin

385

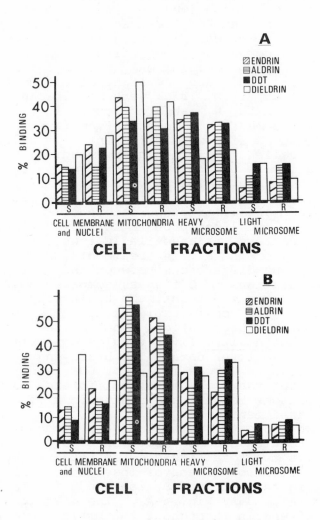

Figure 3. Binding of ^{14}C-endrin, ^{14}C-aldrin, ^{14}C-DDT and ^{14}C-dieldrin to insecticide-resistant (R) and susceptible (S) brain fractions following (A) in vivo treatment and (B) in vitro treatment. Binding is expressed as the percent of the total insecticide retained (Wells and Yarbrough, 1972a,b).

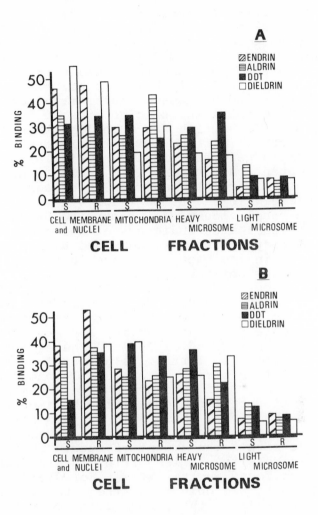

Figure 4. Binding of ^{14}C-endrin, ^{14}C-aldrin, ^{14}C-DDT and ^{14}C-dieldrin to insecticide-resistant (R) and susceptible (S) liver fractions following (A) in vivo treatment and (B) in vitro treatment. Binding is expressed as the percent of the total insecticide retained (Wells and Yarbrough, 1972a,b).

in the brain preparations of R fish than in S
fish. The increased retention by the cell membrane barrier in R fish. Essentially this same
pattern is seen for the DDT treatment. However,
there is an equal distribution of DDT in the brain
fractions of both S and R fish mitochondria and
H-microsomes. There are essentially no differences
between S fish and R fish in the percent retention
of aldrin by the various cellular fractions,
although the total insecticide present in the brain
preparations of R fish was much less than in brain
preparations of S fish. Dieldrin retention patterns
in the brain cell fractions were similar to the
endrin retention patterns in S and R fish. Both S
and R fish liver cell membrane fractions had the
highest dieldrin retention (Fig. 4-A).

The total amount of insecticide present in the
organs investigated indicates either a difference
in total body uptake between S and R fish or a
difference in the rate of uptake into liver and
brain tissues between the two populations. If we
look at insecticide levels in liver and compare
those to brain levels, a definite brain barrier is
apparent in R fish which is much less effective in
S fish (Table 5). This barrier appears to be most
effective for DDT and dieldrin. The effectiveness
of this barrier is further illustrated by the fact
that the R fish brain contained only one-fourteenth
the amount of DDT found in the liver, whereas the
S fish brain contained one-fifth the amount of DDT
found in the liver. This same pattern was seen for
endrin, in which the R fish brain contained only
about one-eighth the amount of endrin found in the
liver, whereas the S fish brain contained one-third
the amount found in the liver. For dieldrin, the
R brain contained only 2% of the total contained in
the liver, whereas the S fish brain contained 56%.

In vitro insecticide treatment of liver and
brain from both S and R fish consistently showed
higher retention of the insecticides in brain than
in liver preparations. Brain retention of DDT and
endrin was almost twice that of liver. This would
reinforce the functional brain barrier concept.
In most cases, the liver and brain from S fish had

388

Table 5. In vivo organochlorine insecticide brain to liver ratios in insecticide-resistant and susceptible mosquitofish.[a]

Insecticide[b]	Susceptible	Resistant
	Brain/Liver	Brain/Liver
[14]C-DDT	0.21	0.07
[14]C-Endrin	0.32	0.14
[14]C-Endrin	0.32	
[14]C-Aldrin	0.23	0.10
[14]C-Dieldrin	0.62	0.08

[a] Wells, 1971.

[b] Insecticide treatments consisted of: 75 ppb ^{14}C-p, p-DDT, 5 hr; 2 ppb ^{14}C-endrin, 6 hr; 150 ppb ^{14}C-aldrin, 4 hr; and 24 ppb ^{14}C-dieldrin, 4 hr.

higher insecticide concentrations than the liver and brain from R fish.

In general it would appear that cell membranes of R fish either prevent or slow insecticide entry into the cell at comparable treatment levels. There is less insecticide in the body organs of R fish than in the body organs of S fish. This indicates reduction in total whole body uptake in R fish. Therefore, what is seen at the cell level is reinforced by a decreased total whole body and organ uptake.

The pattern of retention by cellular fractions and uptake by organs of R fish is essentially similar for all four insecticides studied. The relationship between retention, uptake and toxicity is unclear. For example, of the four organochlorine compounds used, DDT is the most toxic to R fish (LC_{50} 96 ppb/48 hrs), while aldrin (LC_{50} 2,558 ppb/ 48 hrs) is least toxic, with endrin (LC_{50} 314 ppb/ 48 hrs) and dieldrin (LC_{50} 434 ppb/48 hrs) being intermediate. Yet, on the basis of total brain homogenates, the S/R ratios for three of the four

insecticides are the same. There is 2.34 times
as much DDT in the S fish as in the R fish preparations. This is true for endrin (2.92) and aldrin
(2.74). The dieldrin S/R ration is greater (3.54)
and also shows the highest S/R ratios for the cell
fractions.

These studies clearly indicate a significant
difference between the uptake of DDT, endrin,
aldrin and dieldrin in S and R fish tissues, and
point to a membrane barrier and/or a brain barrier
to organochlorine insecticides in R fish. If
central nervous tissue is representative of peripheral nervous tissue, then these studies would be
indicative of a protective barrier at the site of
action for R fish that is either absent or less
effective for S fish.

Insecticide Uptake

Ferguson et al. (1966) reported endrin uptake
in susceptible (S) and resistant (R) mosquitofish
to be the same and proposed that a "physiological
tolerance" of the toxicant within the body was a
major mechanism of endrin resistance. Fabacher
and Chambers (1971) reported that, at high concentrations, endrin entered nervous tissue at a slower
rate in R fish than in S fish. They suggested that
binding to non-essential proteins in R fish might
be a factor in resistance.

Since our work with mitochondrial preparations
and insecticide retention in cellular fractions
definitely indicated a membrane barrier, it seemed
logical to investigate insecticide uptake. For this
study endrin uptake was determined in test animals
exposed to endrin and categorized as either exhibiting symptoms of poisoning (symptomatic) or not
exhibiting symptoms of poisoning (asymptomatic).
Three tissue preparations were used: brain, divided
into three parts, prosencephalon (forebrain),
mesencephalon (midbrain), and rhombencephalon
(hindbrain); liver; and muscle. The concentrations
used were 10 ppb and 1500 ppb endrin. The 1500 ppb
level was necessary to produce symptoms of poisoning
in R fish within a reasonable time period. All

390

comparisons were made between fish exposed for essentially the same time periods. The exposure periods were between 3-9 hrs.

In general, there were lower endrin concentrations in tissues of symptomatic S fish than in tissues of asymptomatic S fish. This was the reverse of what was seen in R fish. In all cases the symptomatic R fish had higher tissue endrin concentrations than the tissues of asymptomatic R fish.

At the 10 ppb treatment, when comparisons were made between tissues of symptomatic S fish and tissues from asymptomatic S fish, there was little significant difference (Table 6). However, comparisons between symptomatic S fish and asymptomatic R fish showed significant differences for all tissue comparisons (P < 0.01). For the most part, the tissues from $\bar{S}$ fish had about three times as much endrin as tissues from R fish. When comparisons were made between endrin tissue concentrations of asymptomatic S fish and endrin tissue concentrations of asymptomatic R fish, there was from 4 to 5 times as much endrin in the brain parts and liver of S fish as in the brain parts of R fish. It is difficult to explain why the ratios of endrin tissue levels from asymptomatic S fish compared to endrin tissue levels of asymptomatic R fish show increases. It might indicate a decrease in sensitivity to endrin within the more tolerant individuals in both populations.

The higher endrin concentraions in the S as compared to the R fish indicate that there is an effective barrier in the R population. However, there does not appear to be a functional barrier in the more tolerant S fish as compared to the less tolerant S fish. Apparently the S fish tolerance is related to factors other than a membrane barrier, such as sensitivity to the toxicant.

At the 1500 ppb treatment all S fish were exhibiting symptoms of poisoning, while in the R fish population some were and some were not exhibiting symptoms. Therefore, at the highest endrin level, comparisons are between R fish that are less insecticide tolerant to R fish that are more

Table 6. Tissue concentration ratios of endrin in insecticide susceptible (S) and resistant (R) mosquitofish exhibiting symptoms (s) and not exhibiting symptoms (a) of poisoning.[a]

	10 ppb Endrin			1500 ppb Endrin		
	Ss/Sa[b]	Ss/Ra[b]	Sa/Ra[b]	Ss/Rs[b]	Rs/Ra[b]	Ss/Ra[b]
Forebrain	0.60	3.07++	5.09++	0.47++	3.70++	1.73+
Midbrain	0.65	2.87++	4.44++	0.45++	4.76+++	2.16+
Hindbrain	0.62+	3.05++	4.94++	0.44++	4.43+++	1.95
Liver	0.67	3.11+	4.66++	0.30++	6.50+++	1.94+
Muscle	1.03	3.15++	3.06++	0.49++	2.03++	1.00

a Scales (1973).

b Significant difference between S and R comparisons at $p < 0.05$ (+), $p < 0.01$ (++) or $p < 0.001$ (+++) as determined by t test.

insecticide tolerant. When this comparison is made the R fish ratios are highly significant at all levels (P < 0.01, or P < 0.001) with the exception of muscle (P < 0.05). This definitely indicates a barrier to endrin that is more effective in the more tolerant R fish. It is important to note that at the 1500 ppb endrin treatment the endrin tissue levels (µg/mg protein) were increased by 100 fold over the endrin tissue levels of the 10 ppb treatment (ng/mg protein).

Since peripheral nervous tissue is believed to be the site of organochlorine insecticide action, and muscle tissue has the highest peripheral nerve tissue concentration of our tissue preparations, the muscle ratios should provide indirect information on the effectiveness of the barrier at the site of action. The endrin muscle tissue ratio of symptomatic S fish to asymptomatic S fish is 1. When muscle tissue endrin concentrations from symptomatic R fish are compared to muscle tissue endrin concentrations from asymptomatic R fish the ratio is only 2.0 and is the lowest ratio of all tissue R symptomatic/R asymptomatic comparisons (Table 6). Therefore, there is an apparent insensitivity to endrin at the target site by the more tolerant individuals within both populations. This lack of sensitivity could be expressed as a threshold level which a toxicant must exceed before disruption of nerve function is possible. Thus, in vertebrate resistance, there is both a membrane barrier which is protective at the site of action, and a decrease in the sensitivity of the target tissue of the toxicant.

The barrier is present in both populations, but is most effective in R fish. The barrier, however, is not absolute. The more tolerant R fish seem to have a more effective barrier than the less tolerant R fish. This is consistent with the varying degrees of insecticide tolerance within a population.

The insensitivity of the target tissue to organochlorine insecticides might explain why uptake data and membrane retention studies do not seem to relate directly to toxicity levels (LC_{50} values).

The more tolerant individuals within the R population would probably possess a high insensitivity to
organochlorine insecticides at the target site and
an effective membrane barrier complex. The less
tolerant might possess only one of these factors,
or varying degrees of functional effectiveness of
one or both factors. It is doubtful that individuals
in the S population would contain both factors, or
that the factors would be as functionally effective
as in the individuals in the R population since o
natural selection for a highly tolerant population
has occurred.

Another factor that should be considered is
the rate of uptake. When endrin tissue concentrations from asymptomatic S fish and asymptomatic R
fish after exposure to 10 ppb are compared, there
is a consistently higher level of endrin in the S
fish than in the R fish at all time periods. There
seems to be a general increase in endrin concentration up to 12 hr exposure, followed by a decrease in
uptake rate. In R fish brain (Fig. 5-A), there is
a very dramatic change in the rate of endrin uptake
between the 3-9 and 9-12 hr periods. Again, the
brain barrier is very apparent when endrin levels
in brain of R fish are compared to endrin levels
in brain of S fish. In the liver the same uptake
pattern is seen as that for the brain (Fig. 5-B).
The muscle preparations showed the lowest difference between S and R fish but there was consistently
more endrin in the S fish muscle tissue than in R
fish muscle tissue. The endrin tissue concentrations in asymptomatic R fish after exposure to 1500
ppb were hgher than concentraions in asymptomatic
R fish after exposure to 10 ppb, but the pattern of
uptake was the same (Fig. 5-C).

Membrane Related Properties of Resistance

The obvious difference in the membranes between
resistant (R) and susceptible (S) fish is probably
indicative of not only functional but physicochemical changes as well. There is a possibility
that the membrane lipid content between the two
fish populations is different. Fabacher and

394

Chambers (1971) found that the lipid content of R mosquitofish was 1.8 times that of S mosquitofish, while the lipid content of livers from resistant fish was 1.7 times that of susceptible fish. They found no differences in the lipid content of brains from either fish population.

To investigate the extent of the membrane changes, the physical and physiological nature of the mitochondrial membranes have been investigated by hypotonic swelling experiments (Oakes, 1972). Hypotonic swelling of mitochondrial preparations from S fish and R fish tissues showed that mito-chondria from liver tissue of R fish swell signif-icantly faster ($P < 0.01$) at 30°C than mitochondria from liver tissues of S fish. There is apparently a greater flexibility in mitochondria isolated from R fish tissue than mitochondria from S fish tissue. Two-dimensional thin layer chromatographic analysis of the phospholipid content of mitochondria from R fish tissues and S fish tissues indicates no qualitative differences, but there are apparent quantitative differences in membrane lipids.

In vitro organochlorine retention data indicate a structural difference in myelin in R fish compared to S fish. When retention was compared between S and R fish myelin preparations, the S/R ratios were: 1.35 for endrin; 1.92 for aldrin; and 1.15 for DDT. All were significantly different ($P < 0.01$) (Wells, 1971).

If the primary action of organochlorine com-pounds is disruption of axonic transmission, then the apparent decrease in myelin affinity would offer considerable protection to R fish exposed to organochlorine insecticides.

Acknowledgements

The work reported in this paper was supported by the U.S. Public Health Service National Institutes of Health Grant Number 5RO1ES00412.

The author expresses his appreciation to all his graduate students and a very special thanks to Dr. Janice Chambers and Mr. Phillip Abston for their assistance in the preparation of this manuscript.

395

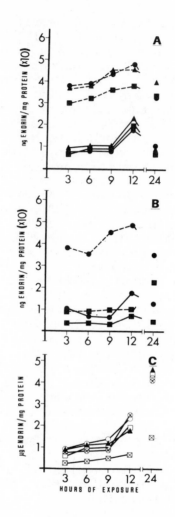

Figure 5. Endrin uptake in tissues of insecticide-resistant (——— R) and susceptible (- - - - S) mosquitofish.
A. 10 ppb endrin treatment (● Forebrain; ▉ Midbrain; and ▲ Hindbrain)
B. 10 ppb endrin treatment (● Liver and ▉ Muscle)
C. 1500 ppb endrin treatment (○ Forebrain; □ Midbrain; ▲ Hindbrain; ⊗ Liver; and ⊠ Muscle).

References

Boyd, C. E. and D. E. Ferguson. 1964a. J. Econ. Entromol. 57:430-431.

Boyd, C. E., and D. E. Ferguson. 1964b. Mosquito News 24:19-21.

Culley, D. D., and D. E. Ferguson. 1969. J. Fish Res. Bd. Canada 26:2395-2401.

Dzuik, L. J., and F. W. Plapp. 1973. Bull. Environ. Contam. Toxicol. 9:15-19.

Fabacher, D. C., and H. Chambers. 1971. Bull. Environ. Contam. Toxicol. 6:372-376.

Ferguson, D. E., and C. E. Boyd. 1964. Copeia 1964: 706.

Ferguson, D. E., D. D. Culley, W. D. Cotton, and R. P. Dodds. 1964. BioScience 14:43-44.

Ferguson, D. E., J. L. Ludke, and G. G. Murphy. 1966. Trans. Amer. Fish. Soc. 95:335-344.

Finley, M. T. 1970. Ph.D. Thesis, Miss. State Univ. 73 p.

Matsumura, F., and M. Hayashi. 1969. Science 153: 757-759.

Moffett, G. B., and J. D. Yarbrough. 1972. J. Agr. Food Chem. 20:558-560.

Mullins, L. J. 1955. Science 122:118-119.

Oakes, E. F. 1972. M.S. Thesis, Miss. State. Univ. 49 p.

O'Brien, R. D., and F. Matsumura. 1964. Science 146:657-658.

Scales, E. H. 1973. M.S. Thesis, Miss. State Univ. 29 p.

Telford, J., and F. Matsumura. 1970. J. Econ. Entomol. 63:795-800.

Vinson, S. B., C. E. Boyd, and D. E. Ferguson. 1963. Science 139:217-218.

Wells, M. R. 1971. Ph.D. Thesis, Miss. State Univ. 41 p.

Wells, M. R., and J. D. Yarbrough. 1972a. Toxicol. Appl. Pharmacol. 22:409-414.

Wells, M. R., and J. D. Yarbrough. 1972b. J. Arg. Food Chem. 20:14-16.

Wells, M. R., and J. D. Yarbrough. 1973. Toxicol. Appl. Pharmacol. 24:190-196.

Yarbrough, J. D., and M. R. Wells. 1971. Bull Environ. Contam. Toxicol. 6:171-176.

INSECTICIDE RESISTANCE IN INSECTS AND ITS ECOLOGICAL AND ECONOMIC THRUST

Albert S. Perry

Vector Biology & Control Branch, Tropical Disease Program, Center for Disease Control, U.S.P.H.S. Atlanta, Georgia

Abstract

Insect resistance to insecticides is an old phenomenon which has been brought into focus with the advent of DDT. It results from the intensive selection of variants in a population carrying preadaptive genes for resistance and is inherited according to Darwinian principles. Further enhancement of resistance can also be brought about by induction due to stresses imparted on the organism by chemicals.

Factors involved in insecticide resistance by insects include the following: Rate of penetration of the toxicant; rates of activation (toxication) and degradation (detoxication) of the chemical to primary metabolites; conjugation and excretion of secondary metabolites; storage of unchanged compound or of metabolites in nonsensitive tissues; degree of sensitivity of nerve tissue and of target enzymes to the toxic agent; binding properties of nerve components with the chemical; nature of lipid barrier surrounding the nerve sheath, and perhaps other factors. Supplementary factors such as lipid content, dietary factors, chemical differences, biotic potential, and behavioral patterns may play a role in resistance but these are of minor importance.

The most important resistance mechanism is the enhanced ability of the resistant insect to detoxify the insecticide at a faster rate and, in many instances, to eliminate it from circulation faster than its susceptible counterpart. Hence, resistance is more a quantitative expression rather than a qualitative difference among organisms of the same species.

DDT-resistant insects have a greater capacity to metabolize DDT via dehydrochlorination which is mediated by the enzyme DDT-dehydrochlorinase, and by hydroxylation of the tertiary carbon through the intermediary of the microsomal enzyme system.

Reistance to BHC is characterized by more extensive degradation of the molecule by the resistant strain involving glutathione-dependent S-alkyltransferase enzymes.

The cyclodiene compounds are activated rather than detoxified. Hence, resistance is not due to degradation of these toxicants. The resistance mechanism is not known.

Organophosphorus (OP) and carbamate insecticides are metabolized by microsomal enzymes requiring NADPH and O_2 and to a lesser extent by hydrolytic enzymes. These biotransformations can result in oxidation to more toxic anticholinesterases and in oxidative and hydrolytic degradation to innocuous derivatives. Resistance is primarily due to a faster rate of degradation of these compounds and accelerated excretion of conjugated metabolites by the resistant organism.

In spite of the tremendous amount of knowledge gained, the resistance problem defies solution. Alternative methods to chemical control of insects are currently being investigated. The ecological implications of extensive usage of tenacious broad-spectrum insecticides are discussed. The economic thrust brought about by resistance is considerable when one considers the debilitating effects of many tropical diseases on vast human populations. An integrated system of insect control could afford a solution to the resistance problem provided other factors such as sanitation, education, and cooperative efforts between agencies can be incorporated into the system.

400

Introduction

The problem of insect resistance to insecticides had been recognized many years ago, perhaps as early as 1887, and the first publication on this phenomenon is credited to Melander (1914) who wrote: "can insects become resistant to sprays?" The early work on insect resistance to lime-sulfur, hydrocyanic acid, tartar emetic, lead arsenate, cryolite, barium fluorosilicate, phenothiazine and other compounds has been reviewed and well documented by Babers and Pratt (1951). However, it was not until the advent of DDT resistance by the housefly in 1946 that this problem gained impetus and received considerable attention from entomolotists, chemists, biochemists, geneticists, and others.

In spite of this tremendous effort no economical solution, other than screening for new insecticides, has been found to counteract this resistance. This endeavor has largely failed because the phenomenon of cross-resistance makes the new compounds short-lived and, consequently, very expensive.

Recently, several new developments have stimulated renewed interest in the resistance problem. The clamor by ecologists, biological control specialists, and scientists in general for a cleaner environment free of persistent pesticide deposits has necessitated a reorientation of our concepts of insect control. Clearly, the control practices of the past three decades have placed emphasis on the applicaton of tenacious broad-spectrum insecticides with complete disregard for selectivity of the target species.

Furthermore, the misconceptions about the feasibility of eradication of certain insect species which are endowed with tremendous biotic potential, and our lack of understanding of pest and pesticide ecology have led to the dramatic acceleration of certain biochemical changes in the insect which, otherwise, might have gone unnoticed over a span of a lifetime. For many insects, these environmental stresses have been so sudden

and overwhelming that they responded with an
effective weapon of their own-a phenomenon known as
resistance.

In the past few years the resistance problem
has experienced another period of rejuvenation.
This resulted from the considerable knowledge
gained from mammalian pharmacology, specifically
from experimental evidence of the role of microsomal mixed-function oxidases in drug metabolism,
the induction of this enzyme system by drugs and
pesticides, and its inhibition by so-called synergists and antioxidants.

The Origin and Characteristics of Resistant Strains

According to most classical geneticists
insecticide resistance by insects results from the
intensive selection of variants in a population
carrying preadaptive genes (Crow, 1957; Kerr
et al., 1957). Because this resistance is inherited, it provides one of the best examples of
Darwinian evolution but at a much accelerated pace,
since the changes brought about in a population
are greatly accentuated by the intensive selection
which precedes the development of resistance.

There is ample evidence to show that the
factors responsible for resistance are present in
wild insect populations. The large increase in
the number of resistant species to the newer insecticides from 1 in 1946 to more than 250 at the
present writing indicates that given sufficient
time and selection pressure resistance becomes the
rule rather than the exception. It can be said
then that many insect populations possess the
elements of survival in the face of continued
environmental stress.

The rate at which resistance develops depends
to a large extent on the frequency of resistant
genes present in the normal population; the nature
of these genes (whether dominant, recessive, or
intermediate); the intensity of selection pressure;
and the biotic potential of the organism (Kerr,
1963). Where the genes for resistance are absent,

402

as may happen occasionally in geographically
isolated areas, resistance will not develop
(Elliott, 1959). Another situation where resistance may fail to develop is among highly inbred
laboratory strains whose gene pool contains no
resistance factors (Cole et al., 1957; Crow, 1966;
D'Allessandro et al., 1949; Harrison, 1952; Merrell
and Underhill, 1956). Yet, most laboratory-
selected strains of houseflies originated from the
highly inbred standard reference lines such as the
MAOD,. CS,A. pr WHO lines. The questions are, what
is the nature of these resistance factors, and are
differences between resistant and susceptible
individuals qualitative or quantitative, or both?

It is also evident that sublethal doses of
insecticides do not induce resistance in susceptible populations of insects (Beard, 1952, 1965;
Brown, 1964), nor do they increase the level of
DDT-dehydrochlorinase (Moorefield, 1958). On the
contrary, daily sublethal amounts of insecticides
exert a cumulative effect and render the insects
more susceptible to their toxic action upon subsequent treatment (Beard, 1952; Hadaway, 1956;
Hoffman et al., 1951).

Toxicological observations clearly indicate
the existence of a dynamic genotypic variability
in response to poisons among most insect
populations.

This graded response to a toxicant is sug-
gestive of quantitative differences in genetic
expression between individuals of various species
or strains. Indeed, with the appearance of new
and extremely sensitive tools at the hands of the
investigator, it is now possible to analyze
individuals rather than groups of insects for the
factors delineating resistance (Oppenoorth and
Voerman, 1965), and differences between strains
can be made more manifest (Grigolo and Oppenoorth,
1966; Oppenoorth, 1965; Khan and Terriere, 1968;
Lovell and Kearns, 1959).

Taken collectively, genetic variability for
resistance, slow development of resistance by inbred lines, failure to induce resistance with sublethal doses of toxicants, or, in some instances,
with dosages causing substantial mortality (Tahori

403

et al., 1969) indicate that insecticides are not mutagenic and that resistance is not caused by alteration of the genetic material.

Perry and Agosin (1974) have proposed that the development of resistance is biphasic. In phase I selection of variants takes place according to genetic principles. Once the level of resistance, commensurate with the gene pool initially present is attained, a further enhancement of that resistance takes place by induction (phase II). The insecticide itself is the inducer. Evidence for this phenomenon comes from extensive investigations on the induction of microsomal mixed-function oxidases in mammals and insects (Agosin, 1971; Gillett, 1971; Ishaaya and Chefurka, 1971; Menzer and Rose, 1971; Remmer, 1971). The induction phase depends on the presence of the toxicant in the organism's environment. Once the chemical is removed from that ecosystem resistance will revert to the preexisting genetic level after selection (phase I). Prolonged breeding in the absence of the toxicant will cause further reversion toward susceptibility, the rate of return being dependent on the resistance genotypes, including the incorporation of modifier genes during the selection process (Crow, 1966; Keiding, 1967; Plapp, 1970). Alternatively, the decline in resistance under field conditions predisposes the population to the rapid recovery of resistance (more rapidly than its emergence originally) on reintroducing the insecticide (Keiding, 1963).

The mechanism of induction in insects is not clearly understood. However, there is sufficient evidence that DDT affects nucleic acid metabolism and protein synthesis in insects (Agosin, 1971; Balazs and Agosin, 1968; Ishaaya and Chefurka, 1968; Litvak and Agosin, 1968) which in turn regulate enzyme synthesis. DDT may act more directly at the genetic level by its action on DNA-dependent RNA polymerase (Agosin, 1971). This induction by DDT can be correlated with certain physiological changes, such as changes in NADP concentration, which may be linked to the action of detoxifying microsomal enzymes (Agosin et al., 1966). Exposure to chemicals can also lead to

404

chemical adaptation and cross adaptation in the metabolism of foreign compounds (Fregly, 1969).

Types of Resistance

By definition "Resistance to insecticides is the development of an ability in a strain of insects to tolerate doses of toxicants which would prove lethal to the majority of individuals in a normal population of the same species" (World Health Organization, 1957). When the resistance is of a low magnitude and is not the result of a specific measurable factor it is termed "tolerance" or "vigor tolerance" (Hoskins and Gordon, 1956). Natural tolerance or natural resistance applies to instances where the insecticide in question is not effective against insect populations before any selection took place.

For the sake of convenience in delineating the factors involved, resistance may be classified as physiologic, morphologic and ecologic-behavioristic. Although behavioristic resistance does not conform with the definition given above, since it involves avoidance of the pesticide rather than tolerance to it, the end result in practical terms is the same, i.e., control failure in the field. The question also has been raised of how great the change in a population response to a chemical must be before it can be classified as resistant. Various figures and interpretations have been given, such as a 5-10 fold increase in the LD_{50} (Knipling, 1950; Decker and Bruce, 1952; Keiding, 1956). These values are based on laboratory testing procedures and are not necessarily applicable to field conditions in terms of an increase in dosage or in frequency of application. The latter practices may ultimately lead to greater resistance and to detrimental ecological consequences on desirable species. To illustrate this point, investigations on the reasons for the failure of DDT to control houseflies in a dairy barn (unpublished work by the author) revealed that, on the average, individual houseflies collected $0.5\mu g$ of DDT from walls sprayed with 200 mg DDT/sq. ft. and 80% of that amount was DDE. The LD_{50} of a susceptible strain of houseflies is 0.2 - 0.3μg of DDT per fly. Hence, control failure can result from only twice the LD_{50} dose.

Physiological Resistance

By far, the most extensive studies on resistance have been those dealing with the metabolic fate of pesticides in resistant insects and their susceptible counterparts. The housefly has been the organism of choice, for it was the housefly which dealt the first blow to our hopes that certain insect control problems should never have gotten out of hand if proper suppressive measures with chemicals were taken. But the development of DDT resistance by the housefly was also a blessing in disguise. It gave impetus to a wide variety of basic and applied research in entomology and in allied scientific disciplines. It also stimulated the chemist to synthesize new classes of compounds with different modes of action.

Resistance to Chlorinated Hydrocarbon (CH) Insecticides

Physiologic resistance is intimately associated with the metabolic fate of insecticides in insects. The first such study with DDT is credited to Ferguson and Kearns (1949) who injected DDT into the large milkweed bug Oncopeltus fasciatus and found that it was completely metabolized within 90 minutes to unidentified metabolites.

The early assumptions that control failure with DDT was due to adulterated insecticide, improper application of the chemical, or to the physical environment were soon dispelled with the simultaneous discovery by Sternburg et al., (1950) and Perry and Hoskins (1950) that houseflies could metabolize DDT to the nontoxic derivative 2,2-bis-(p-chlorophenyl)-1,1-dichloroethylene (DDE). This finding was sooon corroborated by many investigators and it became increasingly evident that resistance to DDT by many insect species was associated, to a large measure, with enhanced detoxication of the chemical (for details see reviews by Perry, 1964; Brown and Pal, 1971; and Perry and Agosin, 1974). Several insect species exhibit natural tolerance for DDT and in these, too, detoxication plays a major role.

In addition to the resistance potential present in most insect populations, DDT has caused the reduction of predator and parasite populations and other nontarget organisms. Interestingly, the lady beetle Coleomegilla maculata, a predator of several insect species, developed a high level of physiological resistance to DDT (Atallah and Nettles, 1966). The same phenomenon has been noted in Macrocentrus ancylivorus, a parasite of the oriental fruit moth (Pilou and Glasser, 1951; Robertson, 1957), in Bracon mellitor, an ectoparasite of the boll weevil (Adams and Cross, 1967) and in several species of mayflies, principally Heptagenia hebe and two Stenonema species (Grant and Brown, 1967).

In general, most DDT-resistant populations investigated so far have the ability to detoxify the insecticide to one or more metabolites. The only exception is the khapra bettle Trogoderma granarium whose natural immunity to DDT is associated with neither detoxication nor with lack of penetration of the toxicant (Gupta et al., 1971).

Another type of DDT breakdown by resistant insects is via oxidation to the corresponding ethanol derivative 2,2-bis-(p-chlorophenyl)-1,1,1-trichloroethanol (dicofol) (Tsukamoto, 1959, 1960; Dinamarca et al., 1962; Agosin et al., 1964; Rowlands and Lloyd, 1969), and to 2,2-bis-(p-chlorophenyl)-1,1-dichloroethanol (FW-152) (Menzel et al., 1961). The body louse Pediculus humanus humanus degrades DDT via dehydrochlorination to DDE, formation of bis-(p-chlorophenyl) acetic acid (DDA) and oxidation to 4,4'-dichlorobenzophenone (DBP). Only the resistant strain metabolizes DDT in vivo. However, homogenates of both susceptible and DDT-resistant lice metabolize DDT in vitro at equal rates and yield the same metabolites (Perry et al., 1963). This dilemma remains unresolved. The various reactions involved in DDT-metabolism are shown in Figure 1.

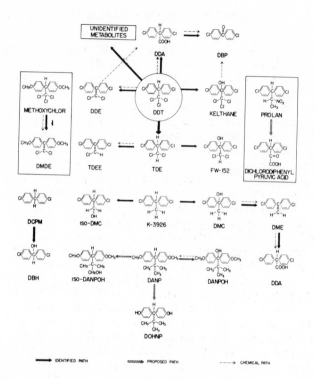

Figure 1.   Pathways of metabolism of DDT, Methoxy-chlor and Prolan in various insects.

The causal relationship between DDT resistance and DDT dehydrochlorination could not be ascertained until the isolation by Sternburg et al., (1953) of the enzyme DDT-dehydrochlorinase (DDTase) which, in the presence of glutathione, catalyzes the breakdown of DDT to DDE (Figure 2).   DDTase has been purified by various procedures (Moorefield, 1956; Lipke and Kearns, 1959a; Dinamarca et al., 1969) and its kinetics have been studied in some detail (Lipke and Kearns, 1959b; Lipke, 1960; Dinamarca et al., 1971).   The enzyme has a tet-rameric structure with each monomer having a molecular weight of 30,000.   The tetramer is formed only in the presence of DDT, possibly because the enzyme is a lipoprotein (Dinamarca et al., 1971). Other DDT isozymes have been described (Goodchild and Smith, 1970) but it is not known if these isozymes are related to the tetrameric forms of DDTase.

Housefly eggs contain no DDTase. The enzyme appears in early larval life and increases progressively in later instars. There is an abrupt drop by as much as 50% as soon as the larva pupates and this lower level of activity is maintained throughout adult life (Moorefield and Kearns, 1957; Figure 3).

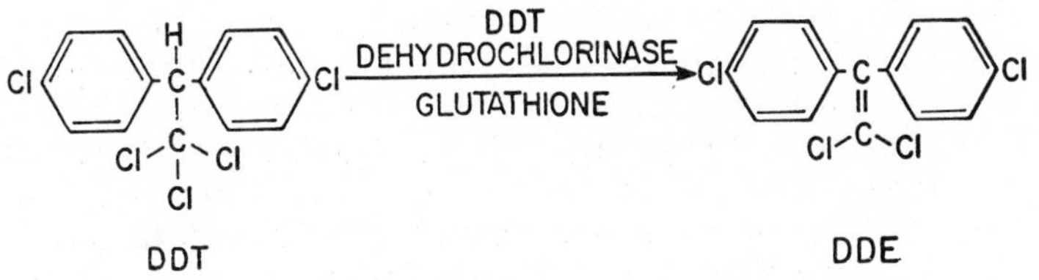

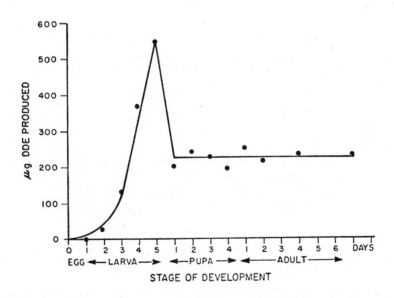

Figure 2. Enzymatic dehydrochlorination of DDT to DDE.

Figure 3. Distribution of DDT-dehydrochlorinase in different stages of development of DDT-resistant houseflies.

High enzyme titers are found in fat body and brain tissue and smaller amounts in other tissues (Miyake et al., 1957). In vivo, DDE/DDT ratios are highest in thoracic and abdominal cuticle, intermediate in alimentary tract, fat body, and nerve cord, and lowest in haemolymph (Sternburg and Kearns, 1950; Lindquist et al., 1951; Hoskins, 1952; Tahori and Hoskins, 1953; Le Roux and Morrison, 1954).

In addition to DDT, DDTase also catalyzes the dehydrochlorination of DDD (TDE) and methoxychlor by the Mexican bean beetle (Chattoraj and Kearns, 1958; Swift and Forgash, 1959; Tombes and Forgash, 1961). However, in this insect, highest concentration of the enzyme is found in the reproductive organs, followed by the alimentary canal, exoskeleton, flight muscle, nervous system, and fat body.

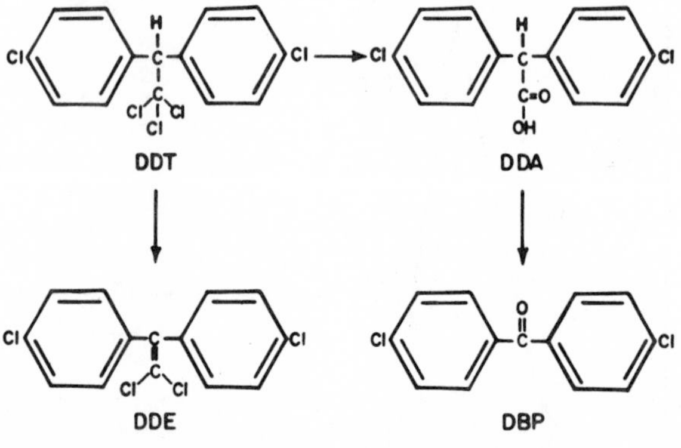

Figure 4. Pathway of DDT metabolism in the body louse Pediculus humanus humanus.

Enzymic degradation of DDT by the body louse yields three metabolites, i.e., DDE, DDA, and DBP. Two of the enzymes responsible for these biotransformations have been isolated and partially purified (Perry et al., 1963; Miller and Perry, 1964). The pathway of DDT metabolism in this insect is shown in Figure 4.

DDTase has also been isolated and characterized from Aedes aegypti (Kimura and Brown, 1964) and its properties have been found to be similar to housefly DDTase. The enzyme activity is roughly proportional to the level of DDT resistance in several strains of this species. On the other hand, such correlation is wanting in certain anopheline species both in vitro (Lipke and Chalkley, 1964) and in vivo (Perry, 1960a).

Another type of enzymic attack on DDT involves hydroxylation of the tertiary carbon. This enzyme system was first isolated and characterized by Agosin et al., (1961). It resides in the microsomal fraction of the cell and requires NADPH and molecular oxygen for activation. The term mixed-function oxidases has been ascribed to this enzyme system which catalyzes the oxidation of a multitude of drugs, insecticides, and other foreign organic compounds.

The role of DDT hydroxylation in resistance was first demonstrated by Morello (1964) who showed that 3-methylcholanthrene increases the hydroxylating capacity of DDT by 5th instar nymphs of Triatoma infestans, whereas SKF 525-A (β-diethylaminoethyl diphenylpropyl acetate) and iproniazid (2-isopropyl-1-isonicotinoyl hydrazine) block this hydroxylation with a concomitant increase in mortality. Earlier, Arias and Terriere (1962) and Schonbrod et al., (1965) showed a higher rate of naphthalene hydroxylation by microsomes of DDT-resistant houseflies than by those of their susceptible counterparts.

Microsomal hydroxylation of DDT has since been shown by a number of other investigators (Tsukamoto and Casida, 1967; Gil et al., 1968; Oppenoorth and Houx, 1968; Plapp and Casida, 1969; Khan et al., 1973) and this reaction now appears to be a major pathway of DDT-detoxication as well as degradation of methoxychlor and methiochlor (Kapoor et al., 1970) in several insects.

Resistance to Hexachlorocylohexane (BHC)

γ-BHC (lindane), which is the toxic isomer, is metabolized more rapidly by resistant insects than by their susceptible counterparts (Oppenoorth, 1954). This is also true for the α-, β-, and δ-isomers which are less toxic (Oppenoorth, 1955; Bradbury and Standen, 1956). The greater metabolic capacity in resistant strains has been implicated in a possible causal relationship to resistance (Bradbury and Standen, 1960) and a good correlation was found between degree of resistance and absorption rate, breakdown capacity, and amount of unchanged toxicant in the housefly (Oppenoorth, 1956).

The ability to metabolize γ-BHC varies greatly among different species. A comparative study (Bradbury, 1957) showed that houseflies are considerably more efficient in this respect than other insects (Table 1).

Table I. Comparative Metabolism of γ-BHC-C^{14} in Various Insects[a]

Species	Dosage µg/gm	External	Internal	Water soluble Metabolites	% Metabolized
		BHC recovered (µg/gm)			
Cockroach	42	10	19	7	22.0
Bean weevil	111	7	94	8	7.7
Grain weevil	34	14	13	1	4.2
Locust	100	16	83	4	4.7
Mosquito	213	17	141	10	5.1
Khapra beetle	166	81	45	11	12.9
House-fly (S)[b]	193	22	54	99	57.9
House-fly (R)[b]	230	13	21	174	80.2

[a]After Bradbury (1957). [b]S=Susceptible; R=Resistant

The metabolites of γ-BHC produced by insects consist of organo-soluble and water-soluble dechlorination products. γ-Pentachlorocyclohexene (PCCH) is a major (Sternburg and Kearns, 1956) or a minor (Bradbury and Standen, 1958; Bridges, 1959) nontoxic metabolite. A second PCCH isomer may be of significance in housefly resistance to lindane (Reed and Forgash, 1968, 1969) and both lindane and the PCCH isomers yield a common metabolite 1,2,4,5-tetrachlorobenzene.

Organo-soluble metabolites are of minor consequence in resistance since water-soluble products predominate in all strains investigated (Reed and Forgash, 1970).

An important contribution in elucidating the mechanism of BHC resistance was the finding that alkaline hydrolysis of BHC metabolites yield dichlorothiophenols (Bradbury and Standen, 1959). This implies the formation of a C-S bond, and the nature of the metabolite suggests a conjugation with aryl mercapturic acid (Bradbury and Standen, 1960). The enzyme catalyzing this reaction requires glutathione for activation and, most likely, belongs to the group of glutathione S-aryltransferases (Clark et al., 1967; Fukami and Shishida, 1966). The same enzyme also converts PCCH to the same water-soluble metabolite (Ishida and Dahm, 1965a, 1965b; Sims and Grover, 1965). The various reactions are depicted in Figure 5.

The causal relationship between detoxication and resistance can further be demonstrated by enzyme inhibition studies using phthaleins and sulfophthaleins (Clark et al., 1969; Balabaskaran et al., 1968) or bromphenol blue (Ishida and Dahm, 1965a). Inhibitors such as these might be used to distinguish between isozymes among different species.

In spite of the extensive investigations made on BHC it is doubtful that a positive correlation exists between detoxication and resistance except, perhaps, in the housefly, for no other insect either resistant or susceptible has shown as great a potential for BHC metabolism as Musca domestica.

413

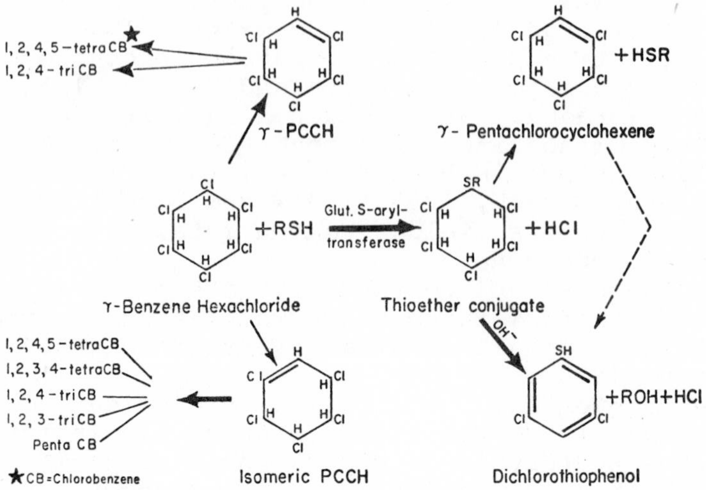

Figure 5. Metabolism of benzene hexachloride by the housefly. Major metabolic routes are designated by heavy arrows.

Resistance to cyclodiene compounds

The cyclodiene insecticides, heptachlor, aldrin, and isodrin, are converted to their respective epoxides; heptachlor epoxide, dieldrin, and endrin. These biotransformations are catalyzed by microsomal mixed-function oxidases in the presence of NADPH and O_2. The epoxides are invariably more toxic than the parent compounds; they are more persistent and less susceptible to attack by insect enzymes.

The cyclodiene compounds have been widely used as broad spectrum insecticides for many years. They have been studied extensively, yet their mode of action is little understood. Many agricultural pests and insect vectors of disease are known to have developed high levels of resistance to the cyclodienes but the mechanism of this resistance is virtually unknown. Obviously, resistance is not due to detoxication of these compounds, so the insect must possess another efficient defense mechanism to protect itself during the initial

414

critical stages of poisoning. The protective
mechanism could reside at the site of action of
dieldrin since the resistant fly shows extreme
tolerance for dieldrin vapors, thus by-passing
cuticular penetration and other barriers (Earle,
1963). There is some evidence that nerve sensitivity to dieldrin is lower in resistant than in
susceptible houseflies (Yamasaki and Narahashi,
1958). A similar characteristic occurs in DDT and
BHC-resistant houseflies. The factor for lower
nerve sensitivity to DDT is inherited as an incom-
pletely recessive gene carried on the 2nd chromosome, but the genetic factor for low nerve sensitivity to γ-BHC is carried on a different linkage
group (Tsukamoto et al., 1965).

Telford and Matsumura (1971), using electron
microscopy and autoradiography, indicated that less
dieldrin is accumulated in nerve tissue of dieldrin-
resistant Blatella germanica, and Sellers and
Guthrie (1971) detected no H^3-dieldrin in gangli-
onic tissue of treated dieldrin-resistant houseflies.

Another physicochemical factor which might be
involved in resistance is the binding of insecticides to subcellular components of nerve tissue.
O'Brien and Matsumura (1964), Matsumura and O'Brien
(1966), and Matsumura and Hayashi (1966a, 1966b)
suggest that DDT and dieldrin form complexes with
lipid components of insect nerve, but Holan (1969)
presents evidence that complex formation is with
protein and not with lipid components. At any
rate, the mode of action of the cyclodiene compounds as well as the mechanism of resistance to
them remain, at present, unresolved. The important
reactions involved in the metabolism of heptachlor
and aldrin are shown in Figures 6 and 7, respectively. In addition, cyclodiene compounds undergo
photolysis under natural conditions and the products of these physicochemical transformations are
of great significance to the ecology. This latter
topic is discussed separately in this symposium.

Resistance to organophosphorus (OP) insecticides

With the ever-increasing number of insect species developing resistance to the chlorinated hydrocarbon insecticides it was hoped that the substitution of OP compounds would overcome the resistance problem. It was soon rediscovered that history has a habit of repeating itself and that given sufficient time and selection pressure, resistance to OP compounds becomes a reality.

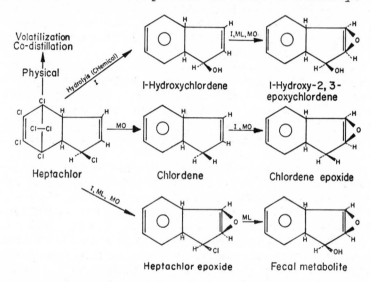

Figure 6. Metabolism of heptachlor by insects (I), mammals (ML), and microorganisms (MO).

Resistance to OP compounds is biochemically limited to levels which are characteristic of the particular insecticide. Cross resistance to other structurally related and unrelated OP compounds is common but the spectrum varies considerably among species and strains. Furthermore, resistance to these insecticides declines fairly rapidly upon removal of the toxicant from the insect's environment (March, 1959, 1960; Busvine, 1959; Oppenoorth, 1959; Mengle and Casida, 1960; Forgash and Hansens,

1962; Van den Heuvel and Cochran, 1965; Bell, 1968).
In many instances, selection with OP compounds
results in cross resistance to carbamates and to
certain chlorohydrocarbon insecticides.

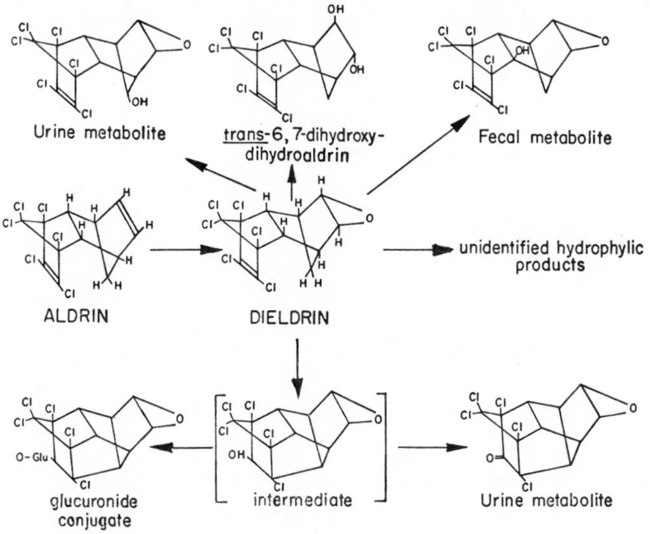

Figure 7. Metabolism of aldrin and dieldrin by insects and mammals.

Resistance to OP compounds is governed largely
by a metabolic balance between rates of activation
and detoxication processes as well as penetration
of the insecticide through the cuticle and sensitivity of the OP receptor at the site of action.
Generally, activation reactions are oxidative
in nature and are catalyzed by microsomal mixed-
function oxidases in the presence of NADPH and O_2.
The products of these reactions (oxon derivatives)
are potent anticholinesterases and possess greater
biological activity than their parent compounds.
The pathways leading to such reactions include:
(a) desulfuration of esters containing P=S groups
to yield the corresponding P=O (oxon) derivatives;
(b) oxidation of aliphatic or aromatic thioethers
to sulfoxides and sulfones; (c) N-oxidation of
phosphoramides; (d) N-dealkylation, e.g., dicrotophos
to monocrotophos; (e) Hydroxylation and cycliza-

tion, e.g., triorthocresyl phosphate; and (f) Dehalogenation, such as the conversion of Dipterex to DDVP. Examples of activation reactions are shown in Figure 8.

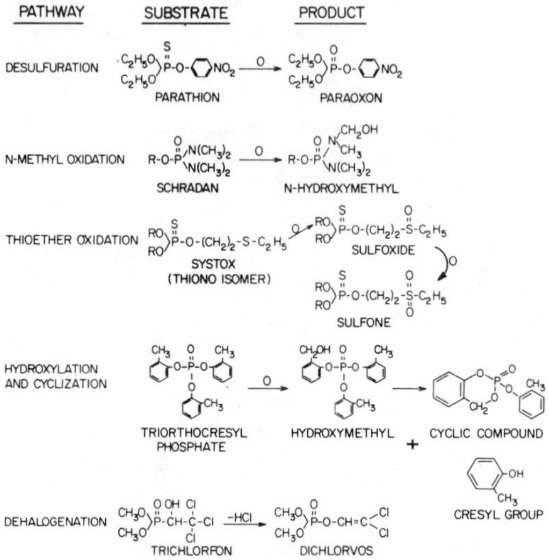

Figure 8. Examples of activation mechanisms of organophosphorus insecticides in insects.

Detoxication of OP compounds leads to products of lower biological activity. The pathways in- volved in such biotransformations include: (a) Transalkylation-conjugation reactions utilizing reduced glutathione and yielding dealkylated metabolites. The enzymes mediating these reactions reside in the soluble fraction and belong to the group of glutathione-S-alkyltransferases. The substrate requirements of this enzyme system seem to favor dimethyl esters of phosphorothioates and phosphates, but aryl groups are also conjugated. (b) Oxidative O-dealkylation and dearylation: Organophosphorus triesters undergo cleavage to diester derivatives, the latter being relatively nontoxic. The O-dealkylated metabolites were pre- sumed to be hydrolytic products of phosphatase attack (Plapp and Casida, 1958) but these reactions are not recognized as being mediated by mixed-

418

function oxidases. (c) S-oxidation: Formation of sulfoxide and sulfone metabolites of lower toxicity. (d) Reactions involving phosphatase enzymes: These reactions have long been designated as hydrolytic reactions (Plapp and Casida, 1958; Heath, 1961; O'Brien, 1960, 1967) attacking the phosphorus ester or the anhydride bond at P-O-C, P-S-C, P-F linkages, etc. Resistance to many OP compounds has been attributed to more rapid hydrolysis and excretion of conjugated products by the resistant insect. It is now apparent that such products of phosphatase action can be obtained by oxidation through the mediation of microsomal mixed-function oxidases (Nakatsugawa et al., 1968; Nakatsugawa et al., 1969; Welling et al., 1971). (e) Carboxyesterases (Aliesterases): These are enzymes hydrolyzing methyl or phenyl butyrate, although their physiological function in insects is not understood. OP compounds and carbamate insecticides inhibit these enzymes, but in some instances these toxicants are hydrolyzed by aliesterases. These observations drew attention to the possible role of aliesterases in OP resistance (van Asperen, 1958). In many strains of houseflies investigated, OP resistance was found to be inversely related to aliesterase activity (van Asperen and Oppenoorth, 1959; Bigley and Plapp, 1960, 1961; Forgash et al., 1962; Matsumura and Sakai, 1968; Collins and Forgash, 1970), although this is not a universal occurence.

Resistant strains of Culex tarsalis and Aedes aegypti contain as much aliesterase activity as their susceptible counterparts (Plapp et al., 1965), and aliesterase activity bears no relation to insecticide resistance in Drosophila melanogaster (Ogita, 1961). In the green rice leafhopper, Hayashi and Hayakawa (1962), Kojima et al., (1963), and Kasai and Ogita (1965) found more aliesterase activity in the malathion-resistant strains.

The hypothesis has been advanced (Oppenoorth and van Asperen, 1960) that the normal carboxyesterase enzyme, whose function in the susceptible strain is to hydrolyze aliphatic esters, is modified to produce an OP-hydrolyzing enzyme in the resistant strain. Its significance has been

419

disputed by O'Brien (1966, 1967) on grounds that the small enzyme activity could not account for the high level of resistance.

The role of carboxyesterases is, nevertheless, quite important in detoxication of certain OP compounds, especially malathion, and there is substantial evidence that resistance to this compound is intimately associated with enhanced carboxyesterase activity as well as with other types of attack. (f) Carboxyamidases: These enzymes participate in the detoxication of OP compounds containing a carboxyamide group such as dimethoate and Imidan. They are more active in mammals than in insects. Examples of detoxication pathways are shown in Figure 9.

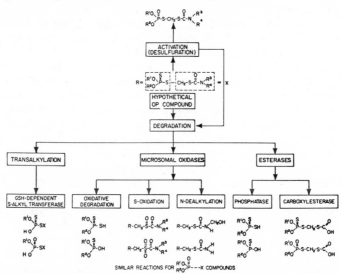

Figure 9. Schematic diagram of detoxication pathways of a hypothetical organophosphorus compound.

Resistance to Carbamate Insecticides

The carbamate insecticides share with the OP compounds the characteristic that they are inhibitors of the enzyme cholinesterase, but they differ from OP compounds in that they are competitive rather than irreversible inhibitors of the enzyme.

Initially, many of the commercially available carbamates proved to be highly effective against a wide variety of resistant insects, but it was soon discovered that these compounds, too, are subject to attack by insect enzymes, notably the microsomal mixed-function oxidases, hydrolases, and conjugative enzymes.

In general, most insects studied show no evidence of qualitative differences in metabolism of carbamates between resistant (R) and susceptible (S) strains. Metcalf et al., (1967) investigated the metabolism of nine carbamates labeled with C^{14} in different parts of the molecule and found that: (a) absorption and metabolism did not vary appreciably between R and S strains of houseflies, (b) rate of conversion to CO_2 was characteristic of the specific carbamate and the position of C^{14} in the molecule, and (c) excretion of metabolites was significantly higher in R strains.

Detoxication of carbamates proceeds via the following pathways: (1) Hydrolysis - such as conversion of carbaryl to 1-naphthol (Eldefrawi et al., 1961; Ku and Bishop, 1967); carbofuran to several hydroxy derivatives which appear mostly in conjugated form (Dorough, 1968; Metcalf et al., 1968). (2) N-Dealkylation - occurs readily with methiocarb (Metcalf et al., 1967) aminocarb, and Zectran (Tsukamoto and Casida, 1967). Several nontoxic metabolites are formed. (3) O-Dealkylation - this reaction is prominent with propoxur which is dealkylated at the isopropoxyphenyl moiety to yield O-depropyl propoxur (Shrivastava et al., 1969, 1970). (4) S-Dealkylation - ordinarily takes place after formation of sulfoxide or sulfone, such as in aldicarb. (5) Ring-C hydroxylation - this is a major pathway in carbamate detoxication, particularly the hydroxylation of propoxur to the 5-hydroxy derivative (Shrivastava et al., 1969, 1970). (6) S-Oxidation - methiocarb is oxidized to the sulfoxide and sulfone derivatives which are less toxic (Metcalf et al., 1967; Tsukamoto and Casida, 1967), but with aldicarb the oxidation products are more toxic to houseflies (Metcalf et al., 1966, 1967) and to bollweevils and tobacco

budworms (Bull et al., 1967). (7) N-Methyl
hydroxylation - this oxidative pathway is common
to many carbamates. For example, homogenates of
the cabbage looper oxidize carbaryl to the
N-hydroxymethyl derivative (Kuhr, 1970); Banol is
oxidized to the N-hydroxymethyl derivative by the
cockroach Blaberus giganteus (Gemrich, 1967) and
the housefly (Tsukamoto and Casida, 1967), and
N-hydroxymethyl propoxur is a major metabolite of
propoxur in spruce budworm larvae and Culex p.
fatigans (Shrivastava et al., 1969, 1970). Similar
products are formed in the metabolism of dimetilan
by cockroaches and houseflies (Zubairi and Casida,
1965). Aromatic N-methyl hydroxylation is a major
oxidative route in Landrin metabolism by houseflies
(Slade and Casida, 1970).

In summary, resistance to carbamates is due,
in many instances, to more rapid rate of metabolism
of the compound and a faster rate of excretion of
conjugated metabolites. The mixed-function oxidase
system is also more active in propoxur-resistant
strains of Anopheles albimanus (Ariaratnam and
Georghiou, 1971) and C. p. fatigans (Shrivastava
et al., 1971).

Resistance to Botanicals
i) Pyrethrins:

Housefly resistance to pyrethrins is an old
phenomenon. The basis for this resistance was,
for many years, thought to be due to hydrolysis of
the ester linkage as a detoxication mechanism.
This was based on the incomplete identification of
chrysanthemumic acid and keto-alcohols resulting
from the in vivo metabolism of pyrethrins by the
American cockroach (Zeid, et al., 1953). Bridges
(1957) and Chang and Kearns (1964) extended this
work and concluded that the metabolic products
were not due to hydrolysis.

There is now convincing evidence that resistance to pyrethrins and allethrins is due to oxidative breakdown rather than hydrolytic cleavage
(Yamamoto and Casida, 1966; Yamamaoto et al., 1969).
It was shown that the metabolites of allethrin
contain the intact acid and alcohol moieties and

the main products are the trans allethrinoic acid, trans allethrinol, and trans allethrinal. The production of allethrinoic acid is associated with greater enzyme activity.

The residual life of pyrethrins is not long lasting. This accounts, perhaps, for its limited use in the field and for the fact that resistance to this insecticide is not widespread. There are, however, reports of field-collected pyrethrum-resistant houseflies (Davies et al., 1958; Keiding, 1969) and laboratory-induced resistance (Fine, 1961). Pyrethrum resistance has also been reported in other insects (Brown & Pal, 1971; Perry & Agosin, 1974).

ii) Rotenone:

Rotenone inhibits mitochondrial respiration by blocking the enzyme system involved in the coupled oxidation of $NADH_2$ and reduction of cytochrome b (Lindahl and Öberg, 1961). In insects, this type of inhibition is equally effective in both susceptible and resistant strains (Fukami et al., 1967). Hence, the selective toxicity of rotenone (being moderately toxic to mammals and highly toxic to fish and some insects) does not involve its site of action but depends primarily on its distribution in various tissues and its rate of detoxication by various organisms (Fukami et al., 1969).

Rotenone is extensively metabolized by the microsomal mixed-function oxidase system yielding several non-toxic hydroxylated products and conjugates, and these reactions are inhibited by methylenedioxyphenyl synergists (Fukami et al., 1969).

iii) Nicotine:

It is remarkable that several species, i.e., the tobacco hornworm, tobacco budworm, tobacco wireworm, green peach aphid, etc., thrive on tobacco plants, yet they are not affected by this plant which contains nicotine, one of the most toxic alkaloids found in nature. The green peach aphid

survives because it selectively feeds on the phloem
of the plant, thus by-passing the nicotine-contain-
ing xylem (Guthrie et al., 1962). On the other
hand, the tobacco hornworm excretes and egests
unchanged nicotine and other alkaloids before it
accumulates a toxic dose (Self et al., 1964a).

Cockroaches, B. germanica and P. americana, are
able to metabolize nicotine to the non-toxic derivative cotinine, and the southern armyworm converts
nicotine to nine other unidentified metabolites
(Guthrie et al., 1957). The tobacco wireworm,
cigarette beetle, differential grasshopper, and the
housefly metabolize nicotine to cotinine and several
other metabolites (Self et al., 1964b). The housefly, however, does not excrete either nicotine or
the metabolic products.

Mammals metabolize nicotine principally to
cotinine and this oxidative reaction is mediated by
the microsomal mixed-function oxidase system in the
liver (Hucker et al., 1960; Stabhandske et al., 1969).
It is quite likely that this metabolic pathway in
insects also proceeds via the mixed-function oxidase
system.

Resistance to other Compounds

Chemosterilants have not yet found wide application in field control operations but, in the
laboratory, it has been possible to induce resistance in Aedes aegypti to apholate (Hazard et al.,
1964), to metepa (Klassen and Matsumura, 1966), to
Hempa (George and Brown, 1967) and in the housefly
to metepa (Sacca and Scirocchi, 1966) and to Hempa
(Akov and Borkovec, 1968; Akov et al., 1968; Chang
and Borkovec, 1969).

In addition to chemosterilants there has been
one report of induced resistance to the toxin of
Bacillus thuringensis (Thuricide) in the housefly
(Harvey and Howell, 1965).

The recent surge in exploration of alternative
methods (other than chemical) for control of insect
pests has led to the synthesis of juvenile hormone
mimics capable of disrupting the normal development
of the insect. It has been suggested (Williams,
1956, 1967) that insects would be unlikely to

424

develop resistance to their own juvenile hormones.
However, Schneiderman et al., (1970) have advanced
arguments that resistance to juvenile hormones is
likely to develop in insects.

Insect control with hormonal insecticides does
not differ much from control with other pesticides.
The hormones must enter the insect's cuticle from
an exogenous source and, consequently, the physiological and biochemical mechanisms involved in
their absorption, transport, and metabolism may be
distinct from analogous systems for the insect's
own endogenous hormone (Schneiderman et al., 1970;
Robbins, 1972). Furthermore, the synthetic hormone
may so differ in structure from the natural hormone
that it may well be considered a xenobiotic, subject
to attack by the same insect enzymes which are
involved in the degradation of other toxicants.
Indeed, studies in vivo and in vitro with the
tobacco hornworm Manduca sexta (Slade and Zibitt,
1972) have shown that the Cecropia juvenile hormone
is extensively metabolized by hydrolysis of the
ester group followed by hydration of the epoxide.
Qualitative differences were found in the hormone
metabolism by Hyalophora cecropia, Schistocerca
vaga and Sarcophaga bullata. Other studies with
rats and the desert locust Schistocerca americana
(Gill et al., 1972) showed extensive metabolism of
the juvenoid, 1-(4'-ethylphenoxy)-6,7-epoxy-3,7-
dimethyl-2-octene (Stauffer R-20458) by microsomal
enzymes in vitro and excretion of several metabolites in vivo.

Lately, resistance to a synthetic juvenile
hormone has been reported in Tribolium castaneum
(Dyte, 1972) and evidence of cross resistance to
the hormone analogue, isopropyl 11-methoxy-3,7,
11-trimethyldodeca-2,4-dienoate (Zoëcon 0515), in
insecticide-resistant houseflies has been presented
(Cerf and Georghiou, 1972). In addition, houseflies
treated with synthetic juvenile hormone exhibited
a 65% increase in microsomal epoxidase activity at
18-24 hours after treatment (Yu and Terriere, 1971).
This induction, most likely, also enhances the
metabolism of the hormone itself.

In spite of the apparent likelihood of resistance development to the juvenile hormones in

insects, the many desirable characteristics of
hormonal compounds, should they continue to hold
true, would be sufficient reason to continue exploration of other juvenile hormones and antihormone
compounds as potential insecticides.

II. Resistance Due to Morphological and Permeability Factors

Practically all reports on the in vivo metabolism of pesticides by resistant and susceptible
insects include some information on penetration of
the insecticide through the insect's cuticle.
Accordingly, numerous attempts have been made to
correlate resistance with slower penetration of the
chemical. There is little doubt that slower rate
of penetration enhances the organism's chances of
survival, especially if the organism possesses an
added protective mechanism such as a pesticide-
detoxifying enzyme. In some instances, reduced
rate of penetration constitutes a major factor in
resistance, for example, in housefly resistance to
diazinon (Forgash et al., 1962; Farnham et al.,
1965; El Bashir, 1967), Aedes aegypti resistance
to malathion (Matsumura and Brown, 1963), housefly
and mosquito resistance to DDT-synergist combinations (Perry, 1958; Pillai and Brown, 1965, respectively), housefly resistance to pyrethrins (Fine
et al., 1967), spotted root maggot resistance to
DDT (Hooper, 1965), and others.
    Reduced absorption of organotin compounds is
controlled by a gene (R-tin) conferring resistance
to these compounds and acting as resistance
intensifier for other insecticides (Plapp and
Hoyer, 1968). A similar phenomenon occurs with a
gene pen (for penetration delaying) which by itself
confers little resistance, but when present with a
factor for dealkylation of OP compounds, the interaction of the two genes enhances the resistance
markedly (Sawicki, 1970).
    Resistance to knockdown in some strains of
houseflies is controlled by a gene kdr (Harrison,
1951; Milani, 1954; Sawicki and Farnham, 1968)
which is associated with reduced penetration of the
toxicant.

426

Housefly resistance to DDT has also been attributed to structural modifications, such as darker pigmentation of the cuticle, stiffer tarsal bristles, and thicker tarsi, pulvilli, and articular membranes of tarsal joints (Wiesmann, 1947; D'Allessandro et al., 1949).

III. Other Factors

Additional factors which could enhance resistance by supplementing a major mechanism already present include higher lipid content, dietary factors, miscellaneous chemical differences, late pupation, late emergence, longer larval life cycle, etc.

IV. Behavioristic Resistance

Resistance due to changes in insect behavior are characteristically escape or avoidance mechanisms. Hence, the term behavioristic resistance is a misnomer because a change in behavior might be a consequence of sublethal intoxication. However, the end result, namely, control failure is the same.

Behavioral changes in mosquitoes have particularly been a source of considerable trouble in malaria eradication programs by the World Health Organization (Mattingly, 1962; Brown and Pal, 1971). These changes are brought about by increased irritability of adult mosquitoes contacting a residual insecticide deposit such as DDT. However, these changes may not be due to the selective effect of the insecticide (Gerold and Laarman, 1967; Gerold 1970a, 1970b).

Experiments by Mouchet and Cavalie (cited by Winteringham, 1966) and a critical survey of the literature by Muirhead-Thomson (1960, 1968) failed to reveal any convincing evidence of behavioristic resistance in mosquitoes, i.e., instances in which irritability and avoidance have resulted from the selective effect of continuous insecticide pressure. On the other hand, Hooper and Brown (1965a, 1965b) have reported clear evidence of behavioristic resistance to OP compounds in a laboratory-selected strain of <u>Euxesta notata</u>. Behavior can readily be influenced by many external factors such as temperature, adult age, length of exposure, testing apparatus, species and strain, etc., (Coluzzi, 1962, 1963; Kaschef, 1970; Brown and Pal, 1971). Hence, ascertaining the existence of a behavioral-type resistance is often a difficult task.

Table II. Numbers of Species with Resistances to Various Classes of Insecticides[1]

	DDT	Cyclo-dienes	OP	Carb.	Other	Total
Diptera	44	68	14	12	3	88
Lepidoptera	14	14	6	10	5	40
Hemiptera	10	15	14	5	4	38
Coleoptera	5	19	1	1	4	23
Acarina	3	7	16	–	1	28
Other orders	15	12	3	–	2	20
Total	91	135	54	28	19	237

[1]Modified from Brown, A.W.A. (1968)

ECOLOGICAL AND ECONOMIC IMPACT OF RESISTANCE

The remarkable effectiveness of DDT and the cyclodiene insecticides as residual insecticides has led to the hope that agricultural pests and vectors of insect-borne diseases were to become a thing of the past. However, the appearance of DDT resistance and the more intense resistance to cyclodienes have spelled a serious warning against a false sense of security regarding the control or eradication of insect pests. This is evident from the distribution of insect species with resistances to various insecticides as shown in Table II, and from the variety of resistant species attacking major agricultural crops (Table III) and stored products (Table IV).

Table III. Resistant Insects of Major Crops[1]

Major Crop	Species	Insecticides	Country
Cocoa	Distantiella theobroma	γ-BHC	Ghana
Cotton	Spodoptera littoralis	Toxaphene	Egypt
Cotton	Anthonomus grandis	Endrin	U.S.A.
Sugar cane	Aeneolamia varia	γ-BHC	Trinidad
Rice	Chilo suppressalis	γ-BHC, OP	Japan
Apple	Carpocapsa pomonella	DDT	U.S.A. & B.C.
Spruce	Choristoneura fumiferana	DDT	U.S.A.
Cattle	Boophilus microplus	Dld, OP	Australia

After Brown, A.W.A. (1968).

Table IV. Resistance to Insecticides by Stored-Product Insects[1]

Species	Insecticide
Sitophilus oryzae	γ-BHC, DDT, Carbaryl
S. granarius	γ-BHC, Pyrethrins, Arprocarb
S. Zea-mays	γ-BHC
Tribolium castaneum	γ-BHC, DDT, Malathion
Dermestes maculatus	Malathion
D. lardarius	Malathion
Ephestia cautella	Malathion
Plodia interpunctella	Malathion

[1]Modified from Brown, A.W.A. (1968).

The initial successes of DDT, BHC and chlordane in abating the incidence of certain gastro-enteric and ophthalmic diseases were soon nullified by the appearance of resistance of the vectors, resulting in a recrudescence of dysentery, trachoma and conjunctivitis.

By far, resistance has had its greatest impact on malaria eradication campaigns promoted by WHO (Brown and Pal, 1971; Brown, 1972). The consequences of resistance have been particularly serious with Anopheles saccharovi in Greece, An. gambiae in West Africa, and An. stephensi in Iran, Iraq, and parts of India, where malaria epidemics erupted following the failure of DDT and dieldrin to control these species. Serious problems have also been encountered in Central America where double resistance to DDT and dieldrin has prevented the eradication of malaria transmitted by An. albimanus. In Ceylon, malaria was practically eliminated following the use of DDT. However, several years ago the disease reappeared explosively. Out of a total population of 13 million, Ceylon has had an estimated 2 million malaria cases in 1967-1968. This was partly due to a record-year abundance of An. culicifacies.

The campaign to eradicate yellow fever from certain parts of the Americas suffered a setback principally because of the development of DDT resistance in Aedes aegypti, and the campaign failure against filariasis in India was due primarily to natural or acquired DDT and dieldrin resistance by Culex pipiens fatigans.

Aedes taeniorhynchus resistance to malathion in Florida and Ae. nigromaculis and Culex tarsalis resistance to several OP compounds in California are becoming serious problems. Culex tarsalis carries encephalitis of a kind that can be fatal to humans.

DDT and BHC resistance in the oriental rat fleas Xenopsylla cheopis and X. astia increased the incidence of plague in India and South Vietnam. The body louse Pediculus humanus humanus, which was effectively controlled with DDT powders, has subsequently developed resistance to DDT and BHC.

430

The recent occurrence of body louse resistance to malathion in the Burundi strain of equatorial Africa spells a serious threat to typhus control in that area (Fabrikant et al., 1973).

Resistance has appeared in several species of blackflies (Simulium) but, fortunately, the vector of onchocerciasis, Simulium damnosum, is still susceptible to chlorinated hydrocarbons, although use of the latter has been discontinued in favor of the less persistent OP compound Abate.

Sandflies (Phlebotomus), carriers of leishmaniasis, sandfly fever and other diseases, and Triatoma and Rhodnius, vectors of Chagas' disease

Table V. Resistance in Arthropods of Public Health Importance[1]

Species	Insecticides
LICE	
Pediculus h. humanus	DDT, Dld, γ-BHC, Pyrethrins, Malathion
COCKROACHES	
Blattella germanica	DDT, Dld, γ-BHC, OP, Carb.
Blatta orientalis	DDT, Dld
Periplaneta americana	DDT
P. brunnea	Dld, OP
BED BUGS	
Cimex lectularius	DDT, Dld, γ-BHC, OP
C. hemipterus	DDT, Dld, γ-BHC
FLEAS	
Xenopsylla cheopis	DDT, Dld, γ-BHC
X. astia	DDT, γ-BHC
Pulex irritans	DDT, Dld
OTHER INSECTS	
Simulium ornatum	DDT, OP
S. damnosum & other species	DDT
Triatoma infestans	DDT, Dld
Rhodnius prolixus	Dld
Musca sorbens	DDT, γ-BHC (?)
M. d. vicina	DDT, γ-BHC (?)

[1]After Brown and Pal (1971)

are still susceptible to insecticides, but predictably could become resistant if intensive control measures are undertaken against these species.
    The important species among arthropods of
public health and veterinary importance which have
developed resistance to one or more insecticides
are shown in Tables V and VI, respectively.

Table VI. Resistance in Arthropods of Veterinary
Importance

Species	Insecticide

LICE[1]

Linognathus vituli	DDT
L. africanus	Dld, γ-BHC
L. stenopsis	Dld, γ-BHC
Haematopinus eurysternus	DDT, γ-BHC, OP
Bovicola caprae	Toxaphene, Dld
B. limbata	Toxaphene, Dld

FLEAS[1]

Ctenocephalides canis	DDT, Dld
C. felis	DDT, Dld

TICKS[2]

Boophilus microplus	DDT, γ-BHC, Dld, OP, Pyr, Carb.
B. decoloratus	DDT, γ-BHC, Dld, OP
Amblyomma americana	Dld
Rhipicephalus evertsi	Dld, Toxaphene
R. appendiculatus	Dld, Toxaphene
R. sanguineus	Dld

---

[1]After Brown and Pal (1971). [2]After Harrison et al.,
(1973).

Taken collectively, all the instances mentioned above emphasize the fact that resistance is a very important public health problem, and gives scientists of all disciplines engaged in vector control a mandate to find other effective non-persistent insecticides or to substitute other proven methods of control.

Disease is often overlooked as an obstacle to economic progress. In the underdeveloped countries millions of potentially productive people suffer the debilitating effects of malaria, trachoma, schistosomiasis, filariasis, etc., with a tremendous loss in manpower and economic growth.

The situation in agriculture is also acute. The occurrence of resistance in many pests of important crops has often led to an increase in dosage of insecticide per treatment or in frequency of application, or both. This practice has resulted in considerable damage to the environment including a rise in mortality of fish and wildlife. According to the National Research Council of the National Academy of Sciences as much as 25% of all DDT compounds produced to date may have been transferred to the sea. On the other hand, the poor nations of the world would suffer most from disease and hunger if all pesticides were banned. U.S. Department of Agriculture experts predict that agricultural production in the U.S.A. would drop about 30% in the absence of pesticide usage.

The replacement of persistent chlorohydrocarbon insecticides by the less stable organophosphorus and carbamate compounds has had some beneficial effect. Though they are not as persistent, some OP compounds are less safe than the organochlorines and their detrimental effects tend to be acute rather than chronic. They also tend to suppress insect predator and parasite populations. However, from an ecological standpoint, the net effect should be on the positive side in favor of the less persistent toxicants.

So far, we have learned a great deal about the chemistry, physiology and biochemistry of resistance. It is obvious that, to date, no solution has been found to remedy the situation other than substituting other toxicants for those

433

which are no longer effective. At best, this is only a stop-gap measure, and from the pesticide manufacturer's standpoint it is a very expensive and unprofitable venture.

It is doubtful that a panacea would ever be found for insect control regardless of the method used. There are alternatives to pesticide usage currently being investigated; such as the use of insect pathogens, attractants and traps, populalation control by sterilization, hormones which disrupt insect development, genetic manipulation, varieties of plants resistant to insect attack, and biological control methods. All of these methods are useful and their adoption in control programs merits their utmost consideration wherever a particular method is applicable.

Future Prospects

The fact that insect resistance to pesticides is brought about partly by selection pressure with a toxicant indicates that to avoid resistance one must slow down the process of selection. This is almost impossible under present practices of the continuous use of pesticides, for to stop the selection process is tantamount to stopping evolution. Since pesticides are still our first line of defense the selection pressure must be minimized through a system of integrated control.

In integrated control systems natural enemies are protected and utilized as fully as possible by applying pesticides only in those areas with economic populations of pests (Smith and van den Bosch, 1967). Hence, the selective action by the pesticide is directed against a smaller portion of the population, and in conjunction with other control methods producing different environmental stresses on the organism, the use of pesticides can be minimized.

The important facts in integrated control are the establishment of economic injury levels in determining pesticide treatment, and supervised control in delimiting the areas requiring treatment (Smith, 1969). This type of selective treatment of localized infested areas becomes important

in obviating the development of resistance.
Details of the integrated control concept have
been published by Stern et al., (1959) and Smith
and van den Bosch (1967). The importance of
integrated control in dealing with the resistance
problem has been reviewed by Waterhouse (1969).

Although the concept of integrated control
may find its greatest usefulness in agriculture,
its application in public health would require
several modifications such as the introduction of
sanitation, education and social reform. It is
here that the scientist would be faced with his
greatest challenge.

References

Adams, C. H., and W. H. Cross. 1967. J. Econ.
Entomol. 60: 1016.

Agosin, M. 1971. In: Proc. 2nd Int. IUPAC Congr.
Pesticide Chemistry (A. S. Tahori, ed.), Vol. II,
Gordon and Breach, New York, N.Y. 29 pp.

Agosin, M., D. Michaeli, R. Miskus, S. Nagasawa,
and W. M. Hoskins. 1961. J. Econ. Entomol. 54:
340.

Agosin, M., A. Morello, N. Sacramelli. 1964. J.
Econ. Entomol. 64: 974.

Agosin, M., B. C. Fine, N. Scaramelli, J. Ilivicky,
and L. Aravena. 1966. Comp. Biochem. Physiol.
19: 339.

Akov, Shoshana, and A. B. Borkovec. 1968. Life Sci.
7 (Pt. II): 1215.

Akov, Shoshana, J. E. Oliver, and A. B. Borkovec.
1968. Life Sci. 7 (Pt. II): 1207.

Ariaratnam, V., and G. P. Georghiou. 1971. Nature
232: 642.

Arias, R. O., and L. C. Terriere. 1962. J. Econ.
Entomol. 55: 925.

Atallah, Y. H. and W. C., Nettles, Jr. 1966. J.
Econ. Entomol. 59: 560.

Babers, F. H. and J. J. Pratt, Jr. 1951. U.S.D.A.,
Bur. Entomol. Plant Quar. E-818.

Balabaskaran, S., A. G. Clark, A. Cundell, and
J. N. Smith. 1968. Australas. J. Pharmacol. 49
(Suppl.): 66.

Balazs, I., and M. Agosin. 1968. Biochim. Biophys. Acta 157: 1.

Beard, R. L. 1952. J. Econ. Entomol. 45: 561.

Beard, R. L. 1965. Entomol. Exptl. Appl. 8: 193.

Bell, J. D. 1968. Bull. Entomol. Res. 58: 137.

Bigley, W. S., and F. W. Plapp, Jr., 1960. Ann. Entomol. Soc. Am. 53: 360.

Bigley, W. S., and F. W. Plapp, Jr. 1961. J. Econ. Entomol. 54: 904.

Bradbury, F. R. 1957. J. Sci. Food Agr. 8: 90.

Bradbury, F. R., and H. Standen. 1956. J. Sci. Food Agr. 7: 389.

Bradbury, F. R., and H. Standen. 1958. J. Sci. Food Agr. 9: 203.

Bradbury, F. R., and H. Standen. 1959. Nature 183: 983.

Bradbury, F. R., and H. Standen. 1960. J. Sci. Food Agr. 11: 92.

Bridges, P. M. 1957. Biochem. J. 66: 316.

Bridges, R. G. 1959. Nature 184: 1337.

Brown, A.W.A. 1964. In: D. B. Dill (ed.) Handbook of Physiology p. 773-793, Williams & Wilkins, Baltimore.

Brown, A.W.A. 1968. Bull. Entomol. Soc. Am. 14: 3.

Brown, A.W.A. 1972. Amer. J. Trop. Med. Hyg. 21: 829.

Brown, A.W.A. and R. Pal. 1971. Insecticide resistance in arthropods. World Health Organizations Monograph Series No. 38, 2nd ed., Geneva, Switzerland.

Bull, D. L., D. A. Lindquist, and J. R. Coppedge. 1967. J. Agr. Food Chem. 15: 610.

Busvine, J. R. 1959. Entomol. Explt. Appl. 2: 58.

Cerf, D. C., and G. P. Georghiou, 1972. Nature, 239: 401.

Chang, S. C., and A. B. Borkovec. 1969. J. Econ. Entomol. 62: 1417.

Chang, S. C., and C. W. Kearns. 1964. J. Econ. Entomol. 57: 397.

Chattoraj, A. N., and C. W. Kearns. 1958. Bull. Entomol. Soc. Am. 4: 95.

Clark, A. G., F. J. Darby, and J. N. Smith. 1967. Biochem. J. 103: 49.

Clark, A. G., Sue Murphy, and J. N. Smith. 1969. Biochem. J. 113: 89.

Cole. M. M., M. D. Couch, G. S. Burden, and I. H.
  Gilbert. 1957. J. Econ. Entomol. 50: 556.
Collins, W. J., and A. J. Forgash. 1970. J. Econ.
  Entomol. 63: 394.
Coluzzi, M. 1962. Unpublished document Wld. Hlth.
  Org./Mal. 329. WHO/Insecticides/130.
Coluzzi, M. 1963. Riv. Malariol. 42: 189.
Crow, J. F. 1957. Ann. Rev. Entomol. 2: 227.
Crow, J. F. 1966. In: "Scientific Aspects of Pest
  Control", p. 263-275. National Academy of
  Sciences, Publication No. 1402, Washington, D.C.
D'Allessandro, G., G. Catalano, M. Mariani,
  E. Scerrino, C. Smiraglia, and G. Valguarnera.
  1949. Sicilia Medica 6: 15.
Davies, M., J. Keiding, and C. G. vonHofsten. 1958.
  Nature 182: 1816.
Decker, G. C. and W. N. Bruce. 1952. Am. J. Trop.
  Med. Hyg. 1: 395.
Dinamarca, Maria L. M. Agosin, and A. Neghme. 1962.
  Exptl. Parasitol. 12: 61.
Dinamarca, Maria L., I. Saavedra, and E. Valdes.
  1969. Comp. Biochem. Physiol. 31: 269.
Dinamarca, Maria L., L. Levenbook, and E. Valdes.
  1971. Arch. Biochem. Biophys. 147: 374.
Dorough, H. W. 1968. J. Agr. Food Chem. 16: 319.
Dyte, C. E. 1972. Nature, 238: 48.
Earle, N. 1963. J. Agr. food Chem. 11: 281.
El Bashir, S. 1967. Entomol. Exptl. Appl. 10: 111.
Eldefrawi, M. E., and W. M. Hoskins. 1961. J. Econ.
  Entomol. 54: 401.
Elliott, R. 1959. Bull. Wld. Hlth. Org. 20: 777.
Fabrikant, Irene B., C. L., Wisseman, Jr.,
  R. N. Miller, and A. Verschueren. 1973. In:
  "Proc. Int. Symposium on Control of Lice and
  Louse-Borne Diseases. Washington, D.C. Pan Am.
  Hlth. Org. Sci. Publ. 263, 229.
Farnham, A. W., K. A. Lord, and R. M. Sawicki.
  1965. J. Insect Physiol. 11: 1475.
Ferguson, W. C., and C. W. Kearns. 1949. J. Econ.
  Entomol. 42: 810.
Fine, B. C. 1961. Nature 191: 884.
Fine, B. C., P. J. Godin, E. M. Thain, and
  T. B. Marks. 1967. J. Sci. Food Agr. 18: 220.
Forgash, A. J., and E. J. Hansens. 1962. J. Econ.
  Entomol. 55: 679.

Forgash, A. J., B. J. Cook, and R. C. Riley. 1962. J. Econ. Entomol. 55: 544.

Fregly, M. J. 1969. Env. Res. 2: 435.

Fukami, J., and T. Shishido. 1966. J. Econ. Entomol. 59: 1338.

Fukami, J. I., I. Yamamoto, and J. E. Casida. 1967. Science 155: 713.

Fukami, J. I., T. Shishido, K. Fukunaga, and J. E. Casida. 1969. J. Agr. Food Chem. 17: 1217.

George, J. A., and A.W.A. Brown. 1967. J. Econ. Entomol. 60: 974.

Gemrich, E. G. 1967. J. Agr. Food Chem. 15: 617.

Gerold, J. L. 1970a. Inf. Circ. Resistance, Wld. Hlth. Org. VBC/IRG/70.9 p. 34.

Gerold, J. L. 1970b. Inf. Circ. Resistance, Wld. Org. VBC/IRG/70.11 p. 25.

Gerold, J. L., and Laarman, J. J. 1967. Nature 215: 518.

Gil, L., B. C. Fine, M. L. Dinamarca, I. Balazs, J. R. Busvine, and M. Agosin. 1968. Ent. Exptl. Appl. 11: 15.

Gill, S. S., B. D. Hammock, I. Yamamoto, and J. E. Casida. 1972. In: "Insect Juvenile Hormones: Chemistry and Action". J. J. Menn and M. Beroza (eds.) p. 177-190. Academic Press, New York.

Gillett, J. W. 1971. Induction in different species. p. 197-235. In A. S. Tahori (ed.) Proc. 2nd Int. IUPAC Congr. Pesticide Chemistry, Vol. II, Gordon and Breach, New York, N.Y.

Goodchild, B., and J. N. Smith. 1970. Biochem. J. 117: 1005.

Grant, C. D., and A.W.A. Brown. 1967. Canad. Entomologist, 99: 1040.

Grigolo, A., and F. J. Oppenoorth. 1966. Genetica 37: 159.

Gupta, B., H. C. Agarwal, and K.K.K. Pillai. 1971. Pesticide Biochem. Physiol. 1: 180.

Guthrie, F. E., R. L. Ringler, and T. G. Bowery. 1957. J. Econ. Entomol. 50: 821.

Guthrie, F. E., W. V. Campbell, and R. L. Baron. 1962. Ann. Entomol. Soc. Am. 55: 42.

Hadaway, A. B. 1956. Nature 178: 149.

Harrison, C. M. 1951. Nature 167: 855.

Harrison, C. M. 1952. Bull. Entomol. Res. 42: 761.

Harrison, I. R., B. H. Palmer, and E. C. Wilmhurst.
1973. Pesticide Sci. 4: 531.
Harvey, T. L., and D. E. Howell. 1965. J. Invertebr.
Pathol. 7: 92.
Hayashi, M., and M. Hayakawa. 1962. Japan J. Appl.
Entomol. Zool. 6: 250.
Hazard, E. I., C. S. Lofgren, D. B. Woodard, H. R.
Ford, and B. M. Glancey. 1964. Science 145: 500.
Heath, D. F. 1961. Organophosphorus Poisons.
Pergamon Press, Inc. New York.
Holan, G. 1969. Nature 221: 1025.
Hooper, G.S.H. 1965. J. Econ. Entomol. 58: 608.
Hooper, G.S.H., and A.W.A. Brown. 1965a. Bull. Wld.
Hlth. Org. 32: 131.
Hooper, G.S.H., and A.W.A. Brown. 1965b. Ectomol.
Exptl. Appl. 8: 263.
Hoskins, W. M. 1952. In: "Proceedings of the Third
International Congress of Phytopharmacy," Paris,
Vol. 2, 443-450.
Hoskins, W. M. and H. T. Gordon. 1956. Ann. Rev.
Entomol. 1: 89.
Hucker, H. B., J. R. Gillette, and B. B. Brodie.
1960. J. Pharmacol. Exptl. Therap. 137: 103.
Ishaaya, I., and W. Chefurka. 1968. Riv. Parassitol.
29: 289.
Ishaaya, I., and W. Chefurka. 1971. Induction of
RNA and protein biosynthesis in the housefly
microsomes after DDT treatment. p. 267-280. In
A. S. Tahori (ed.) Proc. 2nd Int. IUPAC Congr.
Pesticide Chemistry, Vol. II, Gordon and Breach,
New York, N.Y.
Ishida, M., and P. A. Dahm. 1965a J. Econ. Entomol.
58: 383.
Ishida, M., and P. A. Dahm. 1965b. J. Econ. Entomol.
58: 602.
Kapoor, I. P., R. L. Metcalf, R. F. Nystrom, and
G. K. Sangha. 1970. J. Agr. Food Chem. 18: 1145.
Kasai, T., and Z. Ogita. 1965. SABCO J.1, 130.
Kaschef, A. H. 1970. Bull. Wld. Hlth. Org. 42: 917.
Keiding, J. 1956. Science, 123: 1173.
Keiding, J. 1963. Bull. Wld. Hlth. Org. 29: 51.
Keiding, J. 1967. Wld. Rev. Pest Control 6: 115.

Keiding, J. 1969. Annual Report, Government Pest Infestation Laboratory, Lyngby, Denmark.

Kerr, R. W. 1963. J. Austr. Inst. Agr. Sci. 29: 31.

Kerr, R. W. D. G. Venables, W. J. Roulston, and H. J. Schnitzerling, 1957. Nature 180: 1132.

Khan, M.A.Q., R. J. Morimoto, J. P. Bederka, Jr., and J. M. Runnels. 1973. Biochem. Gen. 10: 243.

Khan, M.A.Q. and L. C. Terriere. 1968. J. Econ. Entomol. 61: 732.

Kimura, T., and A.W.A. Brown. 1964. J. Econ. Entomol. 57: 710.

Klassen, W., and F. Matsumura. 1966. Nature 209: 1155.

Knipling, E. F. 1950. Soap Sanit. Chem. 26:87.

Kojima, K., T. Ishizuka, A. Shiino, and S. Kitakata. 1963. Japan. J. Appl. Zool. 7: 63.

Ku, T. Y., and J. L. Bishop. 1967. J. Econ. Entomol. 60: 1328.

Kuhr, R. J. 1970. J. Agr. Food Chem. 18: 1023.

LeRoux, E. J., and F. O. Morrison. 1954. J. Econ. Entomol. 47: 1058.

Lindahl, P. E., and K. E. Oberg, 1961. Exptl. Cell Res. 23: 221.

Lindquist, A. W., A. R. Roth, and R. A. Hoffman. 1951. J. Econ. Entomol. 44: 931.

Lipke, H. 1960. J. Econ. Entomol. 53: 31.

Lipke, H., and J. Chalkley. 1964. Bull. Wld. Hlth. Org. 30: 57.

Lipke, H., and C. W. Kearns. 1959a. J. Biol. Chem. 234: 2123.

Lipke, H., and C. W. Kearns. 1959b. J. Biol. Chem. 234: 2129.

Litvak, S., and M. Agosin. 1968. Biochemistry 7: 1560.

Lovell, J. B., and C. W. Kearns. 1959. J. Econ. Entomol. 52: 931.

March, R. B. 1959. Entomol. Soc. Am. Misc. Publ. 1: 13.

March, R. B. 1960. Entomol. Soc. Am. Misc. Publ. 2: 139.

Matsumura, F., and A.W.A. Brown. 1963. Mosquito News 23: 26.

Matsumura, F., and M. Hayashi. 1966a. Science 153: 757.

Matsumura, F., and M. Hayashi. 1966b. Mosquito News 26: 190.

Matsumura, F., and R. D. O'Brien. 1966. J. Agr. Food Chem. 14: 36.

Matsumura, F. and K. Sakai. 1968. J. Econ. Entomol. 61: 598.

Mattingly, P. F. 1962. Ann. Rev. Entomol. 7: 419.

Melander, A. L. 1914. J. Econ. Entomol. 7: 167.

Mengle, D. C., and J. E. Casida. 1960. J. Agr. Food Chem. 8: 431.

Menzel, D. B., S. M. Smith, R. Miskus, and W. M. Hoskins. 1961. J. Econ. Entomol. 54: 9.

Menzer, R. E., and J. A. Rose. 1971. Effect of enzyme-inducing agents on fat storage and toxicity of insecticides. p. 257-266. In: A. S. Tahori (ed.) Proc. 2nd Int. IUPAC Congr. Pesticide Chemistry, Vol. II, Gordon and Breach, New York, N.Y.

Merrell, D. J., and J. C. Underhill. 1956. J. Econ. Entomol. 49: 300.

Metcalf, R. L., T. R. Fukuto, C. Collins, K. Borck, J. Burk, H. T. Reynolds, and M. F. Osman. 1966. J. Agr. Food Chem. 14: 579.

Metcalf, R. L., M. F. Osman, and T. R. Fukuto. 1967. J. Econ. Entomol. 60: 445.

Metcalf, R. L., T. R. Fukuto, C. Collins, K. Borck, S. Abd-El-Aziz, R. Munoz, and C. C. Cassil. 1968. J. Agr. Food Chem. 16: 300.

Milani, R. 1954. Riv. Parassitol. 15: 513.

Miller, S., and A. S. Perry, 1964. J. Agr. Food Chem. 12: 167.

Miyake, S. S., C. W. Kearns, and H. Lipke. 1957. J. Econ. Entomol. 50: 359.

Moorefield, H. H. 1956. Contrib. Boyce Thompson Inst. 18: 303.

Moorefield, H. H. 1958. Contrib. Boyce Thompson Inst. 19: 501.

Moorefield, H. H., and C. W. Kearns, 1957. J. Econ. Entomol. 50: 11.

Morello, A. 1964. Nature 203: 785.

Muirhead-Thomson, R. C. 1960. Bull. Wld. Hlth. Org. 22: 721.

Muirhead-Thomson, R. C. 1968. "Ecology of Insect Vector Populations." Academic Press, London, New York.

Nakatsugawa, T., N. M. Tolman, and P. A. Dahm. 1968. Biochem. Pharmacol. 17: 1517.

Nakatsugawa, T., N. M. Tolman, and P. A. Dahm. 1969. Biochem. Pharmacol. 18: 1103.

O'Brien, R. D. 1960. "Toxic Phosphorous Esters; Chemistry, Metabolism, and Biological Effects." Academic Press, New York.

O'Brien, R. D. 1966. Ann. Rev. Entomol. 11: 369.

O'Brien, R. D. 1967. "Insecticides. Action and Metabolism." Academic Press, New York.

O'Brien, R. D., and F. Matsumura. 1964. Science 146: 657.

Ogita, Z. 1961. Botyu-Kagaku 26: 93.

Oppenoorth, F. J. 1954. Nature 173: 1001.

Oppenoorth, F. J. 1955. Nature 175: 124.

Oppenoorth, F. J. 1956. Arch, Neerl. Zool. 12: 1.

Oppenoorth, F. J. 1959. Entomol. Exptl. Appl. 2: 304.

Oppenoorth, F. J. 1965. Ann. Rev. Ent. 10: 185.

Oppenoorth, F. J., and N.W.H. Houx. 1968. Entomol. Exptl. Appl. 11: 81.

Oppenoorth, F. J. and K. Van Asperen. 1960. Science 132: 298.

Oppenoorth, F. J., and S. Voerman. 1965. Entomol. Exptl. Appl. 8: 293.

Perry, A. S. 1958. Proc. Int. Congr. Entomol. 10th, Montreal, 2: 157.

Perry, A. S. 1960. Bull. Wld Hlth. Org. 22: 743.

Perry, A. S. 1960a. Entomol Soc. Amer. Miscell. Publ. 2: 119.

Perry, A. S. 1964. In: The Physiology of Insecta M. Rockstein (ed.), Vol. 3, Academic Press, New York.

Perry, A. S., and M. Agosin. 1974. In: The Physiology of Insecta M. Rockstein (ed.) 2nd ed. Vol. 6. Academic Press, New York.

Perry, A. S. and W. M. Hoskins. 1950. Science 111: 600.

Perry, A. S., S. Miller, and Annette J. Buckner. 1963. J. Agr. Food Chem. 11: 457.

Pillai, M.K.K., and A.W.A. Brown. 1965. J. Econ. Entomol. 58: 255.

Pilou, D. P., and R. E. Glasser. 1951. Canad. J. Zool. 29: 90.

Plapp, F. W., Jr. 1970. In: "Biochemical Toxicol-

ogy of Insecticides: (R. D. O'Brien and
I. Yamamoto, eds.), pp. 179-192, Academic Press,
New York.

Plapp, F. W. Jr., and J. E. Casida. 1958. J. Econ.
Entomol. 51: 800.

Plapp, F. W., Jr., and J. E. Casida. 1969. J. Econ.
Entomol. 62: 1174.

Plapp, F. W. Jr., and R. F. Hoyer. 1968. J. Econ.
Entomol. 61: 1298.

Plapp, F. W. Jr. G. A. Chapman, and J. W. Morgan.
1965. J. Econ. Entomol. 58: 1064.

Reed, W. T., and A. J. Forgash. 1968. Science 160:
1232.

Reed, W. T., and A. J. Forgash. 1969. J. Agr. Food
Chem. 17: 896.

Reed, W. T., and A. J. Forgash. 1970. J. Agr. Food
Chem. 18: 475.

Remmer, H. 1971. Enzyme induction phenomenon: In:
Proc. 2nd Int. IUPAC Congr. Pesticide Chemistry
(A. S. Tahori, ed.), Vol. II, Gordon and Breach,
New York, N.Y.

Robbins, W. E. 1972. In: "Pest Control Strategies
for the Future" p. 172-196. Natl. Acad. Sci.
Washingtion, D.C.

Robertson, J. G. 1957. Canad. J. Zool. 35: 629.

Rowlands, D. G., and C. J. Lloyd. 1969. J. Stored
Prod. Res. 5: 413.

Sacca, G., and A. Scirocchi. 1966. Wld. Hlth. Org.
Mimeo. pub. WHO/Victor Control/66. 192.

Sawicki, R. M. 1970. Pesticide Sci. 1: 84.

Sawicki, R. M., and A. W. Farnham. 1968. Entomol.
Exptl. Appl. 11: 133.

Schneiderman, H. A., A. Krishnakumaran, P. J. Bryant,
and F. Sehnal. 1970. Agr. Sci. Rev. 8: 13.

Schonbrod, R. D., W. W. Philleo, and L. C. Terriere.
1965. J. Econ. Entomol. 58: 74.

Self, L. S., F. E. Guthrie, and E. Hodgson. 1964a.
J. Insect Physiol. 10: 907.

Self, L. S., F. E. Guthrie, and E. Hodgson. 1964b.
Nature 204: 300.

Sellers, L. G., and F. Guthrie. 1971. J. Econ.
Entomol. 64: 352.

Shrivastava, S. P., M. Tsukamoto, and J. E. Casida.
1969. J. Econ. Entomol. 62: 483.

Shrivastava, S. P. G. P. Georghiou, R. L. Metcalf, and T. R. Fukuto. 1970. Bull. Wld. Hlth. Org. 42: 931.

Shrivastava, S. P., G. P. Georghiou, and T. R. Fukuto. 1971. Entomol. Exp. Appl. 14: 333.

Sims, P., and P. L. Grover. 1965. Biochem. J. 95: 156.

Slade, M., and J. E. Casida. 1970. J. Agr. Food Chem. 18: 467.

Slade, M., and C. H. Zibitt. 1972. In: "Insect Juvenile Hormones: Chemistry and Action." J. J. Menn and M. Beroza (eds.) p. 155-176. Academic Press, New York.

Smith, R. F. 1969. Qual. Plant Mater. Veg. 17: 81.

Smith, R. F. and R. van den Bosch. 1967. In: "Pest Control. Biological, Physical and Selected Chemical Methods." W. W. Kilgore and R. L. Doutt (eds.) p. 295-340. Academic Press, New York.

Stalhandske, T., P. Slanina, H. Tjalve, E. Hansson, and C. G. Schmiterlow. 1969. Acta Pharmacol. Toxicol. 27: 363.

Stern, V. M., R. F. Smith, R. van den Bosch, and K. S. Hagen. 1959. Hilgardia, 29 (2): 81.

Sternburg, J., and C. W. Kearns. 1950. Ann. Entomol. Soc. Am. 43: 444.

Sternburg, J., and C. W. Kearns. 1956. J. Econ. Entomol. 49: 548.

Sternburg, J. C. W. Kearns, and W. N. Bruce. 1950. J. Econ. Entomol. 43: 214.

Sternburg, J., E. B. Vinson, and C. W. Kearns. 1953. J. Econ. Entomol. 46: 513.

Street, J. C., F. M. Urry, D. J. Wagstaff, and S. E. Blau, In: Proc. 2nd Int. IUPAC Congr. Pesticide Chemistry A. S. Tahori ed., Vol. II, Gordon and Breach, New York, N.Y.

Swift, F. C., and A. J. Forgash. 1959. Entomol. Soc. Am. Cotton States Branch, 33rd Annual Meeting, p. 4.

Tahori, A. S., and W. M. Hoskins. 1953. J. Econ. Entomol. 46: 302 and 829.

Tahori, A. S. Z. Sobel, and M. Soller. 1969. Ent. Exp. Appl. 12: 85.

Telford, J. N., and F. Matsumura. 1971. J. Econ. Entomol. 64: 230.

Tombes, A. S., and A. J. Forgash. 1961. J. Insect
    Physiol. 7: 216.
Tsukamoto, M. 1959. Botyu-Kagaku 24: 141.
Tsukamoto, M. 1960. Botyu-Kagaku 25: 156.
Tsukamoto, M., and J. E. Casida. 1967. Nature 213:
    49.
Tsukamoto, M., T. Narahashi, and T. Yamasaki. 1965.
    Botyu-Kagaku 30: 128.
van Asperen, K. 1958. Nature 181: 355.
van Asperen, K., and F. J. Oppenoorth. 1959. Entomol.
    Exptl. Appl. 2: 48.
van den Heuvel, M. J., and D. G. Cochran. 1965. J.
    Econ. Entomol. 58: 872.
Waterhouse, D. F. 1969. FAO Symposium on Pest Resis-
    tance, Rome, Italy, Sept. 1969.
Welling, W., P. Blaakmeer, G. J. Vink, and S. Voerman.
    1971. Pest. Biochem. Physiol. 1: 61.
Wiesmann, R. 1947. Mitt. schweiz. entomol. Ges. 20:
    484.
Williams, C. M. 1956. Nature, 178: 212.
Williams, C. M. 1967. Sci. Am. 217: 13.
Winteringham, F.P.W. 1966. Proc. FAO Symposium
    Integrated Pest Control 1, 25.
World Health Organization. 1957. Expert Committee on
    Insecticides. 7th Report. Tech. Rep. Ser.125.
Yamamoto, I., and J. E. Casida. 1966. J. Econ.
    Entomol. 59: 1542.
Yamamoto, I., E. C. Kimmel, and J. E. Casida. 1969.
    J. Agr. Food Chem. 17: 1227.
Yamasaki, T., and T. Narahashi. 1958. Botyu-Kagaku,
    23: 146.
Yu, S. J., and L. C. Terriere. 1971. Life Sci. 10
    (II): 1173.
Zeid, M., P. Dahm, R. Hein, and R. McFarland. 1953.
    J. Econ. Entomol. 46: 324.
Zubairi, M. Y., and J. E. Casida. 1965. J. Econ.
    Entomol. 58: 403.

COSTS AND BENEFITS OF PESTICIDES: AN OVERVIEW

George C. Decker

Principal Scientist and Head, Emeritus
Section of Economic Entomology
Illinois Natural History Survey and
Illinois Agricultural Experiment Station, Urbana

Perspective

When the Indians migrated to North America some 10 to 20 thousand years ago, many of our present-day pests were already present and well adjusted to their environment. No doubt, the Indians brought a few new pests with them, but consistent with their mode of life and with a population of only about one million in North America, they had little cause to be concerned about the pests that attack plants. In fact, history records that when insects became abundant, they were harvested and dried for food and the same was no doubt true of some plants now regarded as weeds.

Centuries later the white man arrived and he brought with him many Old World crops having little or no resistance to or tolerance for America's indigenous pests. (Of the 70 or so basic crops now grown in the USA, less than a dozen are indigenous to North America.) He also brought with him many Old World pests and each century thereafter, he introduced more and more foreign pests so that the present-day American farmer must combat the literally hundreds of species of insects, mites, nematodes, weeds, and plant diseases imported from abroad as well as those native to North America.

The early settlers were a hardy, self-sufficient, and determined lot who took pride in the fact that they were more or less skilled in most of the agricultural arts of their day. At the same time they readily admitted the problem of coping with the many insects and other pests that destroyed their crops. They sought the aid of neighbors, and the available amateur naturalists, as well as the counsel and advice of the few entomologists located in New England and the Atlantic coastal states. When these sources of information proved

447

inadequate they appealed to the state legislatures to appropriate funds and appoint State Entomologists and other practical scientists to study what appeared to be the most perplexing of all their problems. As the clamor for help increased to a crescendo, the public came to realize that there was something in the environment that would have to be changed. Either man or the pests would have to yield to the other. Even legislative bodies and politicians began to listen and to act:

(1) The federal government appointed Townsend Glover as entomologist in the U. S. Patent Office in 1854; (2) created the U. S. Department of Agriculture in 1862; (3) chartered the Land-Grant Colleges in 1862; and (4) established the system of State Agricultural Experiment Stations in 1877. Almost simultaneously at least a half-dozen states created offices of state entomologist or departments of plant protection.

Historically, most entomologists, plant pathologists, and other scientists have always insisted that insofar as possible pest control should be largely biological and ecological in nature. Actually, for many years entomologists generally devoted most of their research time to biological and ecological studies. In fact, until about 1870, ecological, cultural, and mechanical control measures dominated all pest-control activities. It is often said, at times by scientists who should know better, that up until the 1880's pest control was largely attained, achieved, or accomplished by natural, cultural and/or biological practices and methods. Such assertions, intentionally or otherwise, seem to imply that a reasonable degree of practical insect control was attained, when in many, if not indeed most cases, this was not in accord with the facts. It is suggested that those who wish to challenge this assertion read the pertinent literature of the day: (1) The Prairie Farmer; (2) The Country Gentleman; (3) other farm journals; (4) The American Entomologist, Vol. 1-3; (5) The Practical Entomologist, Vol. 1 & 2; (6) Experiment Station Bulletins; (7) USDA Publications; and (8) in particular the Proceedings of State Horticultural and Agricultural Society Meetings. The author has reviewed such data in previous papers (Decker, 1954, 1958, 1964).

Actually, it was only after such methods as were available proved to be entirely inadequate and the need for better insect control became imperative that the potato growers in 1867, followed by other vegetable and fruit growers in the 1870's and 80's, turned to the use of the arsenical compounds and other chemicals. Then, as exemplified by my illustrious predecessor in Illinois, S. A. Forbes (1880), the entomologists more or

less reluctantly followed the farmers' lead. A similar chance
discovery by a French vine dresser, who observed that Bordeaux
mixture would control mildew on grapes in 1887, led to many
other uses for this and other fungicides. Thus, entomology
and plant pathology became involved in the chemical control of
pests in the latter days of the 19th century.

I realize it may be difficult for some people to understand how or why I and many of my colleagues, who have for
half a century insisted that man should be able to outwit insects and that chemicals should be regarded as firefighting
equipment to be used only when natural control measures are
lacking or ineffective, continue to recommend the use of chemical insecticides in 1973. The answers are clear if not
simple. (1) A man who has, as a child, spent 4-8 hours a day
for weeks on end hand-picking hornworms on tomato vines, hand-
picking potato beetles or beating their larvae into pails of
oil and water, herding the old-fashioned potato beetles (blis-
ter beetles) out of a field by walking back and forth while
constantly beating a tin pan and waving the green bough of a
spruce tree can hardly think back on those days as the glor-
ious age of natural insect control. (2) In those days, state
and federal legislative bodies were not about to appropriate
funds to support the extensive basic research needed as an
absolute prerequisite to any possible hope for success in the
area of biological control. If you doubt this, ask the man
who was a research worker in a state experiment station and
had an operative budget of less than $1,000 a year during the
great depression and for several years after that. (3) The
farmers were desperate and both they and the politicians who
made our meager funds available were pressing the Experiment
Stations and the USDA for immediate results. They came to us
with their problems and they expected us to deliver some
reasonably effective and practical control measure to protect
next year's crop. Let me say to you, chemical pesticides
posed the only hope of meeting such demands. We had not yet
reached the point where state and federal employees, misguided
critics, propagandists, and outright scientific agnostics could
stand up and tell the Legislature, the Congress, in fact the
world, to "go to hell" and get away with it.

Introduction

Many fruit and vegetable crops have not been successfully
produced commercially without the use of insecticides since
about 1880 (Tables 1 and 2). Thus, it would seem to be both

Table 1. The percentage of apples in Illinois orchards damaged by codling moth.

Year	Unsprayed	Chemical	Sprayed
1885	68	Paris green	21.0
1886	40	Paris green	12.0
1915–18	45	Lead arsenate–nicotine	4.4
1956–58	69	DDT and related synthetics	2.2

Table 2. Spraying practices in relation to the yield of apples and peaches.

	Bushel per tree of bearing age	
No. of sprays	Apples	Peaches
0	1.6	0.5
1–4	0.7	0.6
5–9	5.3	2.2
10–14	6.3	2.5
15+	8.3	2.8

Taken from Apple and Peach Survey 1962; Illinois Agricultural Statistics, Illinois Crop Reporting Service (Supplement to 63–5) 1963.

fitting and proper for us to briefly look at the history and current status of a couple of classic examples of crops in these two categories. Let us begin with the Irish potato where the large scale use of pesticides had its beginning. In the 1860's the Colorado potato beetle came close to eliminating potato production in the United States, but the timely discovery that this pest could be controlled by the use of an arsenical paint pigment called Paris green saved the day. From 1867 to 1910 with the potato beetle at least controllable, if indeed only partially controlled, potato yields remained rather close to 5,000 pounds per acre. With improved application equipment and better arsenical compounds plus the use of Bordeaus mixture for disease and leafhopper control, yields increased to 6,000 pounds by 1920 and to about 8,500 pounds

450

by 1945, at which point potato growers thought they had about reached the pinnacle of success. Then came DDT and the other new synthetic insecticides and fungicides. As shown in Table 3, with better control of all pests and reduced foliage damage caused by the arsenical and copper compounds, potato yields jumped by 62% in 5 years, and 88% in 10 years. With soil insecticides to control wireworms and grubs, yields jumped another 31% in the next 5 years and roughly 20% more each year thereafter so that each acre of potatoes grown in 1971 produced 2.5 times as much marketable produce as did the same acre in 1945 and 3.5 times that produced prior to 1910.

Orchard productivity

Conservatively, a good mature apple tree should produce about 10 bushels of apples per year, but a study of statistics on apple production in Illinois reveals that at the time of World War I, 7½ million trees produced about 7½ million bushels of apples (many not marketable by 1973 standards), or about one bushel per tree. In other words, apple growers were sharecropping with pests on a 9:1 basis. By 1962, apple production had increased to about 6.5 bushels per tree, and its quality was unsurpassed anywhere in the world.

How did all this come about? Well, the early fruit growers complained that the codling moth, the apple maggot, apple and plum curculio, by attacking the fruit, caused most of it to fall to the ground prematurely and that apple scab and other diseases rendered much of the remaining fruit unattractive, if not indeed unsalable. This was the condition of Illinois apples 100 years ago when infested fruit was of necessity acceptable in interstate commerce. If this were not true, how can we account for B. D. Walsh's finding 200 codling moth cocoons in one apple barrel shipped from Ohio? Success with Paris green on potatoes led to the use of Paris green and other arsenical compounds on apples and eventually on peaches and many other fruits and vegetables. As time passed and more and more effective insect control measures were perfected, the quality of the fruit was improved and the yields of marketable fruit per tree rose. Eventually the housewife demanded clean, sound, high-quality fruit and would no longer accept inferior home-grown fruit.

Of course, there are orchards that do much better than the 6.5 bushel per tree average, and each year 25 to 30 or more Illinois orchardists qualify for the 95% Clean Apple Club. In other words, many efficient orchardists produce 10 or more

Table 3.   Average (U.S.) per acre crop yields for five years
use in 1946.

		Average Annual Yields					
Crop	Units	1941 1945	1947 1951	1952 1956	1957 1961	1962 1966	1967 1971
Timothy seed	lb	154.6	141.0	142.8	146.6	148.4	168.8
Broom corn	lb	330.0	282.4	234.5	330.2	313.4	292.4
Oats	Bu	32.2	34.3	34.2	41.2	45.7	52.1
Barley	Bu	24.1	26.1	28.3	30.3	37.4	43.4
Sugar beets	Tons	12.4	14.5	16.1	17.4	17.3	18.4
Field corn	Bu	32.8	36.5	41.0	50.1	68.3	79.9
Peanuts	lb	674.2	780.0	959.0	1151.6	1496.4	1875.4
Potatoes	Cwt	84.9	137.6	159.7	185.9	202.4	220.6

bushels of apples per tree, and 95 to 99% of their fruit is
free of blemishes due to any insect or plant disease.

Pesticides and the economics of vegetable production

Dr. George McNew (1963) provided two excellent examples
of the value of fungicides used on tomatoes and peas. Data
presented in Table 4 show that spraying alone increased tomato
yields by 42%; fertilizer alone increased yields by 81%, and
where both were applied, the increased yield was 153%. The
cash returns were even more spectacular. The corresponding
values were 75, 106, and 263. Obviously, there must have
been an increase in quality as well as yield. In the case of
the peas, the fungicide seed treatment produced a 43% yield
increase whereas a fertilizer application increased the yeild
by only 25% and the application of manure actually reduced the
yield. It is worthy of note that in both studies, yield increases resulting from combined fungicide-fertilizer treatment far exceeded the sum of the two treatments alone.

before and at five-year intervals after DDT came into general

% Deviation						Degree of Usage	
1941 1945	1947 1951	1952 1956	1957 1961	1962 1966	1967 1971	Insecti- cide	Herbi- cide
0	-9	-8	-5	-4	9	Scant	Scant
0	-15	-29	0	-5	-11	Scant	Scant
0	7	6	28	42	62	Light	Heavy
0	9	18	26	55	80	Light	Heavy
0	17	30 ·	41	39	48	Mod.	Mod.
0	11	25	55	108	144	Mod-H*	Heavy
0	16	42	71	122	176	Heavy**	Mod.
0	62	88	119	138	160	Heavy**	Mod.

*Moderate foliar and moderate to heavy soil treatment after 1956.
**Heavy foliar and moderate to heavy soil treatment after 1956.

Crop yields and pesticide use

In the light of what pesticides did for apple, potato, tomato, and pea production, let us now look at some apparent correlations between modern pesticide (post-1946) usage and crop yields. Comparisons are based upon the average for the five years 1941-45, immediately preceding the rather large-scale use of DDT in 1946. As is evident in Table 3, there seems to be a positive correlation between the extent to which DDT and other pesticides were used on the various crops listed and the increase in crop yield with the passing of time. One might, with good reason, question the validity of such correlations if it were not for the fact that they are supported by overwhelming circumstantial evidence, e.g., (1) the absence of comparable gains in previous decades; (2) the fact that the upward trends coincide with the advent of DDT

Table 4. Yield and cash returns for tomatoes grown in a
commercial field where early blight was severe;
when: sprayed, unsprayed, fertilized, not fertilized, both or neither.[1]

Category		Treatment		
	Check	Sprayed only	Fertilized only	Sprayed & fertilized
Yield data:				
Tons per acre	7.59	10.74	13.77	19.22
Gain in tons	0	3.15	6.18	11.63
Gain in percent	0	42	81	153
Cash Returns:				
Dollars per acre	128	224	264	464
Gain in Dollars	0	96	136	336
Gain in percent	0	75	106	263

[1] Data as presented by McNew (1963).

and other modern pesticides; (3) the close relationship between the magnitude of increased yields and the extent of
pesticide usage on the crops involved; and (4) their general
agreement with voluminous data obtained on experimental plots.
     Timothy seed and broomcorn crops, on which insecticides
are rarely used, have shown no gains, and in fact, some losses
since 1945. Oats and barley, crops on which insecticides are
used only occasionally and then lightly, showed gains of 6
and 18% in the first 10 years, but with the extensive use of
herbicides, yields increased by 20 to 30% each 5 years so that
1967-71 yields were 62 to 80% above those of 1941-45. Such
crops as sugar beets and field corn on which pesticides were
used quite frequently and in moderate amounts, showed gains
of 30 and 25% in the first 10 years and then with a moderate
increase in pesticide usage, sugar beet yields made continued
moderate gains to a 48% increase over 1945 by 1971. On the
other hand, as we shall see later, corn with spectacular
pesticide use made some spectacular gains, more than doubling
yields in less than 20 years. Finally, as was to be expected,
such crops as peanuts and potatoes, on which all three of the
major classes of pesticides (insecticides, herbicides, and

454

fungicides) are quite extensively used, showed the greatest gains, ranging up to 176 and 160%. In other words, yields of 276 and 260% of their pre-DDT levels were attained in 25 years.

It is also noteworthy that crops like potatoes and sugar beets, on which the new insecticides were used extensively at an early date, made sizable gains in the first five-year period, 1947-1951, whereas field corn with only moderate foliar treatment made the greatest gains in the last 15 years for reasons we shall see shortly. In general the same general trends held true for the other important vegetable crops. On the other hand, in two seperate studies data accumulated by the United States Department of Agriculture over periods of 34 and 20 years showed that the omission of insecticide treatments reduced cotton yields 25.5% and 41.8% respectively. Just as the Illinois Agricultural Census in 1962 validated the claims made for pest control on apples, so, too, the U.S. Agricultural Statistics seem to reflect correlations between the use of pesticides and crop yields. Increased yields of fruit and vegetable crops between 1910 and 1944, as shown in Fig. 1, are in line with increases in the use of several insecticides as reported by Shepard (1951). (1) Lead arsenate consumption increased from 5 million pounds in 1908 to 85 million pounds in 1944. (2) Calcium arsenate consumption increased from 3 million pounds in 1919 to 80 million pounds in 1942. (3) Rotenone consumption increased from 5 thousand pounds in 1931 to 13 million pounds in 1947. During this same period, the yields for cereal grain crops showed little or no change. Then with the advent of DDT in 1946 followed by other chlorinated compounds like benzene hexachloride, chlordane, aldrin, dieldrin, and heptachlor and a whole host of herbicides which, as we shall see later, were most extensively used on corn and small grains, yields showed steady and phenomenal increases.

Corn--A special case?

Corn presents an interesting though very complex picture (Fig. 2). For over half a century, corn yields in Illinois remained more or less static at about 35 bushels per acre; then about the mid or late 1930's, the trend turned upward. Annual corn yields in Illinois are now double the 1941-45 average and roughly three times the yields obtained in the 1930's. Fig. 2 reveals that the upward trend was evident before 1946, but appeared to be temporarily accelerated slightly at that point. However, the abrupt climb seemed to

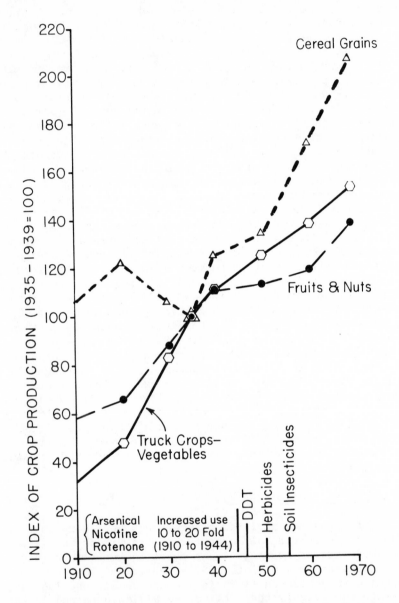

Fig. 1. Indices of crop production for selected classes of
crops in relation to pesticide usage, 1910–1970.
(Indices – 1935–39 = 100).

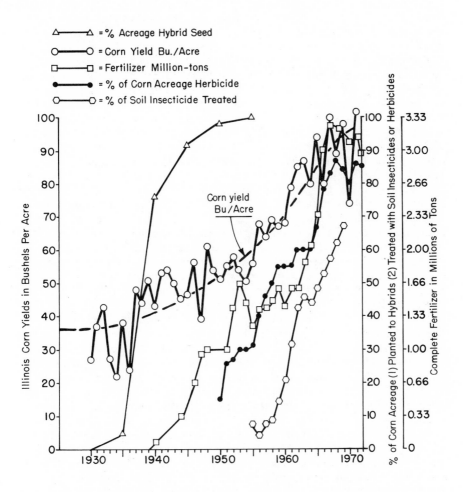

Fig. 2. A comparison of the increased use of hybrid seed, fertilizer, and pesticidal chemicals with rising corn yields in Illinois, 1930-1972.

start about 10 years later, when the U.S. average jumped from 56 bushels per acre in 1955 to 102 bushels per acre in 1971, thus effecting in 17 years a rise almost twice that attained in all of the previous 90 years for which records are available.

To whom or to what are we to credit this apparent progress? The fact that it apparently began in the mid-30's suggests that the introduction of hybrid seed corn was a factor. Fig. 2 also shows that the acreage planted to hybrid corn rose from 15% to 69% in eight years (1939-1946) and then slowed to a walk, increasing only 17% in the next 15 years. With improved methods for the control of grasshoppers, chinch bugs, armyworms, cutworms, weeds, and seed-borne plant diseases, it is reasonable to assume that these advances also contributed something to the increases in corn yields observed between 1935 and 1944. In the following decade (1945-54), with the use of DDT for European corn borer control, toxaphene for armyworms and cutworms, chlordane for grasshoppers and white grubs, inproved fungicides for seed treatment to control seed-borne plant diseases and up to 30% of the corn acreage receiving some herbicide treatment by 1953, it would seem absurd to even suggest that pesticides played little or no role in attaining a 12% gain in corn yields during the decade. Just to cite an example: Luckmann and Petty (1969) showed that over a period of 6 years corn yields in the corn borer control portions of 85 fields under observation ranged from 5.9 to 9.1% and averaged 7.3% higher than the checks. This is only half the story. Most all corn borer treatments are made on early corn in July. They reduce borer populations by 60 to 90% and average 65-75%. There is normally 10 to 50-fold increase in the overall corn borer population by fall (Kuhlman et al., 1973). Thus, with a great reduction in the numbers of first generation moths, the overall benefits to all of the corn fields infested by second generation borers may far exceed those observed in the fields that were treated in July.

The data presented in Fig. 2 seem to suggest a significant positive correlation between the increase in corn yields and the percent of the corn acreage treated with herbicides and that treated with soil insecticides. The validity of such apparent correlations is well supported by the extensive research findings of dozens of research workers in at least a dozen states. Here again, time and space permit only a couple of examples. Bigger and Decker (1966), in summarizing a 10-year study, found that soil treatment resulted in yield increases ranging from 4 to 12 and averaging 7%. Incidentally, the study included a lot of experimental treatments later shown to be quite inferior. Thus, an average increase of 10% would seem to be conservative and in line with the findings in adjacent states.

Unfortunately, I am not familiar with a comparable publication on the value of herbicide treatments, but I do have permission to quote from a private communication by Dr. Fred Slife: "The best data I have pertain to a study still in progress at the University of Illinois Agronomy Farm. The data are for 1966 through 1971. Land planted with corn during this period has received 3 cultivations without herbicide treatment as compared to modern herbicide treatment plus one cultivation. The average yield increase has been 27 bu/A. Figuring all costs involved over the 6-year period, there has been an average increase in return of $26/A over three cultivations alone. This is a net increase after all costs were figured.

"During the same period we have had a study on a corn-corn-soybean rotation. On corn in this rotation we have a complete herbicide treatment with one cultivation compared with 3 cultivations, and the treated corn has averaged 24 bu/A more. Net increase annually has been $22 for herbicide treatment. This is for first-year corn in the rotation. For second-year corn, 25 bu/A, the net increase is $23.

"In a corn-soybean-wheat rotation, corn treated with herbicides showed a 22 bu/A net increase, or $25/A."

On the basis of the apparent correlations and the supporting data, it would be justified in claiming a strong cause and effect relationship between the better than 85% increase in corn yields in the 17-year period (1955-72), and the increased use of soil insecticides (a rise of from 5 to over 60% of the acreage), and herbicides which showed a comparable rise (31 to 85%). We might even be carried away by over-enthusiasm for the value of pesticides if we were not aware that fertilizer consumption has been greatly increased during the same 17-year period.

There is no doubt that hybrid corn, fertilizers, weed control, and insect control have made more or less simultaneous contributions, and there is no reason why any one factor should be singled out for all or even a major part of the credit. In fact, there is an abundance of evidence that they may be mutually interdependent in a sort of symbiotic relationship. Without the support of pest control, the use of fertilizer may be futile, and conversely, without the use of hybrid seed and fertilizer, the yields may be so low as not to warrant the cost of insect, disease, and weed control. In the light of the McNew (1963) paper and some very similiar data related to the value of fertilizers and soil insecticides by Muma et al., (1949) and Floyd et al., (1949), one might well conclude that hybrid seed corn and fertilizers presented really great potentials that could not be realized until pest control allowed such potential to be manifest.

There is another angle to the corn story that has to do with the economics of sweet corn production. With the appearance of the European corn borer in the Midwest, sweet corn, a preferred host, was badly damaged. Crop losses ran high, but the worst was yet to come. With a high percentage of the ears badly infested, it became physically impossible for the canner to detect and eliminate all the borers, so a few found their way into the canned product, where they were soon detected by the efficient Food and Drug Administration inspectors, and thousands of cases of canned corn were seized and condemned. Threatened with financial ruin, the canners had no choice but to develop an efficient corn borer control program or go out of business. Within two years, insecticides were doing this job and doing it well. Use of insecticides reduced corn borer damage and in turn increased yields. With a lower degree of ear infestation, it took less labor to sort and trim the corn in the canning plant. With less trimming there was another saving--more cases of corn per ton of ears. Finally, with increased efficiency in processing, overhead costs were reduced. Did the canner get rich and live happily ever after? No! As usually happens when an industry achieves an overall economy, shrewd buyers drove prices down to a point where the canners at best made only a nominal profit, but the housewife was able to buy corn for less than 15 cents a can.

Costs--Benefits: Pesticide costs

So far we have considered the value of pesticide usage in terms of crop yields and have not mentioned costs or benefits in terms of cash. Data presented in Table 5 show that costs in terms of dollars and cents vary greatly from class to class (herbicide, fungicide, insecticide, etc.), and of course, from compound to compound, and use to use within each class. They range from an average of $1.95 per acre for herbicides on pasture land to $13.41 for fungicides or $13.68 for nematicides on certain special crops. In 1969, 143 million acres of crops were treated with one or more pesticides at a cost of 756 million dollars or an average of $5.29 per acre. With the total value of all crops produced in 1969 reported as 22.9 billion dollars, the amount spent for pesticides amounts to 3.3% of the value of the crop produced.

Data presented in Table 6 show that special pesticide requirements of specific crops pose the major variable in

Table 5. Pesticides used in crops and on livestock and poultry, acreages treated and cost of treatment. United States, 1969.[1]

Pesticide	ACRES 1,000	DOLLARS 1,000	DOLLARS per acre
Herbicide			
Pasture	4,967	9,679	1.95
Other	84,914	345,684	4.07
ALL	89,881	355,363	
Insecticide			
Hay	2,180	8,628	3.96
Other	39,882	296,971	7.45
ALL	42,062	305,599	
Fungicide	4,088	54,803	13.41
Nematicide	1,267	17,335	13.68
Plant Defoliators & Regulators	5,781	23,096	4.00
TOTAL CROP USES	143,079	756,196	5.29
Livestock & Poultry		26,428	
		782,624	

[1] From Table 13. The Pesticide Review 1972 U.S.D.A., June 1973.

per-acre costs, ranging from 61 cents in the case of wheat to $54.80 in the case of apples which required several applications of both insecticides and fungicides. Just as per-acre costs are influenced by the variables just mentioned, so, too, per-acre costs vary from state to state. California with large acreages of cotton, fruits and vegetables ranks No. 1 (over 7 million acres treated at a cost of nearly 105 million dollars or $14.48 per acre). Illinois, a typical corn belt state with some 9 million acres treated with herbicides and nearly 5 million treated with insecticides, ranked more nearly

461

average (14 million acres treated at a cost of nearly 55 million dollars for an average of $3.91 per acre). North Dakota,
typical of the Northern Great Plains where the use of herbicides on grain exceeds all other uses, ranks low (with 7.6
million acres treated at a cost of $7.5 million dollars or
only 99 cents per acre).

In each case the figures cited above are for the purchase
of chemicals only. Data on the cost of application for pesticides are harder to come by. While estimates by individuals

Table 6. Extent of use and cost per acre for the use of pesticides on specific crops in 1966.[1]

| Crop | Percent treated[2] | Expenditures in dollars per acre | | | |
		Fungicide	Herbicide	Insecticide	All
Apple	93	23.83	9.26	23.39	54.80
Tobacco	91	6.41	7.63	10.38	21.70
Citrus	97	3.10	3.27	14.61	18.82
Cotton	74	7.60	5.33	10.30	11.73
Vegetables	78	5.35	9.42	8.49	10.94
Irish potato	96	10.47	2.22	5.56	6.67
Soybean	30	N	4.16	1.83	3.95
Alfalfa	8	-0-	3.40	3.71	3.11
Corn	67	N	2.49	1.81	3.01
Wheat	30	N	0.59	0.78	0.61

[1] Data taken from Tables 5 and 11--Farmers Pesticide Expenditures in 1966. Agr. Econ. Report 192, Econ. Res. Ser.
USDA, September 1970.

[2] Percent of the acreage of each crop that was treated with
one or more pesticides.

vary from about one-third to three times the costs of chemicals, the majority of all those asked to supply figures ended up by saying "by and large" or "all told", the costs are about equal or 50-50. Thus, to be on the conservative side, I will suggest that those interested in estimates of overall costs just double the costs given for chemicals alone. I say this with full knowledge of the fact that a USDA study of: "Farmers expenditures for Custom Pesticide Services in 1964," indicated that application costs were about one-half the cost of the chemicals or only about one-third the total cost of pesticide treatments.

Costs--Benefits: Monetary return

The magnitude of economic returns like costs are variable. Many farmers would tell you pesticides do not cost: "They pay dividends much higher than those paid by preferred stocks and bonds." On the other hand as shown in Table 6, there are undoubtedly some growers of soybeans, alfalfa, small grains, and perhaps a few other crops who rarely find it necessary to treat these crops, and they may even question either the necessity or the value of using pesticides. If we accept the data released by the Minnesota Agricultural Extension Service, it would appear that perhaps no farm operation pays greater dividends than proper pest control, as illustrated by the cost and return values obtained in the weed control data presented in Table 7. Here increased costs ranged from $1.05 to $10.24 per acre, and net returns due to weed control ranged from $1.72 to $41.05, with net profits of $0.39 to $34.52. While the $0.39 per acre profit seems small, one may note it amounted to 29% interest on a $1.33 investment. Looking further, we see that some flax growers obtained profits of over $20.00 per acre, which represented about a 1,000% interest on a $2.00 investment for 6 months.

While it is not summarized as beautifully as the Minnesota data on weed control, H. B. Petty and his associates have over a period of 25 years collected and preserved a mass of otherwise unpublished and unavailable data on the extent and value of the use of insecticides in Illinois, in the annual Summaries of Presentations of the Custom Spray Operators Training School (1949-73). I would like to draw upon this bank account. In 1958, J. H. Bigger said: "We continue to recommend the use of 1.5 lbs of either aldrin or heptachlor per acre broadcast and disced in ahead of planting. Data show that the treatment pays for itself 66% of the time and that it pays 100% or more

Table 7. Monetary return over and above cost of production (per acre) for weedy and weed-free crops. Per acre difference in net return and production costs; profit per acre and percent return on weed control investment.[1]

Crop	Return over cost per acre		Difference between plots, weed-free and weedy		Profit per acre	Percent return on weed control investment
	Weed-free	Weedy	Net return	Cost		
Corn	$35.65	$27.63	$8.02	$1.84	$6.18	336
	35.65	27.07	8.58	1.92	6.66	347
	35.65	-5.60	41.05	6.53	34.52	529
Soybeans	30.54	26.00	4.54	3.44	1.10	32
	17.21	4.35	12.86	10.24	2.62	26
Oats	-1.29	-3.01	1.72	1.33	.39	29
	21.98	6.49	15.49	3.56	11.93	335
	1.21	-9.37	10.58	2.77	7.81	282
Barley	-3.08	-5.09	2.01	1.05	.96	91
	13.87	3.07	10.80	1.87	8.93	477
	3.94	-3.55	7.49	5.69	1.80	32
Wheat	17.02	10.79	6.23	1.29	4.94	383
	25.08	5.47	19.61	2.44	17.17	704
	17.92	2.09	15.83	5.35	10.48	196
Flax	17.78	-4.64	22.42	1.95	20.47	1,004
	16.23	-14.60	30.83	2.32	28.51	1,229
	10.93	4.03	14.96	6.16	8.80	143

[1] Data from Tables 81–86, Special Report No. 13, Minn. Agr. Ext. Ser., 1964.

464

dividends 43% of the time and 200% or more dividends 25% of the time." Knowing the data as I do, there is no doubt that the last 5% saved 20 to 30 or more bushels per acre which means 800 to 1,000% dividends on their $3.00 investment.

In 1973, Kuhlman et al. summarized net profits from the use of insecticides on field crops as shown in Table 8. You will note an annual net profit of nearly 28 million dollars. A check of the individual items in the 10 volumes involved shows that roughly 90% of this profit was due to soil treatment to control the subterranean insects that attack corn. Tabulating such estimates for a period of 20 years (1953-72), I find estimated profits over and above costs (in terms of dollars per acre) varied from year to year as follows: (1) soil insect complex 2 to 6 dollars per acre profit; (2) cutworms 4 to 7 dollars; (3) European corn borer 3 to 8 dollars; and (4) grasshoppers 2 to 6 dollars.

We have previously noted dollar values mentioned by Drs. Slife and McNew.

Table 8. Estimated annual profits from using insecticides to control insects in field crops, Illinois, 1963-1972.[1]

Year	Profits ($1,000)
1963	23,197
1964	18,776
1965	27,660
1966	29,593
1967	34,261
1968	33,937
1969	36,413
1970	27,502
1971	23,093
1972	23,765
TOTAL	278,197

[1] Data by Kuhlman et al., p. 109, 25th Custom Spray Manual, 1973.

Costs--Benefits: Environmental economics

Insofar as fruit and vegetable crops are concerned it is not a question of a profit of so many dollars per acre or percent return on the investment. Since most fruits and vegetables can not be commercially produced without the use of pesticides, the question is how to get maximum efficiency with maximum safety. All of the evidence presented so far may be open to criticism on the basis that the author is biased. In this day and age anyone familiar with the facts of life is suspect--"conflict of interest." With that thought, I would like to cite two indepen-

465

dent views. In summarizing his research on the economics of
pesticides, Dr. J. C. Headley (1968), an agricultural econo-
mist, said: "Results of this study indicate that the marginal
value of a one-dollar expenditure for chemical pesticides is
approximately $4.00." Incidentally, in the same study the
values for pesticides and fertilizer were almost identical.
A. H. Strickland (1970) indicates a factor of 6 to 1 based
upon conditions prevailing in England.

All of this seems to imply that the farmer is the big,
if not the only, beneficiary of pesticide usage. Nothing is
farther from the truth. Since man seems unable to place
tangible values on human life, health, and comfort, I shall
of necessity concede that the value of pesticides in controlling the vectors of human and animal diseases exceeds all
others. Military values closely related to the former are a
close second. Time and space forced me to by-pass these subjects, but fortunately they have been well covered by Simmons
(1959); Livadas and Athanassatos (1963); and numerous reports
emanating from the W.H.O. Dr. Wayland J. Hayes, Jr., the
internationally famous toxicologist at Vanderbilt University,
is currently completing work on a new book, Toxicology of
Pesticides, which will include an interesting and informative
chapter on "Benefits from Pesticides," which I recommend to
all concerning the contributions of pesticides in the areas
of medicine, the armed services, and agriculture.

Now, back to agriculture. I have been constantly remin-
ded, sometimes by members of my own staff, that under the
economic law of supply and demand the farmer might make more
letting pests run wild, because "he could sell less for more."
They even cite such years as 1947, when a combination of factors reduced corn yields in Illinois from 56 to 39 bu/acre
and the farm price for corn jumped from $1.56 to $2.16; also,
the great corn blight tragedy of 1970, when yields dropped
from 98 to 74 bu/acre and the price rose from $1.15 to $1.33.
Of course, they would also cite the converse situations for
the following years. In 1948, yields jumped from 39 to 61
bu/acre and the price dropped from $2.16 to $1.30 a bushel and
in 1971, yields jumped from 74 to 102 bu/acre and the price
of corn dropped from $1.33 to $1.06. They overlook the fact
that year-to-year fluctuations were incidental to the really
significant factor--an ever-increasing demand due to the increase in the population and foreign markets.

Individual segments of industry made a small profit on
the chemicals they sold, while other segments of the same
industry were going broke. Most farmers, because they were

466

Table 9. Potential U.S. acres saved annually for optional uses during the period 1968-70 as a result of increases in yield since the period 1938-40.

Crop (Units)	1968-70 Production (Millions)	Acres harvested 1968-70 (Millions)	1968-70 yield (Per acre)	1938-40 yield (Per acre)	Acres needed to produce 1968-70 crop at 1938-40 yields (Millions)	Acres saved in 1968-70 through yield increases (Millions)
Hay (tons)	126	62.6	2	1.3	96.9	34.3
Corn, grain (bu.)	4,362	55.9	78	28.4	153.6	97.7
Wheat (bu.)	1,470	48.6	30.1	14.2	103.5	54.9
Soybeans (bu.)	1,121	41.5	27	19.2	58.4	16.9
Oats (bu.)	932	18.0	51.8	31.3	29.8	11.8
Sorghum, gain (bu.)	725	13.7	52.9	13	55.8	42.1
Cotton (bales)	10.3	10.7	0.96	0.5	20.6	9.9
Barley (bu.)	419	9.6	43.5	23	18.2	8.6
Corn, silage (tons)	94	7.9	11.9	7.5	12.5	4.6
Flax (bu.)	30.7	2.5	12.2	9.2	3.3	0.8
Rice (cwt.)	92.5	2.1	44.2	22.7	4.1	2.0
Sugar beets (tons)	25.3	1.4	18.1	12.5	2.0	0.6
Beans, edible (cwt.)	18.6	1.5	12.3	8.9	2.1	0.6
Potatoes (cwt.)	310	1.4	221	75.7	4.1	2.7
Peanuts (cwt.)	26.8	1.4	18.6	7.5	3.6	2.2
Rye (bu.)	31.1	1.3	24.1	12.1	2.5	1.2
Tobacco (lbs.)	1,806	0.9	2,008	947	1.9	1.0
TOTAL		281.0			572.9	291.9

467

able to increase their efficiency by reducing per bushel production costs, while per acre costs were going up under general
pressures of inflation, were still able to sell corn at a
small profit. The fact is, the general public--you, me, the
English, the French, and the Russians, not the farmers--were
the big winners. Despite general inflation during the 5 years
(1966-1970), the average price farmers received for a bushel
of corn was only about 75% of the average price they received
during the 5 years preceding modern pesticides (1946-50).
Since the law of supply and demand can and has induced fluctuations of 25 to 50% in the price of corn on a year-to-year
basis and even double in an emergency as it did in 1973, if
it has any real validity in the long haul, I shudder to con-
template the price of corn, beef, pork, and poultry if average
corn yields were to return to pre-pesticide levels when they
were roughly one half of current levels.

There are those who will argue that any and all damage
to the environment as a whole should be added to generally
accepted costs in assessing the contributions made by pesticides. To the extent such damage can be quantitated I would
agree, but only if and when the now intangible benefits that
accrue to the environment are likewise included in any formula
that is used. In this connection, I would like to refer to
some statistics developed by Dr. John G. Thomas and presented
at a meeting in Louisville, Kentucky, in March, 1973. Presumably, it will appear in the Proceedings of the North-Central
Branch Entomological Society of America. In any case, I have
Dr. Thomas's permission to reproduce his table here (Table 9).
The release of nearly 300 million acres of land for optional
uses might well be regarded as a major contribution to our
overtaxed environment (Thomas, 1974).

Summary

Whether we like it or not, we have reached a point of no
return, and there is no turning back. We cannot now dispense
with modern effective pest control and the other essential
components of Twentieth Century agricultural technology. As
evidence of this fact, let us take a good look at what has
taken place in this country in the course of the last century
(Fig. 3).

In 1850, the United States had a population of 23 million.
Since then it has doubled three times (1875, 1913, and 1962).
In 1850, America boasted 13 acres of farmland per person, 10
acres in 1875, and 9 acres in 1913. Currently the amount is

468

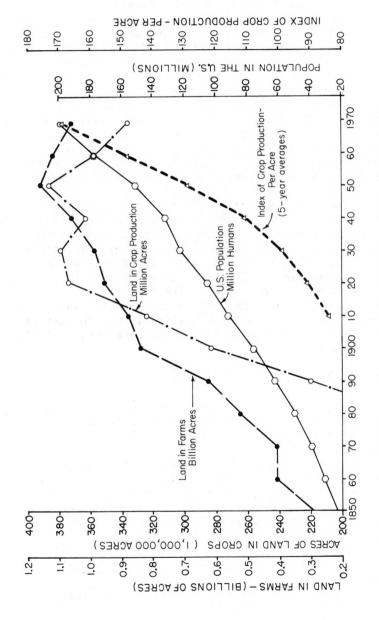

Fig. 3. A graphic presentation of data on acreage of land in farms, the acreage in cultivated crops, and the index of crop production per acre (1935–39 = 100) to illustrate
the possible relationships between trends in agricultural production and the human
population of the United States and its needs.

469

less than 5 acres, of which only about 1.7 acres are devoted
to crop production. The story of how agriculture has been
able to meet the needs of this rapidly expanding population
is most interesting. For some 30 to 40 years the expansion
of agricultural production was attained largely by expansion
into new territory, largely through the Homestead Act. From
about 1890 to 1930, increased production was attained by the
joint action of expansion and intensification--in other words,
more homesteading and the cultivation of more acres per farm.
Since 1930, increased production has been largely dependent
upon advances in technology. In fact, since 1954, at which
time the number of acres in farms and acreage in cultivated
cropt turned downward, all increases have been due to technological progress. It is interesting to note that between
1930 and 1969, per acre production of cultivated crops increased 70%.

Since the acres of available crop land has declined
slightly during the last 40 years, it seems apparent that the
70% increase in production attributable to technology was
needed to keep pace with a 70% increase in the population.
As pointed out by Dr. Thomas, a return to 1938-40 production
methods would require 572.9 million acres of crop land to
produce only the 17 crops listed. The fact is that those
acres are not available; thus, if we are to maintain our current standard of living, we must utilize to the fullest extent
possible all of our modern technological know-how, including
the use of pesticides.

References

Bigger, J. H. 1958. Soil insecticide research. Pages 60-63 in
     Tenth Illinois Custom Spray Operators Training School
     Summaries of Presentations. Coop. Ext. Serv., Univ. of Ill.
     at Urbana-Champaign. 70 pp.
Bigger, J. H., and G. C. Decker. 1966. Controlling root feed-
     ing insects on corn. Ill. Agr. Exp. Sta. Bull. 716, 1-24.
Decker, G. C. 1954. Agr. Chem. 9: 37-9, 111, 113, 115-17.
Decker, G. C. 1958. Economic entomology. Pages 104-26 in: A
     Century of Biological Research, Ill. Natural History Sur-
     vey Bull. 27(2): 85-234.
Decker, G. C. 1964. Bull. Entomol. Soc. Am. 10(1): 8-15.
Floyd, E. H., and C. E. Smith. 1949. J. Econ. Entomol. 42:
     908-10.
Forbes, Stephen A. 1880. On some interactions of organisms.
     Bull. Ill. State Lab. Nat. Hist. 3: 3-17.

Headley, J. C. 1968. Estimating the productivity of agricultural pesticides. Am. J. Agr. Econ. 50: 13-23.

Kuhlman, D. E., Roscoe Randell, and T. A. Cooley. 1973. Insect situation and outbreak, 1973. Pages 109-126 in: Twenty-fifth Illinois Custom Spray Operators Training School Summaries of Presentations. Coop. Ext. Serv., Univ. of Ill. at Urbana-Champaign.

Livadas, G., and D. Athanassatos. 1963. Riv. Malar. 42: 177-187.

Luckmann, W. H., and H. B. Petty. 1969. Controlling corn borers in field corn with insecticides. Univ. of Ill. Coop. Ext. Serv. Cir. 768 (Rev. 1969), 8 pp.

McNew, George L. 1963. Pest control in relation to human society. Pages 1-22 in: New Developments and Problems in the Use of Pesticides. Nat. Acad. Sci.-Nat. Res. Counc. Publ. 1082, pp. 1-82.

Muma, Martin H., Roscoe E. Hill, and Ephriam Hixson. 1949. J. Econ. Entomol. 42: 822-4.

Shepard, Harold H. 1951. The chemistry and action of insecticides. New York, McGraw-Hill Book Co., 503 pp.

Simmons, S. W. 1959. "The use of DDT insecticides in human medicine." DDT, The Insecticide Dichlorodiphenyltrichloroethane and Its Significance, P. Muller (ed.). Birkhauser Verlag, Basel, pp. 251-502.

Strickland, A. H. 1970. Some economic principles of pest management. Pages 30-44 in: Concepts of Pest Management. Proc. of a Conf. held at North Carolina St. Univ., Raleigh, N.C., Mar. 25-27, 1970.

Thomas, John G. 1973. Implementing practical pest control management. Proc. N.C. State Br. E.S.A. 28: 122-130.

BIODEGRADATION OF NITRILOTRIACETIC ACID
AND NTA-METAL ION COMPLEXES:
(The Chemo-biological Life Cycle of a Detergent Builder)

Craig B. Warren

Monsanto Chemical Company

Introduction

Nitrilotriacetic acid (NTA), a relatively simple
symmetrical molecule, was first prepared by Heintz in 1861
from the reaction of chloroacetic acid with
ammonia.

$$N \Longleftarrow \begin{array}{l} CH_2COOH \\ CH_2COOH \\ CH_2COOH \end{array}$$

Relatively little research effort was
expended on the molecule until the early
nineteen thirties at which time NTA was
commercially produced as Trilon A in Germany. The ready
availability of the compound (NTA was the first commercially produced aminopolycarboxylic acid) stimulated the
measurement of the thermodynamic stability constants for a
large number of NTA-metal ion complexes (Sillen and
Martell, 1964 and 1971; Chaberek and Martell, 1959). One
particularly interesting result of the complex work was the
observations that NTA at pH 10 or above could form water
soluble complexes with magnesium and calcium ions.

In 1962 Hampshire Chemical Division of W. R. Grace and
Company patented (Singer and Weissberg, 1962) a process for
the synthesis of NTA based on cyanomethylation of ammonia
that was a modification of earlier work by Ulrich and
Ploetz (1940) and by Eschweiler in 1890. The availability
of both this process and inexpensive by-product HCN from
acrylonitrile production, prompted the commercial development of NTA as a detergent builder which in turn prompted
an intensive research effort into the human and environmental safety of NTA.

In the area of human and environmental safety evaluation, probably more information exists for NTA than for
any other molecule. Thayer and Kensler (1973) have reviewed this literature up to early 1973 in the area of

environmental and human safety of NTA; Mottola (1973) has
reviewed the NTA literature up to Nov., 1972 in the areas
of environmental safety, toxicology, uses, analytical
chemistry and physical chemistry.

It is not the intent of this paper to review the NTA
literature for a third time. Instead, we will gather together published and unpublished literature to provide
answers or at least insight into the following questions:

1.   What is the pathway of NTA biodegradation, i.e., what
     series of biochemical reactions converts NTA into
     universal metabolites?

2.   What are the kinetics and mechanism of NTA biodegrada-
     tion, i.e., how fast is the compound degraded, does
     the permeation process require energy?

3.   What is the biodegradability of NTA metal complexes?

4.   What is the tolerance range of NTA biodegradation?
     Under what range of environmental conditions such as
     pH, temperature, and oxygen concentration does NTA
     biodegrade?

Biodegradation Pathway for NTA

A.   Isolation of Organisms Capable of Degrading NTA

Organisms capable of degrading NTA are ubiquitous in
the environment. This is indicated by the fact that NTA is
biodegraded in sewage facilities (Bouveng, et al., 1968;
Pfeil and Lee, 1968; Rudd and Hamilton, 1972; Shumate et
al., 1973; Swisher et al., 1967; Thompson and Duthie,
1968), soil (Tiedje and Mason, 1973), river water (Warren
and Malec, 1972a, 1972b), lake water (Chau and Shiomi,
1972) (Taylor et al., 1971), sea water (Erickson et al.,
1970), and under anaerobic conditions in mud (Enfors and
Molin, 1973a, 1973b).

Forsberg and Lindqvist (1967a) were first to report
the isolation of a bacterium from sewage that was capable
of utilizing NTA as the sole source of carbon for growth.
Enfors and Molin (1967b) later reported the isolation of
NTA degrading bacteria from several natural waters; one
of the isolated strains was suggested to be a species of
Pseudomonas. Focht and Joseph (1971) isolated a strain of

Pseudomonas from sewage that was able to utilize NTA as the sole source of carbon and nitrogen. Analysis of the biodegradation reaction indicated that NTA was converted to CO_2, H_2O, and NH_3. Wong and coworkers (1972-3) also reported the isolation of a bacterial mutant from sewage that was capable of growth on NTA at concentrations as high as 2.5%. The mutant, identified as a species of Pseudomonas, utilized NTA as the sole source of carbon, nitrogen and energy.

Enfors and Molin (1973a) reported the isolation of a Gram negative, rod-shaped, NTA degrading organism from bottom material obtained from shallow waters. The organism was able to degrade NTA under aerobic conditions and under anaerobic conditions in the presence of nitrate ion.

Tiedje et al., (1973) isolated a strain of Pseudomonas from soil that was capable of growth on NTA. The organism, which could use NTA as the sole source of carbon and nitrogen, converted this compound to CO_2, NH_3, H_2O and bacterial cells. Attempts to detect any biodegradation intermediates even when metabolic inhibitors such as arsenite ion, malonate and dinitrophenol were added to the cell suspensions were unsuccessful.

B. Biodegradation Pathway Work

Pathway work generally proceeds along the following course (a) prediction of possible pathways, (b) isolation of pure bacterial cultures capable of degrading the test compound, (c) Warburg measurements of the ability of the culture to degrade proposed intermediates, (d) preparation of cell extracts and isolation of biodegradation intermediates, and (e) isolation of the enzymes involved in the catabolic process. For the case of NTA the pathway work has progressed to the enzyme isolation stage. Since NTA is the first aminopolycarboxylic acid to undergo such a study, we will briefly trace the study from the prediction stage through the cell extract stage.

1. Prediction of Pathways

The objective of any pathway analysis is the prediction of all reasonably possible biodegradation intermediates. One such scheme is presented in Figure 1. In general, the pathways are relatively simple -- the biodegradation can follow a decarboxylation-demethylation

475

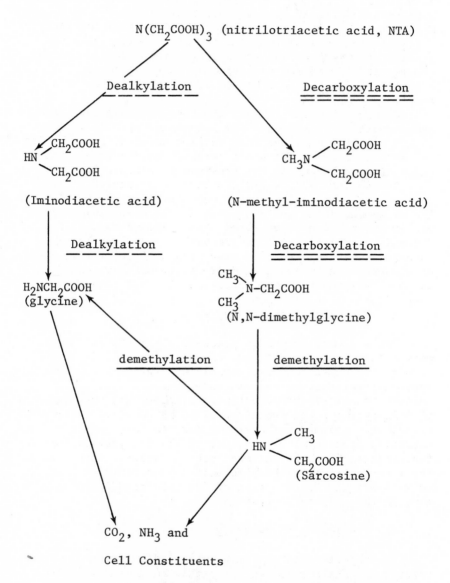

Figure 1. Possible Pathways of NTA Biodegradation

Substrate	Tiedje et al., (1973a) Growth	Oxidation	Focht and Joseph, (1971) Growth	Oxidation
Nitrilotriacetate (NTA)	+	+	+	+
Iminodiacetate (IDA)	+	+	+	+
Glycine	+	+	+	+
Sarcosine	+	Lag	+	Not Measured
N-Methyl-IDA	0	0	+	Lag
N-Nitroso-IDA	0	0	Not Measured	Not Measured
NTA-Amine Oxide	0	0	←	←
N-Oxalyl-IDA	Not Measured	0		
Glyoxylate	+	+		
Glycerate	+	+		
Acetate	+	Lag		

Table 1. Growth on and Oxidation of Several Potential NTA Intermediates by Pseudomonas Isolates

pathway to yield N-methyl-iminodiacetic acid (NMIDA), N,N-dimethyl glycine, sarcosine (SARC) and eventually cell constituents and ammonia. Alternatively, the pathway may be one of dealkylation to yield iminodiacetic acid (IDA) and glycine (GLY). As pointed out by Epstein (1973), sarcosine and iminodiacetic are secondary amines and secondary amines can react with nitrite ions under acidic conditions to produce N-nitrosamines. N-Nitrososarcosine has been shown to be carcinogenic to rats (Druckrey et al., 1963); recent results suggest that N-nitrosoiminodiacetic acid is not carcinogenic to rats (Lijinsky et al., 1973). Thus, it's important to know which secondary amine is formed from NTA breakdown and whether there is any tendency for the compound to leak out of the cell.

2. Warburg Measurements

Warburg measurements provide a relatively rapid source of information about possible biodegradation pathways. These measurements also allow one to differentiate between strains of bacteria that have been isolated with the same compound. Table 1 presents the results of two such studies for NTA degrading pseudomonads. Both strains of bacteria show approximately the same O_2 uptake pattern for NTA, IDA, NMIDA, SARC and GLY. It is interesting to note that the organisms isolated by Tiedje were not able to degrade proposed intermediates such as NTA-amine oxide and N-oxalyl-IDA. In general, the Warburg data indicates that NTA is degraded by C-N cleavage rather than decarboxylation reactions.

$$ON-N(CH_2COOH)_2 \qquad HOOC-\underset{O}{\overset{}{C}}-N(CH_2COOH)_2 \qquad O \leftarrow N(CH_2COOH)_3$$

N-nitroso-IDA   N-oxalyl-IDA   NTA-amine oxide

3. Biodegradation of NTA by Cell Extracts

Tiedje and coworkers (1973) found that a mixture of soluble extract from NTA degrading Pseudomonas, NADH, and O_2 quantitatively converts NTA to IDA. Small amounts of glyoxylate were also detected. When glyoxylate was the substrate glycerate and glycine were formed. In subsequent work Tiedje and Aust (1973) found that addition of Mg^{2+} or Mn^{2+} to the cell extract brought about oxidation also of IDA. Work on the purification of the enzyme responsible

478

for oxidation of the C-N bond of NTA and on the characterization of the IDA oxidation products is underway.

Cripps and Noble (1973) obtained approximately similar results to those of Tiedje. They, too, used a cell extract preparation of <u>Pseudomonas</u>. Oxidation of NTA required in addition to the cell free extract, magnesium ion, thiamine pyrophosphate, and NADH. NTA was converted to glycine and to glyoxylate which was trapped as a dinitrophenylhydrazone derivative. When NADH was omitted glyoxylate was converted to tartronic semialdehyde (trapped as a dinitrophenylhydrazone derivative); addition of NADH resulted in formation of glycerate. Attempts to demonstrate enzymes capable of interconversion of glycine to glyoxylate were unsuccessful. Glycine was metabolized to glycerate by a sequence of reactions not yet elucidated.

The biodegradation pathway for conversion of NTA to universal metabolites suggested by the work of Tiedje et al., 1973a and 1973b and by that of Cripps and Noble, 1972 is presented in Figure 2. Initial oxidation of NTA occurs at the methylene carbon possibly by the action of a mixed function oxidase. The acetic acid side groups of NTA leave as glyoxylate fragments and the pathway of NTA oxidation proceeds through IDA and on to glycine. The only intermediate associated with the pathway that is not a universal metabolite is IDA. IDA, however, is a fleeting intermediate in that it is only observed when cell extract preparations are used and then only when Mg^{2+} or Mn^{2+} are not present.

Kinetics and Mechanism of NTA Biodegradation

A. <u>Nutritional Requirements of Bacteria that Degrade NTA</u>

An idea of the nutritional requirements of a bacterium that can degrade a particular compound may allow for a long range prediction of the biodegradability of the compound. For example, if growth factors or energy sources are required in addition to the compound, the environment in which the compound can be biodegraded becomes more complicated and specific and thus more prone to loss of acclimation. The nutritional requirements for the bacteria that degrade NTA are, however, quite simple. Under aerobic conditions, NTA can serve as the sole source of carbon and nitrogen for energy and growth (Tiedje, 1973a). Under an-

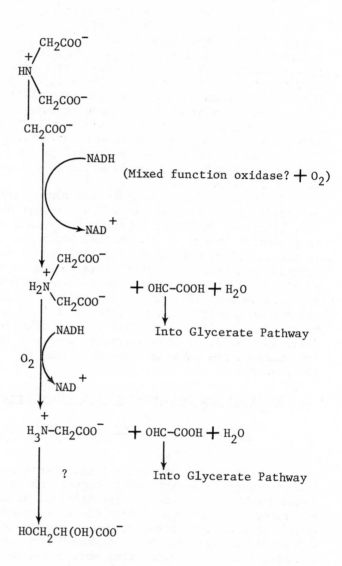

Figure 2.   Biodegradation Pathway for NTA.

aerobic conditions, on the other hand, NTA can serve as the sole source of carbon for energy and growth (Enfors and Molin, 1973a). Since NTA can both stimulate the growth and satisfy all the organic requirements of bacteria found throughout the environment, the prediction is that its removal by biodegradation will not be prone to upset i.e., loss of acclimation.

B. Kinetics of NTA Biodegradation

Wong et al., (1973) have determined the K_m and V_{max} by the method of Lineweaver and Burk for the degradation of NTA by a bacterial mutant. The apparent Michaelis constant (K_m) defined as the substrate concentration required for half-maximal velocity (V_{max}) was 370 ug NTA/hr/(mg dry weight of cells). The high affinity of the enzyme for NTA far exceeded those reported for an amino acid in a marine bacterium (Lijinsky et al., 1973) and for lactose in E. Coli (Kepes and Cohen, 1962).

This high affinity of an acclimated bacterium for NTA also holds for a non-mutant bacterium isolated from soil (Tiedje et al., 1973a). The rate of oxygen uptake during NTA metabolism $(Q_{O_2} = 87$ at 30°C, where Q_{O_2} = ul O_2/mg/hr) reported by Tiedje et al., (1973a) appears to be somewhat faster than that reported by Liu, Wong and Dutka (1973) for their mutant bacterium $(Q_{O_2} = 34$ at 25°C). This higher rate holds even if one corrects for temperature differences by assuming that the rate of oxygen uptake doubles for each 10° rise in temperature.

C. Permeation of NTA into the Cell

Wong et al., (1973) have also determined that energy is required for NTA transport. When their bacterial mutant was treated with 30 mM sodium azide or 10 mM potassium cyanide both the rate and level of ^{14}C-carboxyl-NTA uptake were drastically reduced. These results suggest that energy is involved in NTA transport and that the bacteria have the ability to concentrate NTA from an environment in which the molecule is present in low concentration.

Biodegradation of NTA-Metal Ion Complexes

Since NTA exists in the free acid state only in the pH range of 1 to 2 (Miles, 1965), any discussion of NTA biodegradation has to be a discussion of NTA—metal ion chelate biodegradation. Figure 3 is a simplified flow diagram intended to show the metal ion complexes formed by NTA as it moves from the soap box into the washing machine and subsequently into the environment. In the washing machine, NTA is fully ionized and exists as an equilibrium mixture of Ca^{2+}, Mg^{2+}, and Na^+ metal ion complexes. Once out of the washing machine and into the sewer, soil or aquatic environment, NTA comes in contact with micro-organisms,

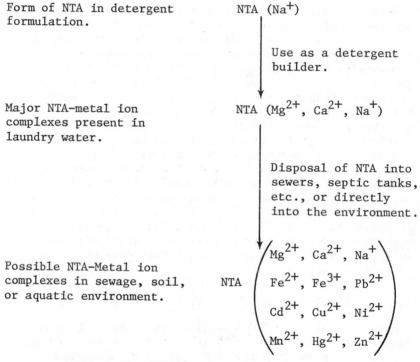

Form of NTA in detergent formulation.

NTA (Na^+)

Use as a detergent builder.

Major NTA—metal ion complexes present in laundry water.

NTA (Mg^{2+}, Ca^{2+}, Na^+)

Disposal of NTA into sewers, septic tanks, etc., or directly into the environment.

Possible NTA—Metal ion complexes in sewage, soil, or aquatic environment.

NTA $\left(\begin{array}{ccc} Mg^{2+}, & Ca^{2+}, & Na^+ \\ Fe^{2+}, & Fe^{3+}, & Pb^{2+} \\ Cd^{2+}, & Cu^{2+}, & Ni^{2+} \\ Mn^{2+}, & Hg^{2+}, & Zn^{2+} \end{array} \right)$

Figure 3. NTA—Metal Chelate Reactions

metal ions and other chelants. Thus, any analysis of the biodegradation of NTA metal ion complexes has to be a systems analysis of a nonequilibrium system made up of the following reactions: (a) NTA—metal exchange reactions in aqueous solutions, (b) NTA—metal ion complex ligand exchange reactions, and (c) NTA—metal ion complex biodegradation. An illustration of this nonequilibrium system is presented in Figure 4; a discussion of the individual components that make up the system follows.

A. Biodegradation of NTA Metal Chelates

The metal ions present at varying concentrations in inland waters are: Ca^{2+}, Na^+, Mg^{2+}, Ba^{2+}, Sr^{2+}, Mn^{2+}, Fe^{3+}, Co^{2+}, Ni^{2+}, Cu^{2+}, Zn^{2+}, Cd^{2+}. At pH 7 the apparent stability constants (K_{M*} defined below) for NTA complexes of the above metals fit into the following groups: (Sillen and Martell, 1964 and 1971; Chabenek and Martell, 1959; Irving and Miles, 1966) (a) Strong complexes (log K_{M*} = 8 to 11) Cu^{2+}, Pb^{2+}, Ni^{2+}, Co^{2+}, Zn^{2+}, Cd^{2+}; (b) weak complexes (log K_{M*} = 2 to 5), $Fe(OH)_2^+$, Mn^{2+}, Ca^{2+}, Ba^{2+}, and Sr^{2+}.

$$M^{2+} + NTA^{3-} \rightleftharpoons (NTA-M)^- \qquad K_M = \frac{[NTA-M]^-}{[M^{2+}][NTA^{-3}]}$$

$K_{M*} = K_M/\alpha$ where

$$\alpha = 1 + [(H^+)/K_3] + [(H^+)^2/K_2K_3] + [(H^+)^3/K_1K_2K_3]$$

K_i (i = 1-3) = Acid dissociation constants for NTA

Work by Miles (1965) indicates that for the strong complexes, NTA exists as a tetradentate ligand, whereas for the weak complexes NTA is protonated on nitrogen and exists as a tridentate ligand.

Warren and Malec (1972a), and Tiedje et al., (1973a) found that biodegradation of NTA yielded no extracellular intermediates. This suggests that extracellular enzymes are not involved in the biodegradation process. Wong et al., (1973) obtained results that suggest that NTA is biodegraded by the membrane fraction of Pseudomonas capable of degrading NTA. Tiedje et al., (1973b), and Cripps and Noble (1972), on the other hand, found that NTA was degraded by the soluble fraction of a cell extract preparation. These results suggest that during the biodegradation process the NTA-metal complex is either degraded by enzymes present in the membrane or must pass through the membrane and come in contact with the enzymes responsible for cleavage of the C-N bond. At some point during the biodegradation of NTA the metal ion originally associated with NTA has to exchange with the metal ion or organic ion associated with the permeation or the bond breaking process. If the equilibrium constant for this ex-

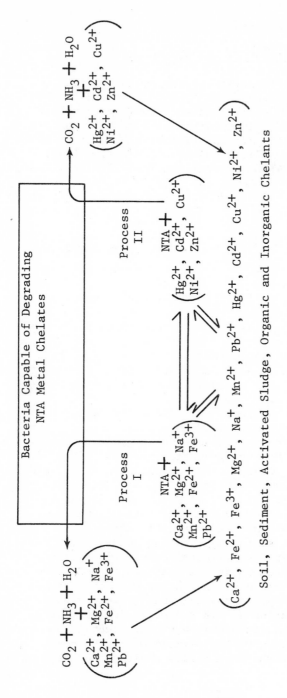

Soil, Sediment, Activated Sludge, Organic and Inorganic Chelants

Process I   Complex readily biodegradable, released metals are not toxic to the NTA biodegrading bacteria.

Process II Complex less biodegradable than those in Process I, released metals are toxic to the NTA biodegrading bacteria.

Figure 4. NTA-Metal Chelate Reactions in the Environment

change favors the original metal ion or if the released
metal ion is toxic to the system, the biodegradation
process is hindered.

The question of the intrinsic biodegradability of
various NTA-metal ion complexes is being considered by the
Tiedje group at Michigan State University. As of the date
of this paper (November, 1973) no definite information is
available. There is available, however, empirical information collected by Swisher et al., (1973), Bjorndal et
al., (1973), Huber and Popp (1972) and Gudernatsch (1970)
on the biodegradation of NTA metal complexes in river water,
BOD water, and activated sludge. Although the experiments
of these workers were not designed to look specifically at
the mechanism of NTA metal complex degradation, information
nevertheless can be extracted that allows for a tentative
classification of NTA-metal ion complex biodegradability.

Bjorndal et al., (1972) found that in minimal media
(inorganic salts) NTA at 3 mg/l in the form of the Cu^{2+},
Zn^{2+}, Ni^{2+} or Cd^{2+} 1:1 complex was not biodegraded by
activated sludge acclimated to NTA. The Fe^{3+} complex however was degraded. Gudernatsch (1970), found that NTA at
25 mg/l in the form of the 1:1 complex with Ni^{2+} or NTA at
30 mg/l in the form of the 1:1 complex with Cu^{2+} were not
biodegraded by activated sludge acclimated to NTA. The 1:1
complexes of NTA-Fe^{2+} and NTA-Mn^{2+} were, however, biodegradable. Swisher, et. al., (1973) studied the biodegradation of 5 mg/l NTA in the presence of varying amounts of
Hg^{2+}, Cd^{2+}, Cu^{2+}, Ni^{2+}, or Zn^{2+}. At metal ion levels where
10% of the 5 mg/l NTA was complexed with any of these met-
als only Hg^{2+}, which was probably in the form of $Hg(OH)_2$
rather than NTA-Hg^{2+} (Bjorndahl et al., 1972), hindered
the biodegradation of NTA. At levels where 30% or more of
available NTA was complexed, biodegradation of NTA was
hindered. Lead II (Pb^{2+}), on the other hand, did not
hinder the biodegradation of NTA.

These data suggest that the presence of Hg^{2+}, Cd^{2+},
Ni^{2+}, Zn^{2+}, or Cu^{2+} hinder the organism's ability to
metabolize NTA. Ca^{2+}, Mg^{2+}, Na^+, Mn^{2+}, Fe^{2+}, Fe^{3+}, and
Pb^{2+}, on the other hand, provide no such hindrance. One
must now differentiate between biodegradation of NTA-metal
ion complexes by pure culture systems and biodegradation by
practical systems such as activated sludge, soil and river
water. In the latter systems, as shown in Figure 3, one
has to consider also the effect of ligand and metal transfer reactions.

485

B. NTA-Metal Ion Exchange Reactions in Solutions

NTA in laundry water is mainly in the form of Ca^{2+}, Mg^{2+}, and Na^+ salts. When this water is discharged into sewers, septic tanks or directly into receiving waters, the pH of the waste water drops from 10 or above to around neutrality and a multitude of metal ions are added to the system. As a first approximation, the distribution of NTA among the various metals will be a function of the stability constants of the NTA-metal ion complexes, the total concentration of NTA and the concentrations of the various metal ions.

Lerman and Childs (1973) have theoretically analyzed the distribution of NTA among the metals in a model fresh water system thought to be a model of Lake Ontario water. At a total NTA concentration of 0.02 mg/l, the principal NTA complexes are those of Cu^{2+}, $FeOH^{2+}$, $Fe(OH)_2^+$, Pb^{2+}, and Zn^{2+}; at a NTA concentration of 0.5 mg/l, 55% of the NTA is in the form of the Cu^{2+} complex, 14% is in the form of the $Fe(OH)_2^+$ complex, and 10% is in the form of the Zn^{2+} complex; at 38 mg/l the principal species is Ca^{2+}-NTA. The calculations show that NTA first partitions among the metals forming the most stable complexes and then partitions among the remaining metals. If one neglects the competition by bottom material and other chelating agents, these results suggest that at predicted environmental levels (0.025 mg/l or less) NTA will exist mainly as complexes of Cu^{2+}, Fe^{3+}, Pb^{2+} and Zn^{2+} (Thayer and Kensler, 1973).

In any system made up of chelants and metal ions, all ions and chelants will be in dynamic equilibrium. Disappearance of any chelant, e.g., by biodegradation, will result in a redistribution of the chelants in the system to accommodate the released metal ions. An example of such a system in operation is provided by Huber and Popp (1972) who found that NTA-Cd^{2+} was not biodegradable. Addition of Ca^{2+} to the system in a Ca to Cd atomic ratio of 710:1 resulted in conversion of 50% of NTA-Cd^{2+} to NTA-Ca^{2+} and biodegradation of NTA. The effect of metal ion transfer reactions on biodegradation of NTA metal complexes is also illustrated by the work both of Swisher et al., (1973) and Bjorndal et al., (1972). Swisher et al., (1973) found that NTA complexed to either Cu^{2+}, Zn^{2+}, Ni^{2+}, Cd^{2+}, Hg^{2+}, or Pb^{2+} biodegraded in river water. Bjorndal et al., (1973) on the other hand, found either zero or poor biodegradation of NTA–Cu^{2+}, NTA–Zn^{2+}, NTA–Ni^{2+}, or NTA–Cd^{2+} in mineral media that had been innoculated with organisms known to degrade NTA. It was subsequently found that the river water contained more Mg^{2+} and Ca^{2+} than the mineral media. Bjorndal increased the concentrations of those two ions and obtained biodegradation of NTA in the presence of Cu^{2+}. The degradation of NTA–Zn^{2+}, NTA–Ni^{2+} and NTA–Cd^{2+} in the presence of increased Mg^{2+} and Ca^{2+} was not investigated.

Thus, biodegradation of NTA metal chelates is a competitive process in which the Mg^{2+}, Ca^{2+}, Fe^{3+}, Mn^{2+} and Na^+ salts of NTA acclimatize and degrade at a faster rate than the corresponding Zn^{2+}, Ni^{2+}, Cd^{2+}, Cu^{2+}, and Hg^{2+} salts. In any medium containing all of the above ions, biodegradation of NTA will funnel through the easier-to-degrade salts. This hypothesis was realized by Swisher, et. al., (1973) who found that the rate of biodegradation of NTA in the presence of Pb^{2+}, Zn^{2+}, Cd^{2+}, Cu^{2+} and Na^+ ions was increased by addition of large amount of Fe^{3+} ions. Analysis of this system by gas chromatography also showed that NTA had degraded without the accumulation of any detectable amounts of intermediates.

C. Ligand Exchange Reactions

In soil, activated sludge river water, or other receiving waters, the metal ions in the system partition between NTA and all other ligands. As a first approximation the concentration of a particular complex will be a function of the stability constant of the complex and the concentration of the ligand. Examples of competing ligands are: (a) inorganic ligands such as carbonate, sulfate, hydroxide ion and orthophosphate; (b) organic ligands such as citrate, ethylenediaminetetraacetic acid (EDTA), humic acid and fulvic acid; and (c) undefined ligands such as undoubtedly occur in activated sludge, soil and bottom materials. These ligands serve several functions. They can participate in ligand exchange reactions and they can serve as acceptors for metals released during the biodegradation of NTA.

1. Exchange with Soil

Tiedje and Mason (1973) found that soil can effectively compete with NTA for metal ions and can serve as a

sink for released metal ions. Thus, NTA at 40.0 ug/g of
soil in the form of either the Cu^{2+}, Fe^{3+}, Mn^{2+}, Zn^{2+},
Pb^{2+}, or Ni^{2+} complex biodegraded at a rate of 8 ug/g/day
in nonacclimated soil and at 10 ug/g/day in the NTA-accli-
matized soil. The Cd^{2+} and Hg^{2+} complexes biodegrade at a
rate of 1.5 ug/g/day in nonacclimatized soil and at 4 ug/g/
day in acclimatized soil. Addition of NTA to soil as the
Cu^{2+} complex and subsequent extraction of the residual NTA
one week later showed that NTA-Cu^{2+} had been converted to
NTA-Fe^{3+}.

2. Exchange with Sediment

Taylor et al., (1971), have found that NTA at concentrations of 20 mg/l in distilled water containing bottom
materials from typical bodies of surface water did not
extract barium, antimony, molybdenum, strontium, chromium,
silver, tin, iron, lead, cadmium, copper, or mercury. Some
extraction of zinc, nickel, manganese and cobalt occurred;
however, the concentrations of these metals (initially
present in the sub-mg/l quantities) never increased by more
than two- or three-fold. Knezak, Mugwira and Ellis (1973),
in a similar study, showed that NTA and EDTA at concentrations of 2 and 20 mg/l solubilized Ni^{2+} and Zn^{2+} from
sediments contaminated with high amounts of these metals.
With sediments low in total Ni^{2+} and Zn^{2+}, small amounts of
Fe^{3+} and Cu^{2+} were solubilized. NTA is biodegradable,
however, whereas EDTA is not and Knezak et al., (1973)
found that the amount of metals extracted by NTA decreased
after 1 to 6 days, whereas the EDTA extracts remained
constant.

The work of Taylor et al., (1971) and of Knezak et
al., (1973) was reinforced by Chau and Shiomi (1972) who
found that NTA, when added at concentrations ranging from
0.5 to 10 mg/l to lake water, released Zn^{2+} and Fe^{3+} from
the bottom material into the water. The concentration of
these materials rapidly declined after the third day,
indicating biodegradation of NTA.

Tiedje (1973) found by Warburg measurements that
NTA-Cu^{2+} was initially biodegraded by _Pseudomonas_. The
initial rate of O_2 uptake rapidly dropped off as the concentration of free Cu^{2+} built up in the flask. Addition of
soil to the flask corrected this problem by absorbing the
released Cu^{2+} and the rate of Cu^{2+}-NTA biodegradation did
not drop off.

3. Exchange with Primary and Secondary Sewage Sludge

Sewage sludge is a complex material made up of biomass and a complex array of organic and inorganic molecules. Unlike soil or sediment this material is in a dynamic state of change and its composition can vary with time and with plant location. Cheng, Patterson and Minear (1973) have measured the relative affinity of secondary sludge (made up mostly of biomass) and other chelating agents for Cu^{2+}. About 10% of the Cu^{2+} was taken up by sludge from complexes of Cu^{2+}-glycine and Cu^{2+}-oxalate whereas the uptake of copper from copper-NTA and copper-EDTA was insignificant. Bjorndal et al., (1972) have studied the exchange of Cu^{2+} -NTA, Ni^{2+}-NTA and Cd^{2+}-NTA with primary sewage sludge (mainly made up of organic matter). Cu^{2+}, Cd^{2+} and Ni^{2+} at concentrations of 1 mg/1 were added to raw unsettled sewage. Copper was adsorbed quite strongly on the settleable solids, but Cd^{2+} and Ni^{2+} were less strongly adsorbed (80, 36, and 33% adsorption, respectively). Addition of NTA at 5.85 mg/1 caused a release of 20% of the Cu^{2+}, 50% of the Cd^{2+}, and all of the Ni^{2+}. These data suggest that unlike soil and sediment, primary and secondary sludge do not compete well with NTA for metal ions.

Preliminary data indicate, however, that activated sludge systems acclimatized to NTA also degrade the metal ion complexes of NTA. Bjorndal et al., (1972), for example, have found that Cu^{2+}- and Cd^{2+}-NTA are completely degraded by sludge, whereas Ni^{2+}-NTA is about 10% biodegraded.

Finally it is not unreasonable to expect situations to develop, e.g., during periods of upset, where there is leakage of NTA-metal ion complexes from septic tanks and sewage treatment plants. The information gathered by Tiedje, and Mason (1973), Swisher et al., (1973), and Knezak et al., (1973), however, show that the residual NTA-metal ion complexes are biodegraded both by soil and by receiving waters.

Tolerance Range for NTA Biodegradation

The tolerance range for NTA biodegradation is the range of external conditions under which NTA will biodegrade. Such conditions can include temperature, moisture, light intensity, pH, osmotic pressure and oxidation-reduction potential (E_h) of the habitat. In this section

we will consider only pH, temperature and oxygen concentration (oxidation-reduction potential).

A. pH Limits

Wong, Liu and Dutka (1972) found that a bacterial
mutant capable of using NTA for growth and energy was able
to grow on NTA in the pH range of 5 to 9. Optimal growth
occurred around a pH of 7 and growth was slightly better at
acidic rather than alkaline pH. Focht and Joseph (1971)
found that their Pseudomonas isolate (from sewage) grew on
NTA media with an initial pH in the range of 6.5 to 8.5.
The isolate would not grow at pH 6.0 or 9.0. Tiedje and
Mason (1973) found that there was no correlation of pH with
biodegradation of NTA in soil. The pH of the soils used in
the experiment ranged from 5.0 to 7.5.
    These data indicate that NTA is biodegraded over the
pH range normally encountered in the environment. The
specific tolerance range of an isolated organism appears to
be dependent on the system from which the organism was
isolated.

B. Temperature

Like any biological process, the biodegradation of NTA
is temperature dependent. The question is whether biodegradation is completely shut off or whether intermediates
accumulate at low temperatures. Swisher and Warren (1971)
have found that Meramec or Detroit River waters at 6°C into
which 5 or 20 mg/l of NTA was added, usually required 6-8
weeks for acclimation, after which NTA disappeared within
3-10 days. Second charges of NTA added at that time required no further acclimation and were all degraded within
another 3-10 days. Analysis of the river water by gas
chromatography during and after acclimation showed no
accumulation of any secondary amine intermediates. Liu,
Wong and Dutka (1973) found that a bacterial mutant isolated at 22° and capable of using NTA for growth and energy
could metabolize the compound over a temperature range of 4
to 50°C. The optimal temperature for degradation was 25°C.
Tiedje and Mason (1973) found that NTA was biodegraded by
the bacteria in soil over the temperature range of 2 to
24°C. For biodegradation to occur at 2°, the soil had to
be acclimated to NTA at 12.5°C. Soil acclimated to 12.5°
degraded NTA at a faster rate at this temperature than soil

acclimated at 24°. These data suggest that a psychrophilic population, distinct from a mesaphilic population may be responsible for NTA degradation in soil acclimatized at 12.5°C. In field studies, an activated sludge system serving a trailer park showed no loss of activity in NTA removal from October through January, giving efficiencies approaching 100% during a particularly cold winter (Renn, 1973). Winter studies in a trickling filter system in Iowa State (Hubley and Cleasby, 1971) showed a NTA biodegradation of 75-87% from an influent level of 8 ppm.

NTA biodegradation appears not to be limited by low temperatures. The work by Tiedje and Mason (1973) and Swisher, and Warren (1971) indicates, however, that efficient removal of NTA at low temperatures requires the development of a psychrophilic population of bacteria. This could readily occur in any practical situation since seasonal temperature changes are gradual.

C. Oxygen Limits

Biodegradation of NTA occurs both under aerobic conditions with O_2 as the electron acceptor and under anaerobic conditions with NO_3^- as the acceptor (Enfors and Molin, 1973a). In situations where oxygen is the limiting nutrient, incomplete oxidation of amines to NO_3^- may occur and NO_2^- may accumulate in the system. It has been suggested (Wong et al., 1972) that NO_2^- may form N-nitrosamines from secondary amines (in particular iminodiacetic acid) resulting from partial breakdown of NTA. This has been tested (Swisher and Warren, 1971) both by direct addition of NO_2^- to bench scale activated sludge units receiving NTA and by addition of large enough amounts of soy peptone to decrease the dissolved oxygen content of the unit to the point that NO_2^- is produced. In both situations no secondary amines or N-nitroso-secondary amines were detected by an analytical method (Warren and Malec, 1972b) capable of detecting 25 ug/l of these compounds.

Tiedje and Mason (1973) have found that biodegradation of NTA by soil (acclimated to aerobic degradation of NTA): (a) does not occur in the absence of O_2, (b) occurs at a hindered rate in an atmosphere containing 0.1% O_2, and (c) occurs at the same rate in 1% O_2 as in air (20% O_2). Warren (1973) has found that Pseudomonas grown on NTA cannot utilize NTA in a nitrogen atmosphere. Conversion of the atmosphere from N_2 to air results in rapid growth of the Pseudomonas and subsequent conversion of NTA to CO_2, H_2O, NH_3 and cell material. Recent work by Enfors and Molin (1973a) on the other hand, suggests that NTA will not accumulate in the bottom materials of lakes and streams. He has isolated organisms from these materials that can utilize NTA for energy and growth under anaerobic conditions.

The fact that NTA is biodegraded aerobically at low O_2 concentrations and anaerobically when NO_3 is present suggests that NTA biodegradations will not be limited by the concentration of oxygen.

Conclusions

In any acceptability study of a detergent component one has to show that the proposed component is nontoxic to humans and presents no hazard to the environment. In this last area, the most important element of an environment study is the demonstration that the test compound is biodegraded to molecules normally found in the environment. This not only insures against a build-up of the compound in the environment, it also protects against any future hazard not originally anticipated. For example, if an unantici- pated hazard appears, a halt to the use of the compound will lead to its complete disappearance from the environ- ment.

Rather than present a laundry list of test results obtained from NTA biodegradation studies, the strategy behind this paper was to use published and unpublished re- search results to obtain answers or at least insight into four questions which were presented in the introduction section of this paper. Our suggested answers to these four questions are presented below.

1. Pathway of NTA Biodegradation: NTA is biodegraded by Pseudomonas to CO_2, NH_3, and H_2O. The only nonuniversal metabolite in the pathway is iminodiacetic acid. Under practical conditions, no intermediates have accumulated from NTA biodegradation even under conditions of low tem- perature, low O_2 concentration, presence of heavy metals, presence of metabolic inhibitors and presence of nitrite ions.

2. Kinetics and Mechanism of NTA Biodegradation: The Michaelis' constants for biodegradation of NTA by a Pseudomonas mutant are: K_m = 82 ug/1, V_{max} = 370 ug NTA/hr/

492

(mg dry weight cells). Comparison of oxygen uptake rates during NTA biodegradation for the above mutant to those obtained for a nonmutant <u>Pseudomonas</u> isolated from soil suggest that the above Michaelis' constants also hold for a nonmutant bacterium. These constants indicate that the enzymes in NTA acclimated bacteria have a very high affinity for NTA.

Permeation of NTA into bacterial cells is an energy consuming process. On the other hand, bacteria can use NTA as the sole source of carbon and nitrogen for energy and growth. These results suggest that bacteria can grow on very dilute solutions of NTA.

3. <u>Biodegradability of NTA Metal Complexes</u>: NTA-metal ion complexes of Ca^{2+}, Mg^{2+}, Na^+, Mn^{2+}, Fe^{2+}, and Pb^{2+} biodegrade rapidly. In comparison biodegradation of NTA-Hg^{2+}, Cd^{2+}, Cu^{2+}, Ni^{2+} and Zn^{2+} is slow. In practical systems such as rivers, lakes and soil, biodegradation of all NTA complexes is quite rapid due to ligand exchange and metal ion exchange reactions which allow NTA biodegradation to funnel through the more readily biodegradable complexes. In activated sludge treatment plants, biodegradation of the difficult to degrade NTA-metal ion complexes appears to occur by means of metal ion exchange reactions since activated sludge does not compete well with NTA for metal ions.

4. <u>Tolerance Range of NTA Biodegradation</u>:

a. pH: The pH range of biodegradation is dependent on the habitat from which the NTA-degrading bacteria have been isolated. Bacteria isolated from sewage degrade NTA in the pH range of 6.5 to 8.5; soils ranging in pH from 5.0 to 7.5 degrade NTA.

b. Temperature: NTA is biodegraded in water at 4° and in soil at 2°. Biodegradation at these temperatures, however, appears to require the development of a psychrophilic population of bacteria.

c. Oxygen concentrations: NTA is biodegraded under aerobic conditions with O_2 as the electron acceptor and under anaerobic conditions with NO_3 as the electron acceptor. NTA biodegrades at the same rate in an atmosphere composed of 1% O_2 as in air (20% O_2).

References

Bjorndal, H., H. O. Bouveng, P. Solyom, and J. Werner, <u>Vatten</u>, 28, 5 (1972).

Bouveng, H. O., G. Davisson, and E. M. Steinberg, Vatten, 24, 348, (1968).

Chaberek, S. and A. E. Martell, "Organic Sequestering Agents," John Wiley and Sons, New York, N.Y., 1959, p. 587.

Chau, Y. K., and M. T. Shiomi, Water, Air, Soil Pollution 1, 149 (1972).

Cheng, M. H., J. W. Patterson, and R. A. Minear, Preprints of Papers Presented at 166th National American Chemical Meeting, Division of Environmental Chemistry, August, 1973, p. 14.

Cripps, R. E., and A. S. Noble, Biochem. J., 130, 31p(1972).

Druckrey, H., R. Preussman, R. Blum, S. Ivankovic, and J. Afkham, Naturwissenshaften, 50, 100 (1963).

Enfors, S. O., and N. Molin, ibid., 7, 889 (1973b).

Enfors, S. O., and N. Molin, Water Res., 7, 881 (1973a).

Epstein, S. S., Staff Report for Committee on Public Works, U. S. Senate, December, 1970. Published in Int. J. Env. Studies, 2, 291; and 3, 13 (1972).

Focht, D. D. and H. A. Joseph, Can. J. Microbiology, 17, 1553 (1971).

Forsburg, C., and G. Lindqvist, Life Sci., 6, 1961 (1967a).

Forsburg, C., and G. Lindqvist, Vatten, 23, 265 (1967b).

Gudernatsch, H., Gas-Wasserfach 111, 511 (1970).

Heintz, W., Justus Liebig Ann der Chemie, 122, 257 (1862).

Huber, W., and K. H. Popp, Fette-Seifen-Anstrichmittel, 74, 166 (1972).

Hubly, D. W., and J. L. Cleasby, "Treatment of Waste Containing NTA in a Trickling Filter," Report of Engineering Research Institute, Iowa State University, Project 849-S, April, 1971. D. W. Hubly, M. S. Thesis, Iowa State Univ., 1971.

Irving, H. M. N. H., and M. G. Miles, J. Chem. Soc. (A) 1268 (1966).

Kepes, A., and G. N. Cohen, "Permeation in the Bacterium," I. C. Gunsalus and R. Y. Stanier, (Ed.), Academic Press, New York, N.Y., 1962, p. 179.

Knezak, B. D., C. M. Mugwira and B. G. Ellis, Report No. PB-220-950, Dept. of Crop and Soil Sciences, Michigan State University, East Lansing, Mich. (1973).

Lerman, A., and C. W. Childs, "Trace Metals and Metal-Organic Interactions in Natural Waters," P. C. Singer, (ed.), Ann Arbor Science Publishers, Inc., Ann Arbor, Mich. 1973, Ch. 7.

Lijinsky, W., M. Gocenblatt, C. Kommineni, J. Nat. Canc.

Inst., 50, 1061 (1973).

Liu, D., P. T. S. Wong and B. J. Dutka, J. Water Pollut. Contr. Fed., 45, 1728 (1973).

Miles, M. G., "The Synthesis of Some New Aminopolycarboxylic Acids and a Study of Their Potentialities as Chelating Agents," Ph.D. Thesis, University of Leeds, (1965).

Mottola, H. A., Toxicological and Env. Chem. Rev., In Press (1973).

Pfeil, B. H., and G. F. Lee, Environ. Sci. Technol., 2, 543 (1968).

Renn, C. E., Unpublished Data, Colgate Company, (1973).

Rudd, J. W. M., and R. D. Hamilton, J. Fish. Res. Bd. Can. 29, 1203 (1972).

Shumate, K. S., J. E. Thompson, J. D. Brookhart, and C. L. Dean, J. Water Pollut. Contr. Fed., 42, 631 (1970).

Sillen, L. G., and A. E. Martell, (Eds.), ibid, Special Publication No. 25, Chemical Society, London (1971).

Sillen, L. G., and A. E. Martell, (Eds.), "Stability Constants of Metal Ion Complexes," Special Publication No. 17, Chemical Society, London (1964).

Singer, J. J., and M. Weisberg, U. S. Patent No. 3,061,628, Oct. 30, 1962.

Swisher, R. D., M. M. Crutchfield and D. W. Caldwell, Environ. Sci. Technol., 1, 820 (1967).

Swisher, R. D., T. A. Taulli, and E. J. Malec, "Trace Metals and Metal-Organic Interactions in Natural Waters," P. C. singer, (Ed.), Ann Arbor Science Publishers, Inc., Ann Arbor, Mich., 1973, Ch. 8.

Swisher, R. D., and C. B. Warren, Unpublished Data, Monsanto Company (1971).

Taylor, L. K., R. Alvarez, R. A. Paulson, T. C. Rains, H. L. Rook, Water Pollution Control Research Series, 16020 GFR 07/71, Environmental Protection Agency (1971).

Thayer, P. S., and C. J. Kensler, CRC Critical Reviews in Environmental Control, 3, 375 (1973).

Thompson, J. E., and J. R. Duthie, J. Water Pollut. Contr. Fed., 40, 306 (1968).

Tiedje, J. M., Unpublished Data, Michigan State University, (1973).

Tiedje, J. M., and S. D. Aust, Unpublished Data, Michigan State University (1973).

Tiedje, J. M., M. K. Firestone, B. B. Mason, and C. B. Warren, Abs. 73rd A.S.M. meeting (1973b).

Tiedje, J. M., and B. B. Mason, Soil Sci. Soc. Am. Proc.,

in press, (1973).

Tiedje, J. M., B. B. Mason, C. B. Warren, E. J. Malec, Appl. Microbiol., 25, 811 (1973a).

Ulrich, H., and E. Ploetz, U. S. Patent No. 2,205,995, June 25, 1940.

Warren, C. B., Unpublished Data, Monsanto Company (1973).

Warren, C. B., and E. J. Malec, J. Chromatog. 64. 219 (1972b).

Warren, C. B., and E. J. Malec, Science, 176, 277 (1972a).

Wong, P. T. S., D. Liu, B. J. Dutka, Water Res., 6, 1577 (1972).

Wong, P. T. S., D. Liu, and D. J. McGirr, Water Res., 7, 1367 (1973).

Wong, P. T. S., J. Thompson, R. A. MacLeod, J. Biol. Chem., 244, 1016 (1969).

ECOLOGICAL AND HEALTH EFFECTS
OF POLLUTANTS IN AUTOMOBILE EXHAUST

D. G. Penney, J. P. Bederka, Jr.,
J. S. McLellan, W. F. Coello,
Z. A. Saleem and M. A. Q. Khan

University of Illinois at Chicago Circle
and Medical Center, Chicago

Introduction

Approximately 200 million tons of man-made pollutants are released into the air over the United States every year. Automobiles contribute about half of these pollutants, which include: carbon monoxide (CO), 64,000,000 tons; hydrocarbons, 17,000,000 tons; nitrogen oxides, 8,000,000 tons; sulfur oxides, 800,000 tons and particulate matter, 1,200,000 tons. Within this latter category is included about 220,000 tons of lead released from the burning of 75 billion gallons of gasoline each year by motor vehicles (Stoker and Seager, 1972; Anonymous, 1967).

The amount of these pollutants from auto-exhaust in any given locale obviously depends upon the number of vehicles present. This in turn depends upon the size and type of community. It is common knowledge to all that the concentrations of these pollutants are higher in cities than in most rural areas. This is true for the reason already mentioned as well as for the fact that cities present both vertical and horizontal barriers to distribution of air pollutants. For example, in cities during rush hour, carbon monoxide concentrations at street level of 100 ppm and above and lead levels of 71 ug/m^3 (Chow, 1973) are not uncommon, whereas rural areas show very much lower concentrations of both pollutants. Thus, humans, their dwellings, animals and vegetation in urban areas are constantly exposed to ever increasing levels of air pollutants. Lead is the more persistent contaminant, while carbon monoxide is the most abundant. It should be borne in mind of course, that these two auto-exhaust contaminants have different dispositions in the environment. This is the case, since about 95% of the CO can be removed from the air by soil micro-organisms, but lead cannot be metabolically degraded by living organisms. The overall annual increase of atmospheric lead content in the U. S. is about 7%. However, some large cities and their suburbs have shown up to 60% increases during the past several years. For example, the overall average of atmospheric lead for the Los Angeles basin increased from 2.32 ug/m^3 in 1961-62 to 3.60 ug/m^3 in 1968-69 (PHS, 1965 and EPA, 1972). Similar increases have been observed in other large American cities (Table 1).

City	Lead Concentration (ug/m^3)
"Natural Atmosphere"	.0006
Chicago, IL	0.5 - 7.8
Cincinnati, OH	1.0 - 11.7
La Jolla, CA	0.42 (annual average)
Los Angeles, CA	
freeway	14 - 38
downtown	
(rush hour)	40
basin: overall ave.	
1961/62	2.32
1968/69	3.60
Miami, FL	1.7
Mojave, CA	0.1 - 0.4
New York, NY	2.5
Pasadena, CA	0.9 - 4.3
Philadelphia, PA	0.3 - 3.4
San Diego, CA	2.1
U.S. National Average	0.1 - 17
downtown	2 - 3
suburban	1 - 2
Japan (11 major cities)	.78 - 11.1
Italy (rush hour)	0 - 40
England:	
Warwick (busy street)	3.5
London (Fleet street)	3.2 - 5.4
U.S.S.R.:	
Novaya Zemlya	0.002

Table 1. Ambient Air Content of Lead in Cities (Chow, 1973; Huang, 1972)

Ecological Effects of Lead in Auto-Exhaust

W. F. Coello, Z. A. Saleem
and M. A. Q. Khan

Department of Biological Sciences
University of Illinois at Chicago Circle

Lead in automobile exhaust and contamination of our environment

The compounds added to gasoline include: tetraethyl
lead, 62%; ethylene dichloride, 18%; ethylene dibromide,
18%; and other miscellaneous additives, 2%. Tetraethyl
lead acts as an antiknock agent for high-compression internal combusion engines. The halogens act as scavengers in
reacting with lead during gasoline combustion. This results in the formation of lead bromochloride and lead
bromochloride-lead oxide ($PbBrCl-2PbO$), both of which are
gaseous at room temperature. These reaction products are
unstable and become converted to the following compounds:
lead carbonate-lead oxide, 30%; lead carbonate, 14%; lead
bromochloride, 12% and lead chloride, 8% (Stoker and Seager,
1972). These are the major lead compounds released into
the atmosphere via auto-exhaust. It is not surprising then
that there is a fairly direct relationship between traffic
count on a given highway and soil content of lead in close
proximity to the highway (Table 2). This is also evident
from the high correlation coefficient ($r=0.941$) seen in Fig.
1 with the average traffic volumes and average soil lead

Cars/Hr.	Soil Lead (ppm)	References
900	2.12	Daines et al., (1970)
1,900	4.34	Daines et al., (1970)
2,400	10.10	Daines et al., (1970)
17,300	565	Khan et al., (1973)
50,400	1,372	Khan et al., (1973)
97,000	2,166	Khan et al., (1973)

Table 2. Relationship of Traffic Volume and Soil Lead
Concentration

499

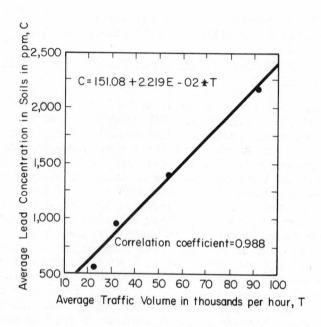

Fig. 1. Correlation between average concentration of lead in soil and average traffic volume

Distance: Feet	Air Lead: ug/m^3	Plant Lead: ppm; Dry Wt
5	5.0	20-60
40	2.3	15
120	1.7	8.4
1,000	–	5

Table 3. Lead Concentration in Grasses (Perennial Rye/Grass) along Highways (1,300 Cars/Hr.)

concentrations. Atmospheric lead concentrations stabilize at low levels approximately 100 feet from the road, probably due to rapid settling of particles larger than 5u in diameter and the downward traverse of smaller particles entrained in the turbulent atmosphere (Habibi, 1970; Mottu et al., 1970). About 85% of the lead in the air between 30 and 1750 feet from the roadway is particulate and under 4u in diameter and about 80% of this is under 2u in diameter (Daines et al., 1970). Lead concentration in the atmosphere decreases rapidly with distance from the highway and this is reflected in the lead content of vegetation at varying distances from heavily trafficed roads as shown in Table 3 and Figure 2. The marked effect of traffic on lead content of air is thus limited to a rather narrow zone within 50 feet of the leeside of the highway (Daines et al., 1970).

Lead is conveyed to the soil from auto-exhaust via the air and we might expect to see a good correlation between air lead concentration and soil lead concentration. This is indeed the case as shown in Figure 3. Some of the airborne lead may however travel long distances before removal by various mechanisms. A number of factors affect the theoretical atmospheric lead contamination from auto-exhaust. These include: volume of traffic, local meteorology, traffic pattern, vehicle condition, driving habits, etc.

Factors affecting environmental concentrations of lead

Lead removal from the air by precipitation in rainwater is a major mechanism. For example, the mean annual deposition of lead via rainwater in New England (19.6 mg/m^2) in 1972 was eighteen times higher than that reported in the mountains of California, but lower than that reported in some urban areas. In rainwater itself current lead concentrations (in ug/l) for various portions of the U.S. are reported to be lowest in California at 1.6 as an overall mean, 18.9 in Illinois overall, while the national median is 10 (Schlesinger et al., 1972). In California urban areas, rainwater lead concentrations, however, may run as high as 200-500 ug/l. It has been estimated that the mean atmospheric residence time for natural lead 210 is 9-16 days (Francis et al., 1970). On the average the soil receives about 1 ug/cm^2/year of lead from precipitation, while

501

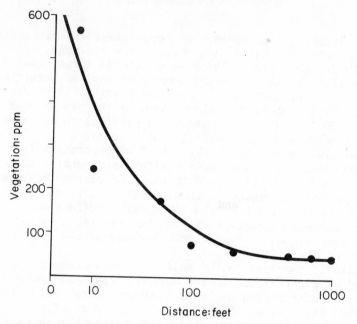

Fig. 2. Plot of variation of lead concentration in vegetation
with distance in feet from a highway

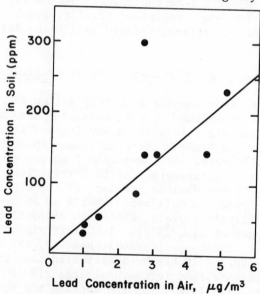

Fig. 3. Relationship between soil lead and atmospheric lead
concentrations (Coello and Khan, unpublished data)

about 0.2 ug/cm^2/year is deposited as dustfall.
Approximately 0.2% of the existing natural burden of soil
lead is added each year from atmospheric sources (Chow,
1973).

As seen earlier, lead concentration depends strongly
upon, among other factors, traffic density and proximity to
the roadway. The measured lead concentrations in surface
soils in certain city parks showed the following lead
levels; Balboa Park, San Diego, 194 ppm; Golden Gate Park,
San Francisco, 560 ppm and McArthur Park, Los Angeles,
3,357 ppm (Zimdahl and Arvik, 1973). Levels of lead in
soils along two of Chicago's expressways are shown in
Table 4. Levels of lead in the soil were as high as 7,600
ppm along the Eisenhower Expressway.

	Distance From Road: Feet	Lead:ppm		
		Soil	Vegetation	Bark
Eisenhower expressway	13-45	60-7,590	0-685	36,670-142,000
Terminal Loop expressway	20	10-2,230	---	1,200- 13,200
Lake Shore Dr.	100	---	(5-202)	(216- 38,855)

Table 4. Ranges of Lead Concentrations in Dried Vegetation
and Soils along Chicago's Three Busy Highways

Lead content of plants

Since traffic density, strength and direction of the
wind and other atmospheric factors affect the transport of
airborne lead, contamination of plants will also depend on
these factors, as well as on the distance of plants from
the road, exposure time of plant organs, exposed surface of
leaves and the distribution and location of leaves. Plants
absorb lead only in its soluble form from the soil through
the roots and there may be a limited translocation to the
shoots. Lead halides in auto-exhaust are relatively soluble and may be carried down into the soil for short
distances. With time these compounds are converted to less
soluble phosphates, carbonates and sulfates, etc. Organic
chelation can also make lead less mobile in the soil and
less available to plants. Thus, most of the lead remains
within the upper 6 inches of the soil, because of its

503

adsorption to organic and inorganic matter and due to its
insolubility (Motto et al., 1970).

Assuming that most of the lead in aerial parts of
plants along highways is due to atmospheric fallout, an inverse relationship between distance from the highway and
vegetation lead concentration should exist. Such a
relationship was noted earlier for rye (Table 3). This has
also been observed for chaff, potato and privet. For example, along a highway with 900 cars/hr the foliage contained
162 ppm lead, while along a highway with 2,700 cars/hr
the foliage showed 570 ppm lead (Zimdahl and Arvik, 1973).
The vegetation within 100 feet of Chicago's Eisenhower
expressway and Lake Shore Drive showed up to 700 ppm lead
as seen in Tables 4 and 5.

Sample 15-55 feet from roadway	Lead Concentration range: ppm (ave.)
Trees	21 - 640 (100)
Grass	0 - 52 (28)
Common garden weed (dandelion):	
whole plant	0 - 685 (64)
leaves	0 - 685 (60)
flowers	14 - 52 (34)
roots	2 - 650 (100)

Table 5. Lead Concentrations in Plants along Chicago's
Eisenhower Expressway (Coello and Khan, unpublished data)

The dry bark of bushes and trees shows very high concentrations of lead (Table 4). Lincoln Park (p. 506)
located 1,000 feet away and downwind from Lake Shore Drive
on Chicago's north side, showed up to 39,000 ppm lead
in the dry bark of trees with an average of 6,350 ppm.
However, similar samples from bushes growing within 15-45
feet of the Eisenhower expressway showed 37,000 to 142,000
ppm lead with an average of 100,000 ppm. Woodshavings
along the terminal loop expressway showed up to 15,000
ppm lead with an average of 7,000 ppm. In contrast,
the bark from trees on the grounds of the Brookfield
Zoological Gardens on Chicago's west side showed a maximum
lead concentration of 400 ppm. In rural areas, the dry
needles of conifers flanking roads with a traffic density
of 1,000 cars/hr have shown lead concentrations as high as
700 ppm. Lead deposited in the annual rings of an elm

tree located 50 feet from a suburban street showed increasing lead concentration with age suggesting the rapid rate at which we are contaminating the environment with lead: 1865-1912, 0.16 ppm; 1940-1947, 0.33 ppm; 1956-1958, 0.74 ppm and 1960 on 3.90 ppm. A one hundred year increase of over 25-fold is seen (Zimdahl and Arvik, 1973).

The lead content of vegetation, especially the edible portions which are consumed by animals and humans must be examined carefully. Table 5 shows the concentrations of lead which have been measured in trees, grasses and various portions of dandelion plants growing along the Eisenhower expressway in Chicago. It can be seen that lead concentrations as high as 600-685 ppm were observed. These lead concentrations in weeds such as the dandelion may be of considerable importance, since they are not uncommonly cooked and eaten by certain ethnic groups in Chicago (Coello and Khan, unpublished data). Vegetation sampled at a number of specific sites over a distance of several miles along this same roadway show similar high lead concentrations (Table 6). Pasture herbage along highways normally shows up to 1.5 ppm lead, except in the fall when concentrations of 30-40 ppm are not uncommon. Similar lead increases in the fall have also been observed in the leaves of some deciduous trees and in wild oats (Rains, 1971). Vegetable samples randomly collected in 1969 contained the following amounts of lead: cabbage leaves, 815 ppm; iceburg lettuce, 915 ppm; tomatoes, 89 ppm; turnip tuber, 58 ppm and potato, 815 ppm (Langerwerff et al., 1973). Corn grown along highways is reported to show up to 25 ppm lead in the leaves, while that grown in wooded areas has a range of 0.3 to 30 ppm. The husk, cob, and kernels of corn grown in air with 1.4 to 3.0 ug lead/m^3 showed no difference in the ratio of lead in cob and kernels as compared with corn grown in filtered air (Zimdahl and Arvik, 1973).

Since airborne lead settles on plant surfaces, leaf size and shape are critical factors in plant contamination. Texture and hairiness of the leaf surface may also be important in this regard (Motto et al., 1970; Bini, 1973; Cannon and Bowles, 1969). Washing can remove 30-60% of the lead from vegetables (Daines et al., 1970). After summer rains, the lead concentration in vegetation along a highway decreased from an average of 77 to 28 ppm. That vegetation closest to the road was most affected by the

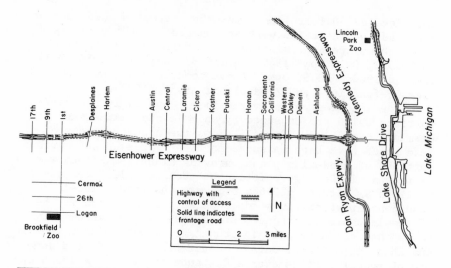

Sampling Site	Lead Concentration and Range: ppm			
	13–25'	26–45'	46–55'	Average
Western Exit	37	116	42	54
	(6– 85)	(14–450)	(6– 77)	(6–450)
California Exit	73	32	57	44
	(0–650)	(0–126)	(0–600)	(0–650)
Cicero Exit	27	99	---	48
	(0– 65)	(66–178)		(0–178)
Oakley/Western	75	---	---	
	(2–130)			
California/Sacramento	47	45	---	
	(0–650)	(0–640)		
Pulaski/Kostner	178	217	---	
Laramie/Cicero	15	99	---	
	(0– 65)	(62–178)		
Laramie/Central	37	54	---	
	(29– 63)	(11–131)		
"Merge/Exits Lane"	---	446	---	
		(51–685)		

Table 6. Lead Concentration in Vegetation along Eisenhower
Expressway Sampled During June–August of 1973,
(13–55 feet from roadway, right hand shoulder,
west bound; Khan et al., 1973)

rainfall (Zimdahl and Arvik, 1973). Similar plant lead
content decreases following rainfall have been observed by
Coello and Khan. Mosses which obtain minerals from precipitation and settled dust, showed an increase from 20 ppm
lead in 1960 to 90 ppm lead in 1968 along Swedish
highways (Bini, 1973). However, in this regard, it is reported that the lichen, Cladonia rangiformis, can absorb
atmospheric lead without showing adverse effects (Zimdahl
and Arvik, 1973). In areas of heavy automobile traffic in
the U.S., mosses growing on trees and bushes probably accumulate much higher lead concentrations than reported in
Sweden.

The amount of lead which can be absorbed from soils by
roots and then translocated to other parts of the plant has
been investigated by several workers (Zimdahl and Arvik,
1973). Root absorption depends not only on total lead in
the soil, but rather on the amount of soluble lead available
and the soil conditions. This in turn is affected by soil
pH, temperature, availability of calcium, heavy metals,
phosphates and silicon. Since most of the lead stays in
the upper 6 inches of the soil and only 0.005% of this is
soluble, root uptake of lead may be critical in plants
whose edible parts are underground and those which do not
have deep roots. Soluble lead nitrate at 100-400 ppm in
the soil quickly accumulates in roots of tomatoes and
potatoes, although the leaves of these plants accumulate
lead more slowly (Bini, 1973). Broad beans, perennial grass,
raddish, tobacco seedlings, lemon cuttings, barley plants
and corn plants all absorb lead rapidly through their roots.
Most of this lead accumulates in the roots. For example,
barley plants and lemon cuttings show 800 to 900 ppm lead
in the roots and only 3 ppm lead in the leaves. However,
corn plants show much higher concentrations of lead in their
leaves in similar studies (Zimdahl and Arvik, 1973).

Lead has been shown to inhibit plant growth and cause
reduction of photosynthesis, water absorption and it may
cause copper deficiency. The French bean, Phaseolus, is
reportedly damaged by 30 ppm lead in solution culture.
Similarily, 3 ppm lead has been shown to be toxic to
fescue. Lead in plants associates with mitochondria and
chloroplasts. In vitro inhibition of succinate oxidation
and stimulation of the oxidation of reduced nicotinamide
adenine dinucleotide (NADH) by lead has been observed in
corn mitochondria (Koeppe and Miller, 1971).

Lead burden in waters

The overall average natural lead level in surface freshwater is approximately 0.5 ug/l. However, this may vary greatly with location as seen in Table 7 (Kehoe, 1966; Chow, 1973). The global mean for lakes and rivers lies between 1 and 10 ug/l, while the maximum lead concentration found in U.S. rivers and lakes is 140 ug/l. Only 2% of the 1,700 samples taken during a

Water	Lead: ug/l
Sea Water	1 - 8
Ground Water	1 - 60
Surface Water	1 - 55
Drinking Water	1 - 500

Table 7. Lead Content of Water

1962-1967 survey contained lead in excess of the 50 ug/l limit set by the U.S. Public Health Service. Nevertheless, concentrations of lead higher than this are common in waters near certain industrial facilities. A study of run-off and chemical loads from the world's largest rivers shows lead to be present at or below 100 ug/l, the median value being 10 ug/l. Since the sea is the final catch basin for most water soluble contaminants, we might expect sea water to contain significant quanties of lead. This is certainly the case as shown in Table 7.

The lead concentration in the public water supplies of the 100 largest cities in the U.S. range from a trace to 500 ug/l. Some of this lead may be contributed by lead pipes in old plumbing systems. However, industrial and mining effluents often contain several hundred ug lead/l. A portion of this contaminant load may be precipitated and settled-out almost immediately, while another portion is carried into the oceans. This is seen in near-shore, shallow sea water in industrialized regions where much higher lead concentrations are found than in deeper water in the open ocean (0.008-0.4 Vs 0.03 ug/l). Even the ice in Greenland now shows 0.2 ug lead per kg (Chow, 1973).

The average lead level in sewage effluents is estimated to be around 100 ug/l, with the sludge containing 2,000-8,000 ppm lead on a dry weight basis. Use of such sludge as a fertilizer could obviously contaminate the top layer of soil and vegetation grown upon it. A schematic representation of the movement of lead through ecosystems is shown in Fig. 4, (p. 512).

Effects of lead on fish and other animals in food chains

The toxicity of lead to several species of freshwater

508

fish has been examined and is shown in Table 8. It appears
that the mechanism of toxicity may be different at high
concentrations and short exposures than at low concentrations and long exposure. As compared with lead, copper was
generally more toxic and chromium less toxic to fishes.
The acute TLm values would cause fish mortality under most
environmental conditions, even during short exposures.
Data on the chronic effects of sub-lethal concentrations of
lead are badly needed. Recent studies show that the goldfish, guppy and minnow are very sensitive to lead while
fishes such as bass and bluegill are quite resistant
(Coello and Khan). The latter species elaborate a mucous
substance on the outer surface which removes the lead from
the integument.

Animals in an area with high atmospheric lead levels
can become contaminated either by inhalation or by feeding
on contaminated food. Earthworms, for example, which in-
gest earth in soils along a highway have been found to
accumulate up to 331 ppm lead. As the concentration of
lead in soils decreases with distance from the roadway so
does the lead in earthworms (Gish and Christensen, 1973).
Such high concentrations of lead may be lethal to animals
feeding on earthworms for extended periods of time. For
example, adult mallards can be killed with 200 ppm lead
in the diet over a long period of time. Dry conditions can
also result in high concentrations of lead in the food of
herbivores as reported for cows fed for 3 weeks on hay which
contained 99 ppm lead and was harvested along a busy highway
in Switzerland. As a result, blood and milk lead levels
were raised nearly 4-fold in relation to those of control
cows. The muscle, kidney, liver, pelvic bones and udders
of cows showed 3, 11, 21 and 19 times more lead than controls
(Zimdahl and Arvik, 1973).

Adult human exposure to lead

Natural foods contain small quantities of lead which
may be increased due to aerial fall-out. The mean dietary
lead intake for adult Americans is about 300 ug/day. Lead
may also enter the human body through the respiratory tract
by inhalation of air contaminated with auto-exhaust. An
urban adult breathing air containing 3 ug lead/m^3 and respiring about 15m^3 of air per day will absorb 20-25 ug of
lead through the respiratory tract everyday. About the

Fish	TLm: mg/1*		
	24 Hr.	48 Hr.	69 Hr.
Flathead Minnow			
soft water	9.84(14.6)	8.75(10.4)	6.46(7.48)
hard water	432	482	482
Bluegills			
soft water	25.9	24.5	23.8
hard water	482	468	442
Goldfish			
soft water	45.4	31.5	31.5
hard water	24.5	24.5	20.6

*Values in parentheses are for lead acetate for the median
limits of tolerance (TLm).

Table 8. Toxicity of Lead Chloride to Fresh Water Fishes
(Pickering and Henderson, 1972)

Type of Population	Mean Blood Lead ug/100ml
Population without known occupational exposures:	
Remote California mountain	12 (9)
Composite Rural U.S.	16 (10)
Suburban Philadelphia	13 (13)
Composite Urban U.S.	21 (16)
Los Angeles Aircraft workers	19 (17)
Pasadena city employees	19 (12)
Downtown Phildelphia	24 (18)
Population with known occupational exposures:	
Cincinnati policeman	25
Cincinnati trafficman	30
Cincinnati automobile test-lane inspectors	31
Cincinnati garage workers	31
Boston Summer-Tunnel employees	30

*U.S. Department of Health, Education, and Welfare, Public
Survey of lead in the Atmosphere of three Urban Com-
munities, Publication #999-AP02 Jan., 1965.
Values in parentheses for females.

Table 9. Blood Lead Levels of Selected Human Populations*

same amount of lead is absorbed via the gut wall from a normal daily dietary intake of about 300 ug. The intake from these two sources of course may be higher in certain communities. The average concentration of lead in Americans in urban populations is increasing due to lead in auto-exhaust (Table 9). Seemingly sublethal quantities of lead are absorbed and at least partly retained over a long period of time. The threshold levels for potential poisoning with delayed toxic effects may thus be exceeded due to this cumulative effect (Robinowitz et al., 1973). The pharmacodymanics of lead in animals (humans) is shown in Fig. 5.

A large part of the dietary inorganic lead is absorbed in the duodenum, but re-excreted in the bile, with a 5-15% net absorption. This and the lead absorbed via the lung alveoli is circulated through the blood stream by binding to erythrocytes and to some diffusible organic ligands. The mean life of lead in blood is 0.27 days, with about 50% of this lead being lost through urinary excretion. Lead is stored in bones and in soft tissues, particularly in the liver and kidney. It is also present in hair, teeth and nails. The organs critically involved in lead intoxication are; hematopoietic tissue, central and peripheral nervous systems and the kidney.

As stated earlier, dietary lead intake results in absorption of about 25 ug of lead/day. An aerosol concentration of 2 ug of lead/m^3 results in absorption of about 26 ug of lead/day. Thus, the total absorption is about 51 ug/day. Isotopic studies show that excretion in urine, nails, hair and sweat is 42 ug/day. About 7 ug of lead enters the skeleton per day from the blood and is stored there. Thus, in atmospheres with lead concentrations higher than 2 ug/m^3, humans will differentially both store and excrete lead absorbed in excess of about 50 ug/day. Such elevated atmospheric concentrations are common in many large cities in the U.S. and other countries and contribute to the blood lead values shown in Tables 9 and 10. Non-urban humans show 10-16 ug of lead per 100 ml of blood, while individuals living near a freeway in California showed an average of 17-23 ug of lead per 100 ml of blood. Traffic policemen, cab drivers, etc., may show even higher blood lead concentrations. There is a continuous turnover of lead in the body, so measured concentrations in the blood tend to reflect the current degree of exposure. The lead in bones may be mobilized during feverish illness, cortisone treatment and old age; however, the biological half-life of lead in the human is 2-3 years.

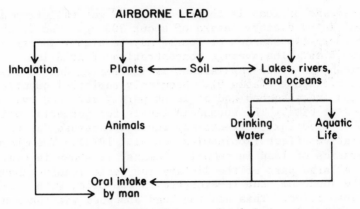

Fig. 4. Transport of airborne lead in ecosystems

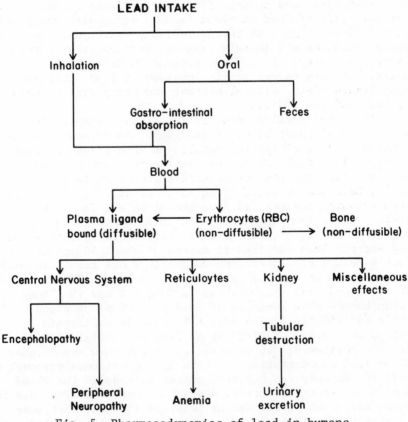

Fig. 5. Pharmacodynamics of lead in humans

A. Lead Effects in the Newborn and Infant

Species	Dose	Effect
Rat	Maternal diet (4% $PbCO_3$) (40 ppm lead in milk)	Hyperactivity (40-90%), aggressiveness, tremors and stereotypies(self-grooming) at four weeks--brain lead(80 ug/g) = 6-9 times controls
Rat	Lead acetate, (orally) 10-3,000 ug/g/day	Death before 30 days of age at 400 ug/g/day--body and brain growth depressed at 50 ug/g/day--CNS hemorrhages at 750 ug/g/day
Mouse	Lead acetate, 10 mg/ml in drinking water	Hyperactivity (100%) at 40-60 days of age--delayed growth and development
Monkey	Lead subacetate, 500 mg, 2X/week for 3 months	CNS capillary destruction
Human	Less than 5 mg/day for several months	Clumsiness, abdominal pain, headache, drowsiness, vomiting, convulsions

B. Maternal - Fetal "Steady States" for Lead

Route and Species	Maternal Dose or Concentration of Lead	Concentration of Lead in Fetus or Newborn
Diet/Rat	0.61 ug/g	0.56 ug/g
	64.0 ug/g	4.2 ug/g
	512.0 ug/g	23.0 ug/g
I.V./Rat	50 ug/ml (6 hrs.)	0.3 ug/g
	705 ug/ml (64 min.)	6.0 ug/g
	1080 ug/ml (64 min.)	53.0 ug/g
I.V./Mouse	30 ug/ml (6 hrs.)	0.02 ug/g
I.V./Goat	26 ug% (0 time)	25 ug%
	45 ug% (200 min. infusion)	25 ug%
Ambient/Human	14 ug% (6-26)	11 ug% (cord blood) (4-24)

Table 10. Lead Concentrations and Biodynamics in some Mammals

Developmental Effects of Lead

J. P. Bederka, Jr. and J. S. McLellan

Department of Pharmacognosy
and Pharmacology
University of Illinois
at the Medical Center

Lead effects in the infant

The incidence of acute lead poisoning in children is inordinately high in regard to their relative contribution to the total population. The reason for this seems to be related to their behavioral characteristic of examining their environment by tasting the various items that they encounter (which behavior may be reinforced by a contributing lead-palliated calcium deficiency). Thus, the use of the term "pica" from the latin for magpie, whose scavenging tendencies are legend. This incidence of acute lead encephalopathy in children is frequently related to urban sites in association with old buildings wherein lead-containing building materials were used. The reason for this apparent site specificity may also be related to the fact that these populations lend themselves to epidemiological-type studies. It is quite likely that many poisonings are also occurring in rural areas, but go undetected and thus unreported, since it is quite certain that the same building materials were used in those sites as well (Snowdon and Sanderson, 1974; Schaplowsky, 1971). Children between the ages of 1 and 6 years with diagnoses of acute lead encephalopathy have been found to have blood lead levels between 100 and 1,000 ug/100 ml of blood (Chisolm, 1970). These elevated lead levels in all cases have been attributed to the ingestion of lead-containing solids or liquids with an added atmospheric lead burden. Developmental studies of these lead poisoned children have shown significant anomalies mostly related to the nervous system. Related studies on children with blood lead levels of 60-140 ug/100 ml have shown no gross developmental

515

defects. Some investigators, however, have reported
behavioral and fine motor abnormalities in these children.
In these human studies, prenatal exposure to lead was not
considered and the populations were selected so as to contain only lead-exposed normals and low-lead normals at the
beginnings of the studies. The conclusion of some of these
investigations is that sublethal concentrations of toxicants in the environment, such as lead, seem to alter the
development of children less than the socioeconomic factors
controlling the environment, in so far as current quantitative measurements can be used to compare the effects of the
two environmental forces (Kotok, 1972). It is assumed that
levels of blood lead below 60 ug/100 ml are without effects
on the population, since chelation therapy is usually begun
only at lead concentrations higher than 60 ug/100 ml. In
fact, the average blood lead levels in many adult and child
populations vary between 5 and 40 ug/100 ml. Thus, maternal
blood lead levels of this magnitude insure that during preg-
nancy the embryo will be exposed to similar concentrations
of lead as shown by Caprio et al. (1974), in Newark, New
Jersey.

Developmental Toxicology of Lead in Mice

Introduction

In studies with mice, certain members of a population
exposed in utero to concentrations of toxicants that are
sublethal to the adult, showed toxicant-mediated developmental anomalies. These teratogenic and/or developmental
effects have been noted at about 10% of the adult toxic
dose for several compounds (Goldstein et al., 1963;
McLellan et al., 1974). Thus a parallel situation may occur with human lead concentration-effects where the in
utero exposure is about 1/10 the childhood toxic dose. The
studies summarized here (previously unpublished) were designed to investigate certain possible developmental
toxicities associated with exposure of the embryo to a lead
insult via the maternal route. Pregnant mice were treated
with a low dose of lead II which corresponded to the equivalent of a body burden of about 100 ug/100 ml and also to a
dose 10-fold higher. If one assumes a total body distribution of the parenterally administered lead, then this low
dose corresponds roughly to the lower limit of blood levels
of lead associated with acute nervous system toxicities in

516

children.

Teratogenic and/or developmental effects

Litter sizes in the lead-treated groups of mice were
normal and the percent dead or resorbed fetuses was the
same as in controls, that is, about 2%. Fetal birth
weights in the high dosage groups were 61% of the control
group and crown-rump length was 86% of the control value.
No macroscopic teratogenic effects were seen in intact and
razor-sectioned 18-day cesarean specimens using a dis-
secting microscope. Microscopic teratogenic and/or develp-
mental anomalies in 15 fetuses included generally incomplete and/or delayed ossification of the phalanges, ster-
nebrae and vertebrae. Similar studies in the rat and
hamster have been reported by Carpenter et al., (1973).

Weight gain

Mean birth weights per litter in the high lead dosage
groups were 61% of the control and low dosage values. However, those animals that survived until day 3 showed no
significant mean weight difference among groups. Beginning
on day 3, the animals were weighed every day until day 10,
and then three times weekly thereafter. Data on rate of
body weight gain in control mice and mice exposed to high
and low dosages of lead are seen in Figure 6. Body weights
in the low dosage and control groups were significantly
different on days 15 and 35 of the study. In the high lead
dosage groups, body weights increased like the controls until about day 11, at which time body weights decreased and
mortality rates increased. Those mice in the high dosage
group that did survive this critical period from day 10 to
about day 18 did not attain the body weights of the controls at 35 days of age. Interestingly, the mean body
weight of the survivors in the low dosage group was only
somewhat greater than the control value on day 35, but
significantly less than the control body weights on day 15;
perhaps, due to a higher mortality of the smaller animals.

Mortality profile

The death rate was different for each of the three
groups. Mortality from day 0-3 was 60% in the high dosage

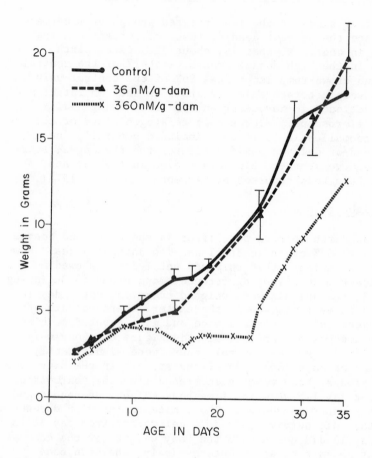

Fig. 6. Growth of mice exposed in utero to lead (II) chloride

group and 25% in both of the other groups. The control group showed only a 25% overall mortality at day 25 of this study, whereas the low and high dosage groups showed 36 and 80% overall mortality, respectively. In the low dosage group, only one litter showed 100% mortality by day 10, while in the high dosage group only one litter had 0% mortality on day 30 and 10 litters had 100% mortality. Four maternal deaths were seen in the high dosage groups 30 or more days postpartum, while no maternal deaths were seen in the other two groups during the 60-day observation period.

Gross motor activity of juvenile mice

Gross motor activity was examined in control mice and mice given both low and high dosages of lead II. The results of these studies are shown in Figure 7. The gross motor activity was quantitated by placing mice in groups of three into a photobeam activity cage and recording the number of counts for a period of 30 mintues. As shown, the control and low dosage groups had similar activities. The high dosage group, however, showed an overall reduction in activity and did not exhibit the normal rate of increase in activity with age. There was a dramatic rise in activity at day 20 in both lead treated groups, the time at which if there were to be deaths they would already have taken place. Yet, after day 20 the surviving mice in the high dosage group still were not as active as the other two groups and at day 35 the mean activity value for the high dosage groups was only 54% of the control, whereas for the low dosage group mean activity was 88% of control.

Summary

Thus, it appears that relatively high levels of lead entering the fetal and, perhaps, neonatal mouse via the maternal route result in microscopic teratogenic effects and decreased fetal birth weight in mice. Effects on post-natal development in the form of increased mortality, slower rate of body weight gain and depressed gross motor activity are also seen during the first 35 days of life in mice. Similar effects upon development at present body levels of lead are possible in the more sensitive members of the human and other species. Any contribution of maternal lead toxicity to the neonatal developmental toxicity remains to be elucidated.

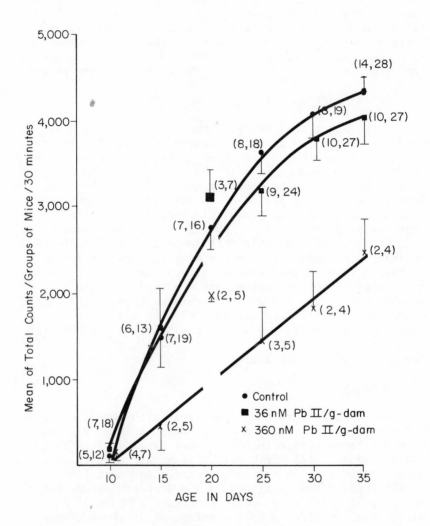

Fig. 7. Gross motor activities of normal and lead (II) chloride-treated mice

Cardiovascular Effects of Carbon Monoxide (CO)

D. G. Penney

Department of Biology
University of Illinois at Chicago Circle

Introduction

Information on the cardiovascular effects of prolonged carbon monoxide-exposure on animals and humans is relatively meager. This is so in spite of the fact that modern man, and more particularly urban man is frequently exposed to relatively high concentrations of this toxic gas. Auto-exhaust represents a major, but by no means the only source of CO contaminating our environment. For example, levels of CO in vehicles in urban rush-hour traffic sometimes exceed 100 ppm (U.S.DHEW, 1970). In air in more confined spaces where heavy use of motor vehicles exists, such as in garages, underground parking areas and vehicular tunnels, CO has been reported to range up to several hundred ppm for extended periods of time (Waller et al., 1965; Chovin, 1967). Thus, traffic policemen, cab drivers and others constantly working in areas of heavy vehicular traffic continually experience some degree of sub-lethal CO poisoning. Of possibly equal importance, it has been estimated that in cigarette smoke inhaled into the lungs the CO concentration reaches as much as 400 ppm (Goldsmith and Landaw, 1968).

CO Thresholds for Polycythemia and Cardiac Enlargement

It has been known for many years that prolonged sublethal CO-poisoning can produce polycythemia (Nasmith and Graham, 1906; Gorbatow and Noro, 1948; Wilkes et al., 1959; Theodore et al., 1971; Jones et al., 1971) and cardiac enlargement (Campbell, 1933; Theodore et al., 1971). To date most studies relating to these responses to CO have been concerned with the effect of either relatively low (100 ppm) or relatively high (400-500 ppm) CO concentrations. At the low concentrations polycythemia and cardiac enlargement are not observed (Stupfel and Bouley, 1970; Preziosi et al., 1970; Eckardt

et al., 1972), while at the high concentrations, alterations
in these parameters is marked (Campbell, 1933; Gorbatow and
Noro, 1948; Theodore et al., 1971). Interestingly enough, no
studies have been carried out at intermediate concentrations
so that threshold levels of CO for these effects might be
determined.

Experiments have recently been carried out in our
laboratory establishing such thresholds (Penny et al., 1974a).
This work consisted of exposing male rats 2 months of age
continuously to CO at concentrations of 100, 200 and 500 ppm.

				heart weight		
		Hb	Body	meas.	pred.	% of
Group	COHb (%)	(g/100ml)	wt.(g)	(g)	(g)	pred.
Control	0.60	15.62	433.3	1.233	1.235	99.83
(13)		±0.20	±10.6	±0.024	±0.031	
CO-ex-	9.26	16.56	435.7	1.281	1.244	102.97
posed	±0.90(8)	±0.23(11)	±15.2	±0.042	±0.004	
(12)						
$p =$	0.001	0.001	0.05	0.05	0.05*	

* measured heart weight vs predicted heart weight

Table 11.   Effect of 46 days continuous exposure to 100
ppm carbon monoxide on carboxyhemoglobin, hemoglobin and heart weight in the rat. Means
given ± S.E.M.

Table 11 shows the effect of exposure to 100 ppm. The
9% carboxyhemoglobin seen in the left-hand column represents
that portion of the hemoglobin which binds CO. This complexed
hemoglobin no longer acts in oxygen transport and is a major
mechanism by which CO-poisoning exerts its lethal effects in
those organisms, such as man, which utilize hemoglobins as an
oxygen transport molecule. Hemoglobin concentration is elevated slightly, but significantly in the animals treated with
CO. From these results as well as studies by others (Preziosi
et al., 1970; Stupfel and Bouley, 1970; Jones et al., 1971;
Eckardt et al., 1972) it appears that a CO concentration near
or slightly below 100 ppm represents the threshold for
measurable polycythemic effects when an animal is exposed
continuously over a period of several weeks. It should also
be noted in the columns labelled heart weight that this

concentration of CO does not result in a significant increase in heart wet weight. In the column labelled predicted heart weight, heart weights of control animals having identical body weights to those of the CO-poisoned animals have been computed using linear regression equations relating heart weight to body weight (Penney et al., 1974b). The slightly larger heart weight of the CO-exposed group than that pre-dicted is also not statistically significant. Apparently 100 ppm CO is below the threshold for measurable cardiac enlargement.

Group	COHb (%)	Hb (g/100ml)	Body wt. (g)
Control	0.66(10)	15.79(10)	459.3(7)
		±0.13	±7.6
CO-ex-posed(7)	15.82 ±0.96	17.87 ±0.07	466.1 ±9.3
p =	0.001	0.001	0.05

Group	measured (g)	predicted (g)	% of predicted
		heart weight	
Control	1.224(7) ±0.011	1.233(7) ±0.017	99.34(7)
CO-ex-posed(7)	1.392 ±0.039	1.249 ±0.021	111.37
p =	0.01	0.01*	

*measured heart weight vs predicted heart weight

Table 12. Effect of 30 days continuous exposure to 200 ppm carbon monoxide on carboxyhemoglobin, hemoglobin and heart weight in the rat. Means given ± S.E.M.

At 200 ppm CO (Table 12) the carboxyhemoglobin con-centration is about twice that at 100 ppm as would be expected from published nomograms relating CO exposure level and carboxyhemoglobin concentration at infinite exposure

times or equilibrium (Forbes et al., 1945). Hemoglobin
concentration is now 2g/100 ml above controls, which is
twice the rise seen at 100 ppm CO. Heart weight of the
CO-poisoned group is now 12% larger than the control group
and is also significantly larger than weights of control
hearts predicted on the basis of body weight. Therefore,
it appears that the threshold for significant cardiac hy-
pertrophic effects of CO lies between 100 and 200 ppm
CO.

Group	COHb (%)	Hb (g/100ml)	Body wt. (g)
Control	0.54(16)	14.93(14)	383.6(16)
		±0.28	±20.9
CO-exposed	41.12(6)	24.98(6)	453.4 (7)
	±4.30	±0.46	±7.8
p =	0.001	0.001	0.05

| | heart weight | | |
Group	measured (g)	predicted (g)	% of predicted
Control	1.119(16)	1.115(16)	100.38(16)
	±0.043	±0.042	
CO-exposed	1.790(7)	1.257(7)	142.44 (7)
	±0.050	±0.015	
p =	0.001	0.001*	

*measured heart weight vs predicted heart weight

Table 13.   Effect of 21-42 days continuous exposure to 500
ppm carbon monoxide on carboxyhemoglobin, hemoglobin and heart weight in the rat. Means
given ± S.E.M.

At 500 ppm CO (Table 13) both the hematologic and
cardiac morphologic effects of CO are very pronounced. The
mortality rate among the semi-adult rats used in this study
was still quite low even at this relatively high CO concen-

tration, thus it still represents a sub-lethal dose. It
should be noted that carboxyhemoglobin now represents about
40% of the circulating hemoglobin. This in turn has
resulted in a more than 60% rise in hemoglobin concentration above controls. Cardiac enlargement is massive
resulting in final heart weights 42% larger than predicted.
The greater final body weight of animals exposed to 500
ppm CO as compared to the control group does not imply
a more rapid rate of body weight gain by the former, since
initial body weights of these two groups were not identical. In fact, the 500 ppm CO-exposed animals gained
weight only slightly less rapidly than controls. Although
data are not available on the effects of such CO-exposure
on human hemoglobin and heart size, the present results may
serve as generally predictive of effects on human hemoglobin and heart size if the CO-exposure of the human is
sufficiently intense and prolonged and not complicated by
other environmentally deleterious factors and if there are
not marked differences in sensitivity to CO between man and
rat.

Time-Course of Blood and Heart Effects

Although it is now well established by this study and
others that long-term severe CO-poisoning results in polycythemia and cardiac enlargement, little information has
been available concerning the precise time-course of
effects of CO on these two parameters, especially effects
on heart size. Experiments have recently been carried out
in our laboratory in this regard (Penney et al., 1974c).
As shown in Figure 8, hemoglobin increase, brought about by
polycythemia, occurs rapidly following onset of CO-exposure.

It was also noted that the heart size of animals
continuously exposed to CO increases rapidly (Figure 8)
and occurs concurrently with the rise in Hb concentration.
It seems possible that the polycythemic blood viscosity
increase and the resulting greater cardiac work required to
propel the blood in CO-exposed animals could be the major
factor in heart weight augmentation. However, other factors may be involved, since heart weight increase appears
to have begun slightly earlier and to have taken place
somewhat faster than the change in hemoglobin. In this regard, it is possible that pulmonary vascular hypertension,
so often described in mammals at high-altitude (Hultgren

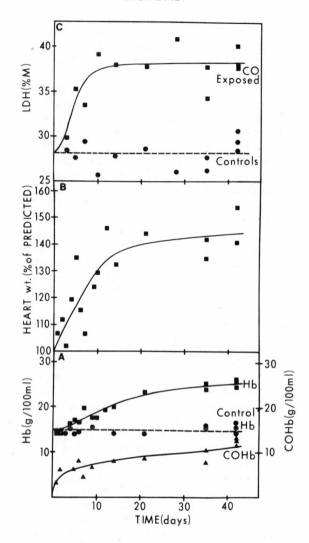

Fig. 8. Effect of 42 days continuous exposure to 500 ppm carbon monoxide in the rat on: A. hemoglobin and carboxyhemoglobin, B. relative heart weight, C. cardiac lactate dehydrogenase M subunit content.

and Grover, 1968), may have played a role in the cardiac hypertrophy, especially of the right heart, observed with CO-exposure.

Mode of CO-induced cardiac Hypertrophy

In experiments designed to compare the effects of hypobaric-hypoxia such as that at high altitude with the effects of chronic CO-exposure (Table 14), the pattern of cardiac enlargement appeared to be quite different (Penney et al., 1974a). Contrary to the pattern in the hearts of hypobarically-exposed animals at a simulated altitude of 5,500 m, seen in the lower third of the table, where cardiac enlargement occurred mainly by hypertrophy of the right ventricle as has been noted by others (Valdivia, 1957), cardiac enlargement in hearts of CO-exposed animals occurred by a more-or-less overall weight increase of both ventricles. This is seen in the similar percentage weight increases of the right and left ventricles in the CO-poisoned animals, and in the unchanging ratio of RV/LV + S ratio in the second column from the right when comparing CO-exposed animals and controls. In contrast, hearts of hypobarically-exposed animals show a RV/LV + S ratio much higher than the controls, reflecting the greater increase in RV weight relative to weight of the LV + S. The lesser degree of right ventricular hypertrophy in the CO-poisoned animals as compared to that of the hypobaric animals suggests that CO-exposure produces considerably less pulmonary vascular hypertension than does simulated altitude hypoxia, since there is reported to be a direct correlation between the size of the right ventricle and pulmonary arterial pressure (Averill et al., 1963; Grover et al., 1963).

Cardiac biochemical effects of CO

Relatively few studies have examined possible cellular level metabolic and biochemical effects of prolonged exposure to CO. It is well known that in most mammalian tissues the glycolytic enzyme lactate dehydrogenase occurs in as many as five isozymic forms with each tissue and cell-type displaying its own particular isozyme pattern. Adult heart characteristically contains mainly anodally migrating LDH components with a high percentage of H subunits and conversely a low percentage of M subunits. We have

Group	Hb (g/100ml)	COHb (%)	body wt. (g)	heart (g)	LV+S (g)
Control (7)	16.13 ±0.21	0.70	392.6 ±20.1	1.147 0.038	0.783 ±0.025
CO-treated (5)	25.34 ±1.05	42.15 ±1.92	371.7 ±27.1	1.631 ±0.083	1.051 ±0.059
p =	0.001		0.05	0.01	0.05
Hypobarical-ly exposed (4) 0	22.06 ±1.08	0	433.4 ±29.9	1.495 ±0.141	0.885 ±0.072
p =	0.001		0.05	0.05	0.05

Group	RV wt. (g)	atrial (g)	RV LV+S	atria LV+S
Control (7)	0.250 ±0.014	0.093 ±0.007	0.320 ±0.013	0.119 ±0.008
CO-treated (5)	0.369 ±0.019	0.169 ±0.013	0.352 ±0.014	0.161 ±0.012
p =	0.01	0.01	0.05	0.05
Hypobarical-ly exposed (4)	0.449 ±0.061	0.127 ±0.012	0.500 ±0.031	0.146 ±0.017
p =	0.05	0.05	0.01	0.05

Means given ± S.E.M.   LV+S = left ventricle + septum;
RV = right ventricle.

Table 14. Effect of 5 weeks continuous exposure to 500
ppm carbon monoxide and 11 weeks continuous
exposure to a simulated altitude of 5,500 m on
hemoglobin, heart weight, left ventricle + septum
weight, right ventricle weight, atria weight,
right ventricle: left ventricle + septum weight
ratio and atria: left ventricle + septum weight
ratio in the rat. Carboxyhemoglobin level also
given for the control and carbon monoxide-exposed
animals.

shown that the M subunit composition of LDH in rat heart is very rapidly altered during the first 10 days of exposure to 500 ppm CO (Penney et al., 1974c;Fig. 8). It is of considerable interest that this change takes place over a very similar time-course to that of the increase in heart weight. A number of other cardiovascular stresses, such as aortic and pulmonary artery constriction (Fox and Reed, 1969; Sobel et al., 1970) coronary artery disease (Ballo and Messer, 1968), hypobaric-exposure (Mager et al., 1968; Anderson and Bullard, 1971) and severe anemia (Penney et al., 1974b) are also known to produce alterations in cardiac LDH isozyme subunit composition. The present data are the first, however, to show that chronic CO-poisoning can produce such cellular biochemical alterations and the first to demonstrate a close correlation between the changes in LDH and the time-course of cardiac enlargement.

Conclusions

The authors have attempted, but in all too brief a manner, to detail some of the dangers to the environment and thus to ourselves of two components of auto-exhaust. Lead concentrations in several segments of the environment have been examined. Air, water, soil, vegetation and animal lead burdens have been determined in relation to automobile exhaust emissions and dietary intake. Absorption after inhalation and ingestion contribute essentially equally to the urban dwellers processing of 40-50 ug of lead per day from a total exposure of over 300 ug/day. Plant growth is significantly altered by the ambient atmospheric lead. Lead-containing waters have, thus far, not been found responsible for fish kills or less toxic episodes. The human, however, seems uniquely challenged by environmental lead. The adult human except for rather rare occupational exposure is seldom found to be acutely poisened by lead. Instead, infants and children up to about age 7 constitute the lead-threatened portion of the population, through purposeful ingestion of lead, rather than via internal combustion engine-generated lead.
Studies on the fetal mouse show that lead levels at about the currently accepted safe blood levels cause developmental deficiencies in certain individuals and that these deficiencies are dose-dependent. Extrapolation of these effects in the mouse to lower doses and other pop-

529

ulations suggests that individuals are being destructively
altered at currently acceptable environmental lead-induced
body lead burdens. It seems clear that this destructive
process could be halted by the immediate elimination of
lead from gasoline and continued public health measures to
identify and remove lead-containing materials from the environment, especially from the environment of children.

It is clear that prolonged exposure to carbon monoxide
does have marked hematologic, cardiac morphologic and biochemical effects on mammalian heart. Concentrations of CO
present in certain industrial facilities, in and around
automobiles and in cigarette smoke may be sufficiently intense after prolonged exposure to produce in humans some
of the effects described. Considerably more research is
needed, however, to better understand the effect of CO on
the human, especially at the tissue and cellular-levels.
Especially informative would be experiments wherein two or
more environmental toxicants, such as lead and carbon
monoxide, would be simultaneously and systematically
studied in animal populations for long periods of time.

Acknowledgements

Studies on the Ecological Effects of Lead in Auto-Exhaust were partially supported by a grant ES-00808 from the
National Institutes of Environmental Health Sciences. Studies
on the Developmental Effects of Lead were supported by a
grant 2-40-37-10-3-01 from the Graduate College Research
Board of the University of Illinois at the Medical Center.
Studies on the Cardiovasculor Effects of Carbon Monoxide
were supported by General Research Funds from the Department
of Biology and the Graduate College Research Board at the
University of Illinois at Chicago Circle. The technical
support of Ms. Meredith Benjamin, Mr. Emmett Dunham and Mr.
Lawrence Bugaisky are gratefully acknowledged.

References

Anderson, G. L. and R. W. Bullard. 1971. Proc. Soc. Exp.
    Biol. Med. 138:441-443.
Anonymous. 1967. The Automobile and Air Pollution. U. S.
    Department of Commerce, October 1967.
Averill, K. H., W. W. Wagner, Jr. and J. H. K. Vogel. 1963.
    Am. Heart J. 66:632-635.
Ballo, J. M. and J. V. Messer. 1968. Biochem. Biophys. Res.

Comm. 33:487-491.

Bini, G. 1973. Internat. J. Environ. Studies 5,59-61.

Campbell, J. A. 1933. J. Physiol. 77:8-9P.

Cannon, H. L. and J. M. Bowles. 1962. Science 137, 765-66.

Caprio, R. J., H. L. Margolis and M. M. Joselow. 1974. Arch. Env. Health 28:195-8.

Carpenter, S. J., V. H. Ferm and T. F. Gale. 1973. Experientia. 29:311-13.

Chisolm, J. J., Jr. 1970. Med. Times 98:92-106.

Chow, T. J. 1973. Our Daily Lead, Chemistry in Britain, Vol. 9, No. 6, 258-263.

Chovin, P. 1967. Environ. Res. 1:198-216.

Coello, W. F. and M. A. Q. Khan. Residues of lead in plants along Chicago's expressways and local highways. To be submitted to Arch. Environ. Cont. Toxicol.

Daines, R. H., H. Motto and D. M. Chilko. 1970. Environ. Sci. Technol. 4, 318-22.

Eckardt, R. E., H. N. MacFarland, Y. C. E. Alarie, and W. H. Busey. 1972. Arch. Environ. Health 25:381-387.

EPA. 1972. Health hazards of lead, summery of information relating to airborne lead. Prepared by Office of Air Programs, Rockville, Md. and N. J. Environmental Health Sciences, Research Triangle, North Carolina.

Forbes, W., F. Sargent, and F. Roughton. 1945. Am. J. Physiol. 143:594-608.

Fox, A. C. and G. E. Reed. 1969. Am. J. Physiol. 216:1026-1033.

Francis, C. W., G. Chestow and L. Haskins. 1970. Environ. Sci. Technol. 4, 586.

Gish, C. D. and R. Christensen. 1973. Environ. Sci. Technol. 7, 1060-62.

Goldsmith, J. R. and S. A. Landaw. 1968. Science 162:1352-1359.

Goldstein, M., M. F. Pinsky and F. C. Fraser. 1963. Genet. Res. (Camb.) 4:258-265.

Gorbatow, O. and L. Noro. 1948. Acta Physiol. Scand. 15:77-87.

Goyo, R. A. 1971. Am. J. Path. 64:167-180.

Grover, R. F., J. T. Reeves, D. H. Will and S. G. Blount, Jr. 1963. J. Appl. Physiol. 18:567-574.

Habibi, K. 1970. Environ. Sci. Technol. 4, 239-48.

Hultgren, H. N. and R. F. Grover. 1968. Ann. Rev. Med. 19: 119-152.

Hwang, J. Y. 1972. Analyt. Chem. 44, 20A-27A.

Jones, R. A., J. A. Strickland, J. A. Stunkard and J. Siegel.

1971. Toxicol. Appl. Pharmacol. 19:46-53.

Kehoe, R. A. 1966. In: Symposium on environmental lead contamination. U. S. Public Health Serv. Publication 1440.

Khan, M. A. Q., W. F. Coello and Z. A. Saleem. 1973. Arch. Environ. Contam. Toxicol. 1, 209-23.

Koeppe, D. E. and R. T. Miller. 1971. Science 167, 1376-77.

Kotok, D. 1972. J. Pediatr. 80:57-61.

Langerwerff, J. W. and A. W. Specht. Environ. Sci. Technol. 4, 583-86.

Lee, D. H. K. 1973. Environ. Res. 6, 121-31.

Mager, M., W. F. Blatt, P. J. Natale, and C. M. Blatteis. 1968. Am. J. Physiol. 215:8-13.

McLellan, J. S., A. W. Von Smolinski, J. P. Bederka, Jr. and B. M. Boalos. 1974. Fed. Proc. 33:479 (Abs).

Motto, H. L., R. H. Daines, D. M. Chilko and C. K. Motto. 1970. Environ. Sci. Technol. 4, 231-37.

Nasmith, G. G. and D. A. L. Graham. 1906. J. Physiol. 35: 32-52.

Penney, D. G., M. Benjamin and E. Dunham. 1974a. J. Appl. Physiol. (in press).

Penney, D. G., L. B. Bugaisky and J. R. Mieszala. 1974b. Biochem. Biophys. Acta 334:24-30.

Penney, D. G., E. Dunham and M. Benjamin. 1974c. Toxicol. Appl. Pharmacol. (in press).

PHS. 1965. Survey of lead in atmosphere of three urban communities. U. S. Public Health Serv. Publication 999-AP-12.

Pickering, Q. H. and C. Henderson. 1972. In: Proceed. 19th Induste. Waste Confer., Purdue University, 578-91.

Preziosi, T. J., R. Lindenberg, D. Levy and M. Christenson. 1970. N. Y. Acad. Sci. 174:369-384.

Rains, D. W. 1971. Nature 233, 210-11.

Robinowitz, M. B. and G. W. Wegherill. 1972. Environ. Sci. Technol. 6, 705-08.

Sanderson, B. A. and C. T. Snowdon. 1974. Science 183:92.

Schaplowsky, A. F. 1970. Public Health Report 85:1109-12.

Schlesinger, W. H., W. A. Reiners and D. S. Knopman. Presented at the 1972 Annual Geological Society of America Meeting, Abstracts with Program, Vol. No. 7, 1972.

Sobel, B. E., P. H. Henry, B. J. Ehrlich and C. M. Bloor. Lab. Invest. 22:23-27.

Stoker, H. S. and S. L. Seager. 1972. Environmental Chemistry: Air and Water Pollution. Scott, Foresman and Co., Ill., 189 pp.

Stupfel, M. and G. Bouley. 1970. N. Y. Acad. Sci. 174:342-368.

Theodore, J., R. D. O'Donnell and K. C. Back. 1971. J. Occup. Med. 13:242-255.

U. S. Department of Health, Education and Welfare. 1970. National Air Pollution Control Administration Publication No. AP-62. pp. 6-22.

Valdivia, E. 1957. Circ. Res. 5:612-616.

Waller, R. E., B. T. Commins and P. J. Lawther. 1965. Brit. J. Indus. Med. 22:128-138.

Wilkes, S. S., J. F. Tomashefski and R. T. Clark, Jr. 1959. J. Appl. Physiol. 14:305-310.

Zimdahl, R. L. and P. B. Arvik. 1973. CRC Critical Reviews in Environmental Control. 3, 213-24.

EPILOGUE

John P. Bederka, Jr.

The phrase "Past is Prologue" may no longer be tenable in terms of continued environmental pollution with the current general popular awareness of and legislation toward the control and elimination of destructive environmental pollution. Or, to perhaps rephrase it "Hope Springs Eternal"!

The Symposium ("Mechanisms of Survival in Toxic Environments") upon which this volume is based was held in Houston, Texas in December of 1973. Of the 21 papers that were presented at the Symposium, 20 are contained herein in their revised and edited forms. These articles when considered topically, include appraisals of models of ecosystems and ecosystems devolving around, humans, birds, fish, estuarine organisms, soil and aquatic microbes, and cells in culture in relation to environmental pollutants and toxicants. The environmental chemistry of pesticides and biochemistry of pesticide metabolism are considered in the detailed presentations in Sections 2 and 3. Section 4 affords some perspective in terms of an overview of pesticides in the environment with cost benefit and environmental economic considerations. In essence, the authors consider many aspects of *successful and unsuccessful* adjustments to toxic environments with only small attempts at prognostication; but, describe many avenues for future research and point out areas for environmental concern.

The theme of Survival in Toxic Environments can be illustrated by the concept of enzyme induction as in the case of decreased toxicity of DDT to certain individuals in some strains of houseflies with extrapolations to humans. Enzyme induction leads to increased metabolism of the environmental toxicant to less toxic intermediates and leads to survival in this new or toxic DDT-containing environment. This ability to survive is not of the nature of an acute or instantaneous effect in that if an entire population is intensively exposed, death would be almost complete for the entire population. Thus, induction and selection (evolution) are on a time scale of days and generations, respectively. Today, with large and concentrated populations, with rapid distribution of chemical products (food, food additives, drugs, and other pollutants), the populations may adapt as in the past, but can least survive acute or brief toxic insults. *It is paramount that society not be exposed to acute toxic insults whereas slowly changing environments must be provided.* In today's highly automated and harmoniously integrated societies, toxicant-mediated interruptions in the activities of the populace are less tolerable than here-to-fore. This acceptable condition of quality of the environment or degree of chemical contamination of the biological reactions in our evolution, can be rationally approached. The route involves the use of extensive modeling with actual intensive testing in human as well as other animal populations of all substances that are to be introduced into our biosphere, the EARTH. Thus, integrated toxicity testing on a national and international scale must be quickly raised to the necessary level and publicized so that the system can be guided in a competitive evolutionary sense. Survival in our toxic environments can, thus, be insured at an acceptable level of human comfort via an integrated and planned approach to environmental monitoring and alteration of our environment toward insuring the continued effectiveness of the human species.

Borrowing from Dr. Khan in his opening remarks, Science and Technology are in a large part the fundamental bases of our (The United States) position in the world today. This is due to our educational and political (funding) programs of about the last 25 years. Perhaps because of an attempt to obtain a balance among the arts or societal activities (science, technology, philosophy, painting, economics, ...), support for science and technology has been ebbing of late, to say the least. In spite of the superior marketability of the products of their efforts, many scientists, engineers, and technicians have turned to even more practical matters of society in recent years, and this is only the beginning of the wave. What seems needed now, in addition to the social move, is an overt political move. Thus, science and technology must have an effective voice. We may still need more political scientists! We do need more scientist-politicians! Not *just* part-*timers!* Funding towards new (perhaps hybrid) careers in environmental economics and environmental law are but two possibilities. Careers must also be changed toward elective office so that scientists will also effectively participate in the highest decisions involving the nature of our societal activities. This is only a reasonable approach to the effective functioning of this most highly developed socioeconomic scientific and technological society in our earthly environment.

536

A

Abate, 41, 335, 342, 431
Acaricidal (acaricides), 145, 146, 155,
    156, 158-160, 162, 164-166, 168,
    170-173
Acarines, 155, 428
Acarol, 161, 163
Acclimation, 110, 112, 114, 115, 119
Accumulation, *see also* Food-web, 87-91,
    103, 132, 147, 148
p-Acetamidophenol, 126
Acetanilide, 158
Acethion, 179
Acetophenetidin, 126
Acetyl glucosamine, 207
2-Acetylamino fluorene, 126
Acetylation, 159, 168-171, 173, 196, 207
Acetylcholine, 321
Acetylcholinesterase, 322, 368
Acids, 33, 43, 128, 131, 135, 137, 145,
    146, 161, 163, 165, 166, 170, 171,
    208, 209, 423, 473, 478, 492
Actinomycin D, 266, 267, 269, 270, 274
Adrenal, 296, 297
Adsorption, 130, 365
Aechmophorus occ., *see* Birds-fish eating
Aedes spp., *see* mosquito
Aerobic, 13, 131, 137
Africa, 430, 431
Agriculture, 19, 68, 69, 432, 435
Air, 46, 497
Alabama, 68
Alcohol de Hase, 300
Alcohols, 136, 138, 165, 230
Aldehydes, 136, 138
Aldicarb, 159, 160, 191, 421
Aldophosphamide, 126

Aldrin, 39, 40, 44, 138, 141, 143, 146,
    191, 192, 294, 335, 340, 345, 346,
    350, 353, 374, 383, 385, 390, 395,
    414, 417, 463
Alfalfa, 462, 463
Algae, 5, 33, 115, 116, 141, 143, 346
Algicides, 131
Aliesterases, 321, 322, 324
Aliphatic, 155, 161, 162, 172, 173, 185
Alkaloids, 128
Alkylamines, 136, 143, 230
Alkylation, 145, 150, 206
Alkylnitrate, 230
Alkyltransferases, 322
Allethrins, 238, 422, 423
Alphanumeric, 56, 57
Aluminum, 39
Amidases, 179
Amides, 207, 230
Aminobenzoic acid, 208, 209
Aminoparaoxon, 157
Aminoparathion, 157
m-Aminophenol, 158
Aminopyrene, 190, 195, 206
Ammonia, 148, 473, 475, 478
Amphibians, 44
Anaerobic, 8, 131, 137, 148
Anhingas, 53-55, 59, 61-63, 64-66,
    71, 75
Aniline, 207, 231, 238, 242
Animals, *see also* mammals and specific
    items, 30, 38, 39, 40, 42, 44, 45, 54,
    87, 89, 92, 94, 96, 101, 102, 105,
    110-112, 128, 130, 133, 136, 143,
    150, 155-157, 160, 161, 165-169,
    202, 213-215, 217, 227, 245, 282,
    461